DRUG CALCULATIONS

Process and Problems for Clinical Practice

SEVENTH EDITION

Meta Brown, RN, MEd

Retired Colonel
U.S. Army Field Hospital;
Former Director, Division of Nursing
Gateway Community College
Phoenix, Arizona

Joyce M. Mulholland, APRN, BC, MA, MS

Nursing Education Consultant
Phoenix, Arizona

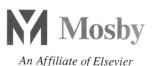

Mosby

An Affiliate of Elsevier

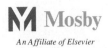

An Affiliate of Elsevier

11830 Westline Industrial Drive
St. Louis, Missouri 63146

Drug Calculations: Process and Problems for Clinical Practice   ISBN 0-323-02562-5

NOTICE

Pharmacology is an ever-changing field. Standard safety precautions must be followed, but as new research and clinical experience broaden our knowledge, changes in treatment and drug therapy may become necessary or appropriate. Readers are advised to check the most current product information provided by the manufacturer of each drug to be administered to verify the recommended dose, the method and duration of administration, and contraindications. It is the responsibility of the licensed prescriber, relying on experience and knowledge of the patient, to determine dosages and the best treatment for each individual patient. Neither the publisher nor the author assumes any liability for any injury and/or damage to persons or property arising from this publication.

Previous editions copyrighted 2000, 1996, 1992, 1988, 1984, 1979

Library of Congress Cataloging-in-Publication Data

Brown, Meta
    Drug calculation : process and problems for clinical practice / Meta Brown, Joyce M. Mulholland.—7th ed.
      p. cm.
    Includes index.
    ISBN 0-323-02562-5 (pbk.)
      1. Pharmaceutical arithmetic—Problems, exercises, etc.   I. Mulholland, Joyce M.   II. Title.
      [DNLM: 1. Pharmaceutical Preparations—administration & dosage—Programmed
Instruction. 2. Mathematics—Programmed Instruction.]
    RS57.B76 2003
    615′.14—dc21

Executive Vice President, Nursing & Health Professions: Sally Schrefer
Acquisitions Editor: Yvonne Alexopoulos
Associate Developmental Editor: Danielle M. Frazier
Publishing Services Manager: Catherine Jackson
Senior Project Manager: Jeff Patterson
Designer: Teresa McBryan Breckwoldt

Printed in the United States of America

Last digit is the print number: 9   8   7   6   5   4   3   2

Reviewers

Janet Tompkins McMahon, RN, MSN
Associate Professor
Department of Nursing
Pennsylvania College of Technology
Williamsport, Pennsylvania

Matthew P. McMahon, RN, NREMT-P, HP
Clinical Instructor
Department of Nursing
Pennsylvania College of Technology
Susquehanna Health System
Williamsport, Pennsylvania

Patricia A. Roper, RN, MS
Professor
Department of Nursing
Columbus State Community College
Columbus, Ohio

Jo A. Voss, RN, PhDc, CNS
Instructor
College of Nursing
South Dakota State University
Rapid City, South Dakota

Robert S. Warner, MS, RN
Assistant Professor
Department of Nursing
Fulton-Montgomery Community College
Johnstown, New York

Preface to Instructors

INTRODUCTION

Drug Calculations was originally designed in the late seventies as a basic practical resource for nursing students and faculty in the classroom and clinical areas. Since then the content has been thoroughly reviewed and expanded to also be useful for refresher courses, practicing nurses in specialty areas, distance-learning students, and nursing students who pursue independent nursing study.

This book primarily presents the Ratio and Proportion method, the easiest provable method of dose calculation for the majority of nursing students to master in a short time, and delivers all the material in a simple to complex sequence with brief rules, succinct examples, and logical steps to understanding and mastery of the underlying concepts.

A comprehensive systematic arithmetic self-assessment quiz allows the student to focus on any basic mathematics areas that may need review in preparation for dose calculations.

The first chapter offers a sufficient review of the basic arithmetic needed to solve all the calculations in the text. Students are referred to a general mathematics text if more practice is desired.

The text presents pharmacology principles and selected illustrations to enhance learning relevant to specific calculation areas. The reader is referred to current pharmacology texts, drug handbooks, and clinical skills manuals for complete coverage of those broad subjects.

As in prior editions, answers are completely worked out in the back of the book for all worksheets so that the learner can pinpoint areas of need. Concepts of the nursing process, logical thinking, and critical thinking are employed throughout the text with highlighted clinical alerts to call the reader's attention to dose-related safety situations in actual practice that have resulted in medication errors. Also, as in prior editions, little emphasis on memorized concepts is encouraged.

Priorities are placed upon patient safety, and proofs and labels are requested for answers to all the basic problems to avoid errors and establish good habits. Use of the calculator is not encouraged for the basic chapters so that the user masters the understanding and the steps necessary to enter data correctly into the calculator. The goal is to be able to function independently without a calculator if that becomes necessary.

NEW FEATURES FOR THE SEVENTH EDITION

- Each chapter has been reviewed and updated for currency and accuracy and expanded to include more labels and new illustrations for realistic practice.
- Chapter Introductions begin each chapter, providing general discussion of content and helping students focus and prepare for learning.

- More problems have been added to the revised chapters to give the student additional practice.
- Two new chapters have been added in response to requests from readers: Total Parenteral Nutrition calculations and a chapter on the Dimensional Analysis method of dose calculations.
- Multiple-choice worksheets have been added near the end of each chapter to prepare the student for the NCLEX test format.
- A new multiple-choice final and an updated comprehensive final are included in this seventh edition along with the answers to both to help the student evaluate progress.
- For reader convenience, abbreviations and formulas are located on the inside front and back covers of the text.

ANCILLARIES

Instructor's Manual and Test Bank for Drug Calculations: Process and Problems for Clinical Practice, Seventh Edition

This manual is a **new** resource specifically geared toward this edition and includes the following:

- Suggestions for classroom and laboratory practice
- Teaching guidelines
- Test bank with over 100 questions
- This resource is also available on CD-ROM and online. To use this great resource online visit the **Evolve** site at http://evolve.elsevier.com/BrownMulholland/.

Romans & Daugherty Dosages and Solutions Computerized Test Bank (Version II)

This generic CTB (CD-ROM format) has been completely updated and is provided as a gratis item to instructors upon adoption of this book. It contains over 700 questions on general math, converting within systems of measurement, oral dosages, parenteral dosages, flow rates, pediatric dosages, IV calculations, and more. This CTB is also available online at the **Evolve** site at http://evolve.elsevier.com/BrownMulholland/.

Daugherty & Romans Dosages and Solutions CD-ROM Companion (Version II)

This updated student tutorial is a user-friendly, interactive program that includes an extensive menu of various topic areas within dosages and solutions. This CD is packaged with the book and provides hundreds of practice problems in the ratio and proportion, formula, dimensional analysis, and fractional equation methods. Engaging animations allow the user to complete interactive exercises and practice problems. This CD also includes a comprehensive posttest. See the next page for sample screenshots.

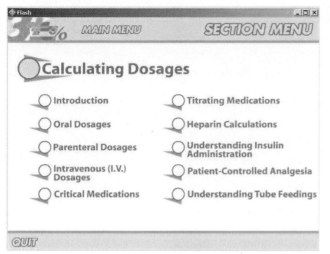

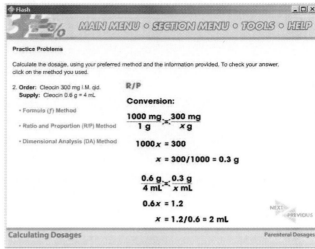

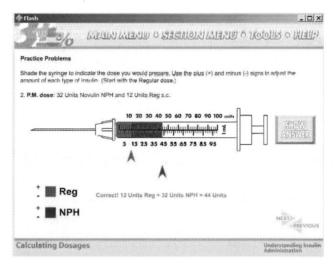

● ACKNOWLEDGMENTS

We hope that the users will find that this edition meets their needs. Our thanks to all the reviewers and users for their thoughts, time, and excellent suggestions. We followed them whenever practical, timely, and consistent with the style of this text and the needs of a majority of practitioners.

We would like to thank Paula Milner, MS, RN, CS, Med/Surg Clinical Educator, Scottsdale Healthcare Osborn, Scottsdale, Arizona; and Jennifer C. Barth, RN, MSN, CDE, Scottsdale Healthcare, Shea Campus, Scottsdale, Arizona, for their input and suggestions.

Meta Brown and Joyce M. Mulholland

Preface to the Student

● DESCRIPTION AND FEATURES

Drug Calculations: Process and Problems for Clinical Practice provides all the information, explanation, and practice needed to competently and confidently calculate drug dosages. It provides exclusive coverage of the ratio and proportion method of drug calculation in a full color workbook format. Take a look at the following features so that you may familiarize yourself with this text and maximize its value:

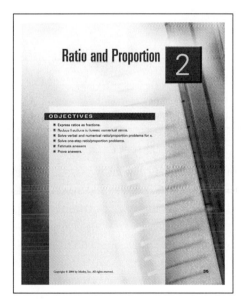

Objectives help guide your approach to learning.

Multiple-choice practice worksheets are designed to prepare you for the NCLEX exam.

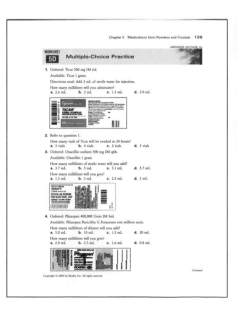

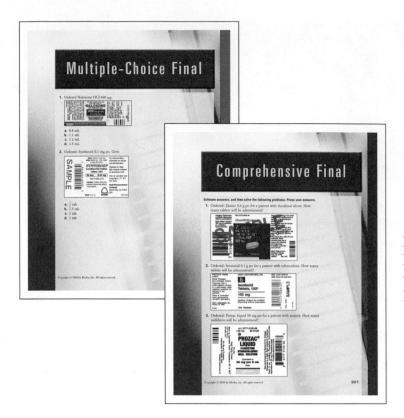

Multiple-Choice and Comprehensive Finals cover topics discussed throughout the book and help you assess total learning of the process of drug calculation.

Daugherty & Romans Dosages and Solutions CD-ROM Companion (Version II) is also included with each text. This updated student tutorial is a user-friendly, interactive program that includes an extensive menu of various topic areas within dosages and solutions. It provides hundreds of practice problems in the ratio and proportion, formula, dimensional analysis, and fractional equation methods. Engaging animations allow the user to complete interactive exercises and practice problems. This CD also includes a comprehensive post-test.

 Look for this icon near the end of the chapters. It will refer you to the *Daugherty & Romans Dosages and Solutions CD-ROM Companion (Version II)* for additional practice problems.

Contents

■ **General Mathematics Self-Assessment**   1

1 **General Mathematics**   3

Fractions, 4
Changing Improper Fractions to Whole or Mixed Numbers, 4
Changing Mixed Numbers to Improper Fractions, 5
Finding a Common Denominator for Two or More Fractions, 6
Changing Fractions to Equivalent Fractions, 7
Reducing Fractions to Lowest Terms, 7
    Changing to Equivalent Fractions Using Higher Terms, 8
Addition of Fractions and Mixed Numbers, 8
Subtraction of Fractions and Mixed Numbers, 10
Multiplication of Fractions and Mixed Numbers, 11
Division of Fractions and Mixed Numbers, 12
Value of Fractions, 13
Value of Decimals, 15
Addition of Decimals, 18
Subtraction of Decimals, 19
Multiplication of Decimals, 20
Division of Decimals, 20
Changing Decimals to Fractions, 24
Changing Common Fractions to Decimals, 25
Rounding Decimals, 26
Percentages, Decimals, and Fractions, 28
    Changing a Percentage to a Fraction, 28
    Changing a Percentage to a Decimal, 28
    Changing a Decimal to a Percentage, 28
    Finding the Percentage, 30
    Multiple-Choice Practice, 31
Chapter 1 Final, 33

2 Ratio and Proportion   35

Ratio, 36
Proportion, 36
   Solving Proportion Problems When One of the Numbers is Unknown,
      or *x*, 37
Setting Up Ratios and Proportions, 40
Multiple-Choice Practice, 43
Chapter 2 Final, 44

3 Patient Safety: Errors, Orders, Labels, and Records   45

Patient Safety, 46
How to Avoid Medication Errors, 46
   Physician's Orders, 47
   Preparation, 48
   Medication Packaging, 48
   Labels, 50
   Calculations, 50
   Administration, 51
   Reporting and Documenting, 51
   Interventions, 52
   Evaluation, 52
Interpreting Medication Labels, 52
   Oral Drug Forms: Solids and Liquids, 53
The 24-Hour Clock: 0000-2400 Hours, 58
Understanding Medication Administration Records (MARs), 60
The Six Rights of Drug Administration, 61
Multiple-Choice Practice, 65
Critical Thinking Exercises, 67

4 Metric System Calculations   69

Metric System, 70
Metric Conversions by Moving Decimals, 71
Rounding Medication Doses, 73
   Rounding Milliliters, 73
   Rounding Drops, 74
One-Step Metric Ratio and Proportion Calculations, 75
Two-Step Metric Ratio and Proportion Calculations, 84
Measuring and Reading Amounts in a Syringe, 89
Multiple-Choice Practice, 100
Critical Thinking Exercises, 101
Chapter 4 Final, 102

5 Medications from Powders and Crystals   105

Measuring Liquid Medications, 106
Reconstituting Medications, 114
    Types of Diluents, 114
Diluting Powders or Crystals in Vials, 115
Reconstitution: Medication Labels, 117
Multiple-Choice Practice, 129
Critical Thinking Exercises, 132
Chapter 5 Final, 133

6 Basic IV Calculations   137

IV Infusions, 138
Types of IV Lines, 138
IV Calculations, 139
    Drop Factor Calculations, 140
Abbreviations for Common Intravenous Solutions, 146
Percentage of Solute in IV Bags, 146
IV Delivery Sets, 153
    Needleless IV Systems, 153
    Gravity Piggyback Infusions, 154
    Piggyback Premixed IVs, 154
    Nurse-Activated Piggyback Systems, 155
    Electronic Infusion Devices, 156
    Piggyback Infusions, 159
Multiple-Choice Practice, 161
Critical Thinking Exercises, 162
Chapter 6 Final, 162

7 Advanced IV Calculations   163

Advanced IV Calculations, 164
Titrated Infusions, 164
    Solving Titrated Infusion Problems, 165
    Hourly Drug and Flow Rate Formula for Titrated Infusions, 165
Direct IV (Bolus) Administration With a Syringe, 176
    Timing IV Push Medications—Method 1, 176
    Timing IV Push Medications—Method 2, 177
Multiple-Choice Practice, 181
Critical Thinking Exercises, 183
Chapter 7 Final, 183

8 Parenteral Nutrition   187

Total Parenteral Nutrition, 188
  Total Grams Per Bag, 190
  Percentage of Concentration Per Bag, 192
  Percentage of Additives, 192
  mL/Hour to Set the Pump, 192
  Kilocalories (Kcal) Per Bag, 192
  Validation of TPN Label With Physician's Order, 193
  Nursing Considerations for TPN, 195
Multiple-Choice Practice, 202
Critical Thinking Exercises, 204
Chapter 8 Final, 204

9 Insulin   205

Insulin, 206
Diabetes Mellitus, 206
Injection Sites, 207
Types of Insulin, 207
Types of U-100 Insulins, 210
  Fast-Acting, 210
  Intermediate-Acting, 210
  Intermediate- and Fast-Acting Mixtures, 211
  Long-Acting, 211
Insulin Syringes, 212
  Types of U-100 Insulin Syringes, 212
Insulin Orders, 213
Mixing Insulin, 219
Sliding Scale Calculations, 224
Intravenous Insulin, 226
Oral Diabetes Medications, 230
Insulin Infusion Devices, 230
Multiple-Choice Practice, 231
Critical Thinking Exercises, 232
Chapter 9 Final, 232

10 Anticoagulants   235

Injectable Anticoagulants, 236
  Subcutaneous Heparin Injections, 238
  IV Flushes, 242
IV Heparin, 243
Oral Anticoagulants, 244
Titrated Heparin, 245
Multiple-Choice Practice, 245
Critical Thinking Exercises, 246
Chapter 10 Final, 247

11 Children's Dosages 249

Dosages Based on Body Weight and Surface Area, 250
The mg/kg Method, 250
    Steps to Solving mg/kg Problems, 250
The BSA Method (mg/m²), 255
    Calculating BSA (m²) Using a Mathematical Formula, 255
Children's IV Medications: Reconstitution, Dilution, and Flow Rate
    Information, 264
Multiple-Choice Practice, 274
Critical Thinking Exercises, 276
Chapter 11 Final, 276

12 Dimensional Analysis 281

Dimensional Analysis, 282
Multiple-Choice Practice, 289
Chapter 12 Final, 291

■ Multiple-Choice Final 293

■ Comprehensive Final 301

■ Answer Key 309

■ Index 411

General Mathematics Self-Assessment

Accurate medication dose calculations build on fundamental mathematics knowledge. Solve these basic problems and check your answers on page 309. Chapter 1, General Mathematics, provides a refresher if needed.

Change to whole or mixed numbers:

1. $\frac{11}{2}$

2. $\frac{36}{7}$

Change to improper fractions:

3. $6\frac{2}{9}$

4. $9\frac{1}{2}$

Find the lowest common denominator in the following fractions:

5. $\frac{4}{11}$ and $\frac{1}{6}$

6. $\frac{2}{5}$ and $\frac{5}{9}$

Add the following:

7. $\frac{1}{5}$, $\frac{1}{6}$, and $\frac{2}{3}$

8. $1\frac{1}{2} + 3\frac{1}{8} + 2\frac{1}{6}$

Subtract the following:

9. $\frac{5}{7} - \frac{1}{4}$

10. $8\frac{1}{4} - 3\frac{3}{8}$

Multiply the following and reduce to lowest terms:

11. $\frac{1}{6} \times \frac{1}{2}$

12. $\frac{2}{8} \times 1\frac{1}{3}$

Divide the following and reduce to lowest terms:

13. $\frac{1}{3} \div \frac{2}{5}$

14. $1\frac{1}{8} \div 2\frac{1}{2}$

Express the following fractions reduced to lowest terms (numbers):

15. $\frac{3}{150}$

16. $\frac{4}{19}$

Write the following as decimals:

17. Fourteen hundredths

18. Three and sixteen thousandths

Add the following:

19. $3.04 + 1.865$

20. $25.7 + 3.008$

Subtract the following:

21. $3 - 0.04$

22. $0.96 - 0.1359$

Multiply the following:

23. 0.003×1.2

24. 3×0.5

Divide the following and carry to the third decimal place:

25. $201.1 \div 20$

26. $20.6 \div 0.21$

Change the following to decimals and carry to the third decimal place:

27. $\frac{23}{43}$

28. $9\frac{1}{8}$

Find the following percentages:

29. 15% of 63

30. 2% of 4210

Change the following decimals to fractions:

31. 0.7

32. 0.492

33. Write 17% as a decimal and as a fraction.

34. Write $\frac{1}{8}$ as a decimal and as a percentage.

35. Write 0.014 as a fraction and as a percentage.

36. Round 0.55 to the nearest tenth.

37. Round 0.8734 to the nearest tenth.

38. Round 0.872 to the nearest hundredth.

39. Round 2.85 to the nearest whole number.

40. Round 4.122 to the nearest whole number.

General Mathematics

1

OBJECTIVES

- Convert fractions into whole and mixed numbers.
- Change mixed numbers into improper fractions.
- Find lowest common denominators in fractions.
- Add fractions and mixed numbers and reduce to lowest terms (reduce fractions).
- Subtract fractions and mixed numbers.
- Multiply fractions and mixed numbers.
- Divide fractions and mixed numbers.
- Determine which of two fractions is larger and which is smaller.
- Distinguish among tenths, hundredths, thousandths, ten-thousandths, and hundred-thousandths in decimal fractions.
- Read whole numbers and decimal fractions.
- Divide decimals to the third decimal place.
- Add, subtract, and divide decimals.
- Change decimals to fractions.
- Find a common denominator.
- Reduce fractions to lowest terms.
- Change fractions to equivalent fractions.
- Change fractions to decimals.
- Change percentages to fractions.
- Round decimals to the nearest tenth, hundredth, and whole number.
- Change percentages to decimals.
- Convert decimals to percentages.
- Find percentages.

INTRODUCTION

This chapter provides a thorough and easy-to-follow review of the arithmetic needed for accurate medication dose calculations. Many examples, practice problems, and answers related to fractions, decimals, and percentages are offered. Your ability to avoid medication errors and solve medication dose-related problems starts with competence in basic arithmetic. If you need further review, refer to a general basic mathematics text. Mastery of these concepts is essential before you proceed to the following chapters and medication-related calculations.

● FRACTIONS

A fraction is part of a whole number. The fraction $\frac{6}{8}$ means that there are 8 parts to the whole number (bottom number, or denominator), but you want to measure only 6 of those parts (top number, or numerator).

The fraction $\frac{6}{8}$ can be reduced by dividing both the numbers by 2.

$$\frac{6 \div 2}{8 \div 2} = \frac{3}{4} \begin{array}{l} \text{numerator} \\ \text{denominator} \end{array}$$

● CHANGING IMPROPER FRACTIONS TO WHOLE OR MIXED NUMBERS

An improper fraction has a numerator that is larger than the denominator, as in $\frac{8}{4}$.

STEPS When the top number (numerator) is larger than the bottom number (denominator), divide the bottom number (denominator) into the top number (numerator).

Write the remainder as a fraction and reduce to lowest terms.

EXAMPLES $\frac{8}{4} = 8 \div 4 = 2$ *Whole number*

$\frac{16}{6} = 16 \div 6 = 2\frac{4}{6} = 2\frac{2}{3}$ This is a *mixed number* because it has a whole number plus a fraction.

ANSWERS ON PAGE 309

WORKSHEET 1A — Changing Improper Fractions to Whole or Mixed Numbers

Change the following to whole numbers or mixed fractions and reduce to lowest terms:

1. $\frac{8}{8} =$ **2.** $\frac{6}{2} =$ **3.** $\frac{13}{4} =$

4. $\frac{14}{9} =$ **5.** $\frac{34}{6} =$ **6.** $\frac{100}{25} =$

7. $\frac{7}{4} =$ **8.** $\frac{120}{64} =$ **9.** $\frac{12}{4} =$

10. $\frac{41}{6} =$

● CHANGING MIXED NUMBERS TO IMPROPER FRACTIONS

STEPS Multiply the whole number by the denominator of the fraction.

Add this to the numerator of the fraction.

Write the sum as the numerator of the fraction; the denominator of the fraction remains the same.

EXAMPLES $2\frac{3}{8} = \frac{8 \times 2 + 3}{8} = \frac{19}{8}$ numerator/denominator

$4\frac{2}{5} = \frac{5 \times 4 + 2}{5} = \frac{22}{5}$ numerator/denominator

ANSWERS ON PAGE 309

WORKSHEET 1B — Changing Mixed Numbers to Improper Fractions

Change the following to improper fractions:

1. $1\frac{1}{5} =$ **2.** $1\frac{1}{4} =$ **3.** $4\frac{3}{8} =$

4. $3\frac{7}{12} =$ **5.** $13\frac{3}{5} =$ **6.** $16\frac{1}{3} =$

7. $3\frac{5}{6} =$ **8.** $2\frac{5}{8} =$ **9.** $10\frac{3}{6} =$

10. $125\frac{2}{3} =$

● FINDING A COMMON DENOMINATOR FOR TWO OR MORE FRACTIONS

To add and subtract fractions, the denominators must be the *same*.

EXAMPLE   Fractions with same denominators

$$\frac{5}{16} - \frac{2}{16} \quad \text{or} \quad \frac{3}{8} + \frac{1}{8} \quad \text{or} \quad \frac{3}{4} + \frac{1}{4}$$

These fractions can be added and subtracted. Each set's value is also easier to compare because of the common denominators.

EXAMPLE   Different denominators in fractions with the same value as the fractions in example A:

$$\frac{5}{16} - \frac{1}{8} \quad \text{or} \quad \frac{3}{8} + \frac{2}{16} \quad \text{or} \quad \frac{3}{4} + \frac{2}{8}$$

These fractions cannot be added or subtracted until they are converted in *equivalent* fractions with a *common* denominator. The relative value of each set is harder to compare. A *common* denominator is a number that can be divided evenly by *all* the denominators in the problem.

> **STEP**   Examine the largest denominator in the group to determine whether the other denominators will divide *evenly* into it.

EXAMPLE $\frac{5}{16}$ and $\frac{1}{8}$: the largest denominator, 16, can be divided by 8 without a remainder. 16 is the common denominator.

EXAMPLE $\frac{2}{8}$ and $\frac{3}{4}$ and $\frac{1}{2}$: the largest denominator, 8, can be divided by 4 and by 2 without a remainder. 8 is the common denominator.

> **STEP**   If any of the denominators will not divide evenly into the largest denominator, examine multiples (greater than one) of the *largest* denominator to find a number that the other denominators will divide into evenly.

EXAMPLE $\frac{3}{8}$ and $\frac{2}{3}$ and $\frac{1}{4}$: 3 will *not* divide evenly into 8.

The largest denominator in the group is **8**.

$8 \times 2 = 16$ 3 will *not* divide evenly into 16.

$8 \times 3 = 24$ Both 3 and 4 will divide evenly into **24**.

$8 \times 4 = 32$ 3 will *not* divide evenly into 32.

$8 \times 5 = 40$ 3 will *not* divide evenly into 40.

$8 \times 6 = 48$ Both 3 and 4 will divide evenly into **48**.

Therefore 24 and 48 are common denominators for $\frac{3}{8}$ and $\frac{2}{3}$ and $\frac{1}{4}$, but 24 is the *lowest* common denominator for the three numbers.

EXAMPLE $\frac{1}{7}, \frac{1}{6}$, and $\frac{1}{3}$

3 and 6 will *not* divide evenly into 7.

Multiples of 7: 14, 21, 28, 35, and 42.
42 is the lowest number that can be divided evenly by 6 and 3. Therefore **42** is a common denominator, the lowest common denominator.

CHANGING FRACTIONS TO EQUIVALENT FRACTIONS

◉◀◀◀◀◀◀RULES Whatever you do to the denominator (multiply or divide by a number), you must do the *same* to the numerator so that the value does not change.

To maintain equivalence, the numerator and the denominator must be divided (or multiplied) by the *same* number.

EXAMPLE $\frac{3}{8}$, and $\frac{2}{3}$, and $\frac{1}{4}$

STEPS Find the common denominator—in this case 24.

Multiply each *numerator* by the *same* number used to obtain the common denominator for that fraction. You multiplied 8 by **3** to arrive at the common denominator 24.

$\frac{3}{8} (\overset{=}{\times 3}) \frac{?}{24}$ $3 \times 3 = 9$ Therefore $\frac{3}{8} = \frac{9}{24}$

$\frac{2}{3} (\overset{=}{\times 8}) \frac{?}{24}$ $2 \times 8 = 16$ $\frac{2}{3} = \frac{16}{24}$

$\frac{1}{4} (\overset{=}{\times 6}) \frac{?}{24}$ $1 \times 6 = 6$ $\frac{1}{4} = \frac{6}{24}$

REDUCING FRACTIONS TO LOWEST TERMS

A fraction is in lowest terms when the numerator and denominator cannot be divided by any other number except one.

◉◀◀◀◀◀◀◀RULE To reduce a fraction to *lowest* terms, **divide** the numerator and denominator by the *largest* same number that will divide evenly into both. When there are no whole numbers that can be used except one, the fraction is in lowest terms.

The fraction $\frac{6}{8}$ is not in lowest terms because it can be reduced by dividing both the numerator and the denominator by 2, a common denominator. $\frac{3}{4}$ is expressed in lowest terms.

EXAMPLE $\frac{6 \div 2 = 3}{8 \div 2 = 4}$ Note that both 6 and 8 are divided by 2.

EXAMPLE $\frac{10 \div 5 = 2}{15 \div 5 = 3}$ Note that both 10 and 15 are divided by 5.

EXAMPLE $\frac{4 \div 4 = 1}{24 \div 4 = 6}$ Note that both 4 and 24 are divided by 4.

$\frac{3}{4}$ and $\frac{2}{3}$ and $\frac{1}{6}$ cannot be further reduced. No other number than one will divide evenly into both the numerator and denominator. They are now in their simplest or *lowest* terms.

Changing to Equivalent Fractions Using Higher Terms

◀◀◀◀◀◀◀◀RULE   To change a fraction to *higher* terms and maintain equivalence, **multiply** both the numerator and the denominator by the *same* number.

EXAMPLE $\dfrac{6 \times 2}{8 \times 2} = \dfrac{12}{16}$ $\dfrac{6}{8} = \dfrac{12}{16}$

The value has not changed because the multiplier 2 is used for both the numerator and the denominator, and $\dfrac{2}{2} = 1$.

Multiplying or dividing numbers by one does *not* change the value. Equivalence is maintained.

ADDITION OF FRACTIONS AND MIXED NUMBERS

◀◀◀◀◀◀◀◀RULE   If fractions have the same denominator, add the numerators, write over the denominator, and reduce.

EXAMPLE

$$\begin{array}{r} \dfrac{1}{5} \\[2mm] + \dfrac{2}{5} \\[1mm] \hline \dfrac{3}{5} \end{array} \qquad\qquad \begin{array}{r} \dfrac{2}{6} \\[2mm] + \dfrac{1}{6} \\[1mm] \hline \dfrac{3}{6} = \dfrac{1}{2} \end{array}$$

◀◀◀◀◀◀◀◀RULE   If fractions have different denominators, convert each fraction to an equivalent fraction using the lowest common denominator and then add the numerators.

EXAMPLE

$$\begin{array}{r} \dfrac{3}{5} = \dfrac{9}{15} \\[2mm] + \dfrac{2}{3} = + \dfrac{10}{15} \\[1mm] \hline \dfrac{19}{15} = 19 \div 15 = 1\dfrac{4}{15} \end{array} \qquad \begin{array}{l} \dfrac{3\,(\times 3)}{5\,(\times 3)} = \dfrac{9}{15} \\[3mm] \dfrac{2\,(\times 5)}{3\,(\times 5)} = \dfrac{10}{15} \end{array}$$

◀◀◀◀◀◀◀◀RULE   To add mixed numbers, first add the fractions by converting to a common denominator and then add this to the sum of the whole numbers.

EXAMPLE

$$\begin{array}{r} 9\dfrac{5}{8} = 9\dfrac{15}{24} \\[2mm] + 6\dfrac{1}{6} = + 6\dfrac{4}{24} \\[1mm] \hline 15\dfrac{19}{24} \end{array} \qquad \begin{array}{l} \dfrac{5\,(\times 3)}{8\,(\times 3)} = \dfrac{15}{24} \\[3mm] \dfrac{1\,(\times 4)}{6\,(\times 4)} = \dfrac{4}{24} \end{array}$$

ANSWERS ON PAGE 310

WORKSHEET 1C Addition of Fractions and Mixed Numbers

Add the following fractions and mixed numbers, using the common denominator and reduce to lowest terms:

1. $\dfrac{1}{5}$
$+ \dfrac{2}{5}$

2. $\dfrac{3}{5}$
$+ \dfrac{2}{3}$

3. $6\dfrac{1}{6}$
$+ 9\dfrac{5}{8}$

4. $2\dfrac{1}{4}$
$+ 3\dfrac{1}{8}$

5. $1\dfrac{3}{8}$
$+ 9\dfrac{9}{10}$

6. $\dfrac{1}{8}$
$\dfrac{1}{4}$
$+ \dfrac{2}{9}$

7. $\dfrac{7}{9}$
$\dfrac{4}{5}$
$+ \dfrac{9}{10}$

8. $3\dfrac{1}{4}$
$+ 9\dfrac{3}{4}$

9. $8\dfrac{2}{5}$
$14\dfrac{7}{10}$
$+ 9\dfrac{9}{10}$

10. $2\dfrac{1}{3}$
$+ 4\dfrac{1}{6}$

● SUBTRACTION OF FRACTIONS AND MIXED NUMBERS

◎◁◁◁◁◁◁◁◁RULE   If fractions have the same denominator, find the difference between the numerators and write it over the common denominator. Reduce the fraction if necessary.

EXAMPLE

$$\begin{array}{r} \frac{27}{32} \\ -\ \frac{18}{32} \\ \hline \frac{9}{32} \end{array}$$

The difference between the numerators (27 minus 18) equals 9. The denominator is 32.

◎◁◁◁◁◁◁◁◁RULE   If fractions have different denominators, find the lowest common denominator and proceed as above.

EXAMPLE

$$\begin{array}{r} \frac{7}{8} = \frac{21}{24} \\ -\ \frac{2}{3} = \frac{16}{24} \\ \hline \frac{5}{24} \end{array}$$

The difference between the numerators (21 minus 16) equals 5. The lowest common denominator is 24.

◎◁◁◁◁◁◁◁◁RULE   To subtract mixed numbers, first subtract the fractions and then find the difference in the whole numbers. If the lower fraction is larger than the upper fraction, you cannot subtract it. *You must borrow from the whole number before subtracting the fraction.*

EXAMPLE

$$\begin{array}{r} 21\frac{7}{16} \\ -\ 7\frac{12}{16} \\ \hline \end{array}$$

You cannot subtract 12 from 7 because 12 is larger than 7. Therefore you must borrow a whole number (1) from the 21, make a fraction out of 1 $\left(\frac{16}{16}\right)$, and add the 7.

$$\frac{16}{16} + \frac{7}{16} = \frac{23}{16}$$

Because you added a whole number to the fraction, you must take a whole number away from 21 and make it 20. The problem is now set up as follows:

$$21\frac{7}{16} = 20\frac{16}{16} + \frac{7}{16} = \quad 20\frac{23}{16}$$
$$-\ 7\frac{12}{16}$$
$$\overline{\qquad 13\frac{11}{16}}$$

◎◁◁◁◁◁◁◁◁RULE   Reduce your answer to lowest terms.

ANSWERS ON PAGE 310

WORKSHEET 1D

Subtraction of Fractions and Mixed Numbers

Subtract fractions and mixed numbers, and reduce the answers to lowest terms:

1. $\dfrac{4}{5}$
$-\dfrac{1}{2}$

2. $\dfrac{27}{32}$
$-\dfrac{18}{32}$

3. $21\dfrac{7}{16}$
$-7\dfrac{12}{16}$

4. $7\dfrac{16}{24}$
$-3\dfrac{1}{8}$

5. $6\dfrac{5}{10}$
$-2\dfrac{1}{5}$

6. $\dfrac{7}{8}$
$-\dfrac{2}{3}$

7. $3\dfrac{5}{8}$
$-1\dfrac{3}{8}$

8. $5\dfrac{3}{7}$
$-1\dfrac{6}{7}$

9. 7
$-1\dfrac{3}{4}$

10. $2\dfrac{7}{8}$
$-\dfrac{3}{4}$

MULTIPLICATION OF FRACTIONS AND MIXED NUMBERS

STEPS Change the mixed number to an improper fraction if necessary.

Cancel, if possible, by dividing the numerators and denominators by the largest common divisor contained in each.

Multiply the remaining numerators to find a result, or product.

Multiply the denominators to find a result, or product.

Reduce the answer to lowest terms.

EXAMPLE $\dfrac{4}{5} \times \dfrac{15}{16} = \dfrac{\cancel{4}^{1}}{\cancel{5}_{1}} \times \dfrac{\cancel{15}^{3}}{\cancel{16}_{4}} = \dfrac{3}{4}$

$4\dfrac{1}{2} \times 2\dfrac{1}{4} = \dfrac{9}{2} \times \dfrac{9}{4} = \dfrac{81}{8} = 10\dfrac{1}{8}$

$6 \times \dfrac{3}{8} = \dfrac{6}{1} \times \dfrac{3}{8} = \dfrac{\cancel{6}^{3}}{1} \times \dfrac{3}{\cancel{8}_{4}} = \dfrac{9}{4} = 2\dfrac{1}{4}$

ANSWERS ON PAGE 311

WORKSHEET 1E Multiplication of Fractions and Mixed Numbers

Multiply the following fractions and mixed numbers, and reduce the answers to lowest terms:

1. $\frac{1}{3} \times \frac{2}{4} =$

2. $\frac{1}{5} \times \frac{1}{3} =$

3. $1\frac{3}{4} \times 3\frac{1}{7} =$

4. $4 \times 3\frac{1}{8} =$

5. $\frac{2}{4} \times 2\frac{1}{6} =$

6. $5\frac{1}{2} \times 3\frac{1}{8} =$

7. $\frac{3}{4} \times \frac{5}{8} =$

8. $\frac{5}{6} \times 1\frac{9}{16} =$

9. $\frac{5}{100} \times 900 =$

10. $2\frac{1}{10} \times 4\frac{1}{3} =$

● DIVISION OF FRACTIONS AND MIXED NUMBERS

STEPS Change mixed numbers to improper fractions if necessary.

Invert the number after the ÷ (division) sign.

Follow the steps for multiplication, and reduce any fractions.

EXAMPLES $\frac{1}{2} \div \frac{5}{8} = \frac{1}{2} \times \frac{8}{5} = \frac{8}{10} = \frac{4}{5}$

$8\frac{3}{4} \div 15 = \frac{35}{4} \times \frac{1}{15} = \frac{\overset{7}{\cancel{35}}}{4} \times \frac{1}{\underset{3}{\cancel{15}}} = \frac{7}{12}$

ANSWERS ON PAGE 311

WORKSHEET 1F Division of Fractions and Mixed Numbers

Divide the following fractions and mixed numbers, and reduce the answers to lowest terms:

1. $\frac{2}{5} \div \frac{5}{8} =$

2. $\frac{1}{3} \div \frac{1}{2} =$

3. $\frac{3}{4} \div \frac{1}{8} =$

4. $\frac{1}{16} \div \frac{1}{4} =$

5. $8\frac{3}{4} \div 15 =$

6. $\frac{3}{4} \div 6 =$

7. $2 \div \frac{1}{5} =$

8. $3\frac{3}{0} \div 4\frac{1}{2} =$

9. $\frac{3}{5} \div \frac{3}{8} =$

10. $4 \div 2\frac{1}{8} =$

● VALUE OF FRACTIONS

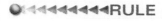**RULE** The smaller the denominator of a fraction, the greater the fraction's value.

EXAMPLE Which would you rather have, $\frac{1}{6}$ or $\frac{1}{9}$ of your favorite candy bar? $\frac{1}{6}$ is greater than $\frac{1}{9}$. It represents a larger part of the whole unit.

$\frac{1}{6}$	$\frac{1}{6}$	$\frac{1}{6}$	$\frac{1}{6}$	$\frac{1}{6}$	$\frac{1}{6}$

$= 6$ parts   Each $\frac{1}{6}$ part is **larger** than the $\frac{1}{9}$ part.

$\frac{1}{9}$	$\frac{1}{9}$	$\frac{1}{9}$	$\frac{1}{9}$	$\frac{1}{9}$	$\frac{1}{9}$	$\frac{1}{9}$	$\frac{1}{9}$	$\frac{1}{9}$

$= 9$ parts   Each $\frac{1}{9}$ part is **smaller** than the $\frac{1}{6}$ part.

ANSWERS ON PAGE 312

WORKSHEET
1G   Value of Fractions

Answer the following questions by circling the correct answer:

1. Which is **greater**? $\frac{1}{3}$ or $\frac{1}{5}$

2. Which is **smaller**? $\frac{1}{100}$ or $\frac{1}{150}$

3. Which is **greater**? $\frac{1}{250}$ or $\frac{1}{300}$

4. Which is **smaller**? $\frac{1}{6}$ or $\frac{1}{8}$

5. Which is **smaller**? $\frac{1}{50}$ or $\frac{1}{200}$

6. Ordered: gr $\frac{1}{300}$. You have gr $\frac{1}{150}$ tablets on hand. Will you need to give *more* or *less* of what is on hand?

    more or less

7. Ordered: gr $\frac{1}{6}$. You have gr $\frac{1}{4}$ tablets on hand. Will you need to give *more* or *less* of what is on hand?

    more or less

8. Ordered: gr $\frac{1}{10}$. You have gr $\frac{1}{4}$ tablets on hand. Will you need to give *more* or *less* of what is on hand?

    more or less

9. Ordered: gr $\frac{1}{100}$. You have gr $\frac{1}{200}$ tablets on hand. Will you need to give *more* or *less* of what is on hand?

    more or less

10. Ordered: gr $\frac{1}{8}$. You have gr $\frac{1}{6}$ tablets on hand. Will you need to give *more* or *less* of what is on hand?

    more or less

VALUE OF DECIMALS

A decimal fraction is a fraction whose denominator (bottom number) is 10, 100, 1000, 10,000, and so on. It differs from a common fraction in that the denominator is *not* written but is expressed by the proper placement of the decimal point.

Observe the scale below. All whole numbers are to the left of the decimal point; all decimal fractions are to the right.

◑◀◀◀◀◀◀◀RULES

All whole numbers are to the left of the decimal; all decimal fractions are to the right of the decimal point.

To read a decimal fraction, read the number to the right of the decimal and use the name that applies to "place value" of the *last* figure other than zero. Decimal fractions read with a *ths* on the end.

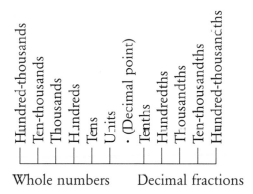

EXAMPLES

0.257 = Two hundred fifty seven thousand*ths*

0.2057 = Two thousand fifty-seven ten-thousand*ths*

0.20057 = Twenty thousand fifty-seven hundred thousand*ths*

◑◀◀◀◀◀◀◀◀RULE

For a whole number and a fraction, read the decimal point as an **and**.

EXAMPLE

327.006 = Three hundred twenty-seven *and* six thousand*ths*

ANSWERS ON PAGE 312

WORKSHEET
1H   **Value of Decimals**

Read the following decimals and write out in words:

1. 0.08   **2.** 0.092

3. 0.0017   **4.** 100.01

5. 0.0006   **6.** 3287.467

Write the following as decimals and decimal fractions:

7. Thirty-six hundredths   _____

8. Three thousandths   _____

9. Eight ten-thousandths   _____

10. Two and seventeen thousandths   _____

11. Five hundredths   _____

12. Four and one tenth   _____

13. Twenty-four and two tenths   _____

14. Fifteen and one hundredth   _____

15. Nine and two ten-thousandths   _____

16. Three and eight thousandths   _____

17. One hundred and eighteen thousandths   _____

18. Eighteen and fifteen hundredths   _____

19. Fifty-five thousandths   _____

20. Thirty-four and one tenth   _____

CLINICAL ALERT!

Make it your habit to always insert a zero (0) in front of decimal fractions when a whole number is absent. This draws attention to the decimal and avoids two potential critical errors: missing the decimal or mistaking it for a number "1."

ANSWERS ON PAGE 312

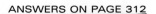

WORKSHEET
11

Comparison of Decimals

One of the keys to avoiding decimal errors when calculating medication doses is to know at a glance whether the amount you will give will be *more* or *less* than the amount provided.

Which is *smaller?* Circle the correct answer:

1. 0.4 or 0.2

2. 0.14 or 1.03

3. 0.68 or 0.8

4. 2.309 or 2.07

5. 1.465 or 1.29

6. 0.5 or 0.37

7. 5.12 or 0.512

8. 0.394 or 0.094

9. 0.005 or 0.015

10. 1.224 or 1.088

Which is *larger?* Circle the correct answer:

11. 0.238 or 1.99

12. 0.07 or 0.7

13. 0.58 or 0.09

14. 0.25 or 0.05

15. 0.001 or 0.10

16. 2.74 or 2.0067

17. 0.147 or 0.31

18. 25.04 or 25.14

19. 0.125 or 0.25

20. 0.75 or 0.075

● ADDITION OF DECIMALS

STEPS Write decimals in a column, keeping the decimal points under each other.

Add as in whole numbers, from right to left.

Place the decimal point in the answer directly under the decimal points in the numbers to be added.

EXAMPLES

$$\begin{array}{r} 0.8 \\ + 0.5 \\ \hline 1.3 \end{array}$$

$$\begin{array}{r} 3.27 \\ + 0.06 \\ \hline 3.33 \end{array}$$

 REMEMBER ● Line up the decimal points.

ANSWERS ON PAGE 313

WORKSHEET

1J   Addition of Decimals

Add the following decimals:

1. 0.8 + 0.5 =

2. 5.01 + 2.999 =

3. 3.27 + 0.06 + 2 =

4. 15.6 + 0.19 + 200 =

5. 210.79 + 2 + 68.4 =

6. 88.6 + 576.46 + 79.0 =

7. 6.77 + 102 + 88.3 =

8. 79.4 + 68.44 + 3.00 =

9. 10.56 + 356.4 =

10. 99.7 + 293.23 =

● SUBTRACTION OF DECIMALS

STEPS Write decimals in a column, keeping the decimal points under each other.

Subtract as in whole numbers, from right to left.

Place the decimal point in the answer directly under the decimal points in the numbers to be subtracted (zeros can be added *after* the decimal point without changing the value).

EXAMPLE $0.6 - 0.524 =$

$$
\begin{array}{r}
0.600 \\
-\ 0.524 \\
\hline
0.076
\end{array}
$$

 REMEMBER ● Line up the decimal points.

ANSWERS ON PAGE 313

WORKSHEET
1K   Subtraction of Decimals

Subtract the following decimals:

1. $98.4 - 66.50 =$

2. $21.78 - 19.88 =$

3. $0.450 - 0.367 =$

4. $108.56 - 5.40 =$

5. $266.44 - 0.56 =$

6. $7.066 - 0.200 =$

7. $34.678 - 0.502 =$

8. $78.567 - 6.77 =$

9. $1.723 - 0.683 =$

10. $0.8100 - 0.6701 =$

● MULTIPLICATION OF DECIMALS

STEPS Multiply as with whole numbers.

Count the total number of decimal places in the multiplier and in the number to be multiplied.

Start from the right and count off the same number of places in the answer.

If the answer does not have enough places, supply as many zeros as needed counting from right to left as illustrated below.

EXAMPLE $2.6 \times 0.0002 =$

$$
\begin{array}{r}
2.6 \quad \text{(1 decimal place)} \\
\times\ 0.0002 \quad \text{(4 decimal places)} \\
\hline
\mathbf{0.00052} \quad \text{(5 decimal places from right to left in the answer)}
\end{array}
$$

ANSWERS ON PAGE 313

WORKSHEET
1L ## Multiplication of Decimals

Multiply the following decimals:

1. $3.14 \times 0.002 =$

2. $95.26 \times 1.125 =$

3. $100 \times 0.5 =$

4. $2.14 \times 0.03 =$

5. $36.8 \times 70.1 =$

6. $200 \times 0.2 =$

7. $88 \times 90.1 =$

8. $2.76 \times 0.003 =$

9. $54.5 \times 21 =$

10. $203.7 \times 28 =$

● DIVISION OF DECIMALS

Examine the divisor—the number you are dividing by. Is it a *whole* number or a *decimal?*

●◀◀◀◀◀◀◀◀RULE If the divisor is a **whole** number, the dividend decimal place is unchanged. Immediately place the decimal point prominently on the answer line directly *above* the decimal point in the dividend. Use zeros in the answer to hold places until you can divide. Prove your answer.

EXAMPLES   ■ $1.20 \div 15$

$$
\begin{array}{r}
0.08 \leftarrow \text{\textbf{Answer}} \\
\text{\textbf{Divisor}} \rightarrow 15\overline{)1.20} \leftarrow \text{\textbf{Dividend}} \\
1\,20
\end{array}
$$

PROOF (Divisor
$\times$ answer
= dividend)

$$
\begin{array}{r}
15 \\
\times\,0.08 \\
\hline
1.20
\end{array}
$$

■ $3.15 \div 7$

$$
\begin{array}{r}
0.45 \\
7\overline{)3.15} \\
2\,8 \\
\hline
35 \\
35
\end{array}
$$

PROOF
$$
\begin{array}{r}
0.45 \\
\times\quad 7 \\
\hline
3.15
\end{array}
$$

RULE   If the divisor has a *decimal,* you must make it a whole number by moving the decimal point to the right. Move the decimal point in the dividend the same number of places to the right and immediately place the decimal point directly above on the answer line. Then divide as with whole numbers. Prove your answer.

EXAMPLE $10 \div 4.4$

$$
\begin{array}{r}
2.27 \\
4.4\,\overline{)10.0\,00} \\
8\,8 \\
\hline
1\,2\,0 \\
8\,8 \\
\hline
3\,20 \\
3\,08 \\
\hline
12\ \text{\textbf{Remainder}}
\end{array}
$$

PROOF
$$
\begin{array}{r}
2.27\ \text{\textbf{(2 decimal places)}} \\
\times\,4.\ \text{\textbf{(1 decimal place)}} \\
\hline
908 \\
908 \\
\hline
9988 \\
+\quad 12\ \text{\textbf{Remainder}} \\
\hline
10.000 \\
3\,2\,1
\end{array}
$$

EXAMPLE $30 \div 5.2$

$$
\begin{array}{r}
5.7 \\
5.2\,\overline{)30.0\,0} \\
26\,0 \\
\hline
4\,0\,0 \\
3\,6\,4 \\
\hline
3\,6\ \text{\textbf{Remainder}}
\end{array}
$$

PROOF
$$
\begin{array}{r}
5.2 \\
\times\,5.7 \\
\hline
36\,4 \\
260 \\
\hline
296\,4 \\
+\,3\,6\ \text{\textbf{Remainder}} \\
\hline
30.00
\end{array}
$$

Note that, as with whole division, a remainder is not just added to the answer in decimal division. Additional division will allow the remainder to be converted to a decimal fraction.

EXAMPLE $2.6 \div 4$

$$
\begin{array}{r}
0.6 \\
4\overline{)2.6} \\
2\,4 \\
\hline
2\ \text{\textbf{Remainder}}
\end{array}
\qquad
\begin{array}{r}
0.65 \\
4\overline{)2.60} \\
2\,4 \\
\hline
20 \\
20
\end{array}
$$

 REMEMBER ● Keep all your decimals dark.

ANSWERS ON PAGE 314

WORKSHEET 1M   Division of Decimals

In the following problems, the divisor is a whole number. Place the decimal point on the answer line as illustrated in red in #1. Do **NOT** do the math in these problems.

1. $60\overline{)1.35}$ (with decimal point placed on answer line)

2. $4\overline{)2.013}$

3. $20\overline{)15.6}$

4. $75\overline{)35}$

5. $19\overline{)10.14}$

6. $304\overline{)95.14}$

7. $7\overline{)60.5}$

8. $15\overline{)25.14}$

9. $25\overline{)35.9}$

10. $100\overline{)75}$

In the following problems, the divisor has a decimal. Make the divisor a whole number, move the decimal place in the dividend, and place the decimal point on the answer line as illustrated in red in #11. Do **NOT** do the math in these problems.

11. $8.4\overline{)1.3\,5}$

12. $0.25\overline{)3.57}$

13. $0.10\overline{)0.5}$

14. $94.5\overline{)0.029}$

15. $4.8\overline{)2.04}$

16. $0.52\overline{)120}$

17. $60.2\overline{)50.923}$

18. $0.75\overline{)0.5}$

19. $4.3\overline{)2.1}$

20. $0.50\overline{)0.25}$

Continue the division in the following problems to one more decimal place in the answer and add it to the answer as illustrated in red in #21. Do not round answers.

21.
$$
\begin{array}{r}
2.2 \\
10\overline{)22.0} \\
20\downarrow \\
\hline
2\,0 \\
2\,0 \\
\hline
\end{array}
$$

22.
$$
\begin{array}{r}
5. \\
50\overline{)255} \\
250 \\
\hline
5 \\
\end{array}
$$

23.
$$
\begin{array}{r}
0.6 \\
75\overline{)50.0} \\
45\,0 \\
\hline
5\,0 \\
\end{array}
$$

24.
$$
\begin{array}{r}
0.3 \\
30\overline{)10.0} \\
9\,0 \\
\hline
1\,0 \\
\end{array}
$$

25.
$$
\begin{array}{r}
4. \\
2.5\overline{)12.0} \\
10\,0 \\
\hline
2\,0 \\
\end{array}
$$

ANSWERS ON PAGE 315

WORKSHEET

1N More Division of Decimals

Divide the following and carry to the *third* decimal place if necessary:

1. $158.4 \div 48 =$

2. $200 \div 6.0 =$

3. $15.06 \div 6 =$

4. $79.4 \div 0.87 =$

5. $670.8 \div 0.78 -$

6. $78.6 \div 2.43 =$

7. $26.78 \div 8.2 =$

8. $266.5 \div 5.78 =$

9. $10.80 \div 6.5 =$

10. $76.53 \div 10 =$

● CHANGING DECIMALS TO FRACTIONS

◐◀◀◀◀◀◀◀◀RULE   The numbers to the *right* of the decimal can be written as a fraction because they are only part of the whole number.

   REMEMBER ● The first number past the decimal to the *right* is ten*ths*, the second is hundred*ths*, the third is thousand*ths*, the fourth is ten-thousand*ths*, and so on.

So if your problem has 3 numbers to the *right* of the decimal, just remove the decimal and put the number over 1000.

EXAMPLES ■ 0.375 has 3 numbers to the *right* of the decimal. To make a fraction out of 0.375 and also get rid of the decimal, place it over 1000.

0.375 written as a fraction is $\frac{375}{1000}$.

It's easy to remember: 3 numbers on top and 3 zeros on the bottom.

■ 0.91 written as a fraction is $\frac{91}{100}$.

The idea is the same as above: 2 numbers on top and 2 zeros on the bottom.

ANSWERS ON PAGE 316

WORKSHEET
10   Changing Decimals to Fractions

Change the following decimals to fractions, and reduce to lowest terms:

1. 0.4 =   **2.** 0.8 =

3. 0.25 =   **4.** 4.08 =

5. 1.32 =   **6.** 0.5 =

7. 0.75 =   **8.** 0.2 =

9. 0.65 =   **10.** 0.7 =

CHANGING COMMON FRACTIONS TO DECIMALS

◉◄◄◄◄◄◄◄◄RULE   To change a common fraction to a decimal, divide the numerator by the denominator and place the decimal point in the proper position on the answer line.

$$\textbf{EXAMPLES}\quad \frac{2}{5} = 5\overline{)2.0}$$
$$\begin{array}{r} 0.4 \\ 5\overline{)2.0} \\ \underline{2\,0} \end{array}$$

$$\frac{1}{8} = 8\overline{)1.000}$$
$$\begin{array}{r} 0.125 \\ 8\overline{)1.000} \\ \underline{8} \\ 20 \\ \underline{16} \\ 40 \\ \underline{40} \end{array}$$

ANSWERS ON PAGE 317

WORKSHEET 1P   ## Changing Common Fractions to Decimals

Carry out the following division problems to the *third* decimal place:

1. $\frac{19}{100} =$

2. $\frac{9}{7} =$

3. $5\frac{9}{16} =$

4. $\frac{1}{5} =$

5. $\frac{2}{3} =$

6. $\frac{1}{2} =$

7. $\frac{1}{12} =$

8. $\frac{6}{8} =$

9. $\frac{15}{200} =$

10. $\frac{20}{8} =$

● ROUNDING DECIMALS

STEPS Calculate *one* decimal place beyond the desired place.

If the final digit is **4** or less, make no adjustment. If the final digit is **5** or more, *increase* the prior digit by one number.

Drop the final digit.

tenths

EXAMPLES
- Round 2.7 to the nearest whole number. Examine the tenths column.
- Because 7 is more than 5, the answer is 3 and 0.7 is dropped.

tenths hundredths

- Round 2.55 to the nearest tenth.
  Examine the second decimal place (hundredths column).
  Because the hundredths column is 5, the 2.5 is rounded up to 2.6 and the final 0.05 (hundredths) is dropped.

- Round 3.762 to the nearest hundredth.
  Examine the third decimal place (thousandths column).
  Because 2 is less than 5, no adjustment will be made in the hundredths column and the 2 is dropped.
  3.76 is the answer.

	NEAREST WHOLE NUMBER	NEAREST TENTH	NEAREST HUNDREDTH
1.689	2	1.7	1.69
204.534	205	204.5	204.53
7.87	8	7.9	7.87
3.366	3	3.4	3.37
0.845*	1	0.8	0.85

*To reduce reading errors, maintain the habit of placing a zero (0) in front of the decimal when a whole number is absent.

⬡ CLINICAL ALERT!

Do *not* round medication dosages to the nearest whole number. This could result in an overdose. For instructions on how to round medication doses, refer to Chapter 4 (p. 73).

ANSWERS ON PAGE 318

WORKSHEET
10   ## Rounding Decimals

Round the decimal to the nearest whole number, the nearest tenth, and the nearest hundredth:

	NEAREST WHOLE NUMBER	NEAREST TENTH	NEAREST HUNDREDTH
1. 93.489			
2. 25.430			
3. 38.10			
4. 57.8888			
5. 0.0092			
6. 3.144			
7. 8.999			
8. 77.788			
9. 12.959			
10. 5.7703			

ANSWERS ON PAGE 318

WORKSHEET
1R   ## Rounding Decimal Products

Multiply or divide the following numbers. Round your answers to the nearest whole number, the nearest tenth, and the nearest hundredth:

	NEAREST WHOLE NUMBER	NEAREST TENTH	NEAREST HUNDREDTH
1. $25.3 \times 4.2 =$			
2. $9.3 \times 2.86 =$			
3. $4.5 \times 7.57 =$			
4. $1.3 \times 9.69 =$			
5. $2.4 \times 5.88 =$			
6. $8 \div 5 =$			
7. $4.1 \div 3 =$			
8. $5 \div 1.2 =$			
9. $9 \div 2.2 =$			
10. $10.2 \div 3 =$			

● PERCENTAGES, DECIMALS, AND FRACTIONS

The term *percent* and its symbol (%) mean *per hundred*. A percent number is a fraction whose numerator is already known and whose denominator is *always* understood to be 100. 25% means 25 *per hundred*.

◨ Changing a Percentage to a Fraction

◉◄◄◄◄◄◄◄RULE The numerator is the percent and the denominator is always 100.

EXAMPLES ■ 5% written as a fraction is $\frac{5}{100}$.

Drop the percent sign when converting 5% to $\frac{5}{100}$.

■ $\frac{1}{2}$% written as a fraction is $\frac{1/2}{100}$. You cannot leave the problem like this. $\frac{1/2}{100}$ means $\frac{1}{2} \div 100 = \frac{1}{2} \times \frac{1}{100} = \frac{1}{200}$.* Thus $\frac{1}{2}$% must be changed to $\frac{1}{200}$.

◨ Changing a Percentage to a Decimal

◉◄◄◄◄◄◄◄RULE A percent number can be changed to a decimal by moving its decimal point 2 places to the *left* to signify hundred*ths* and removing the percent sign.

EXAMPLES ■ 5% written as a decimal is 0.05 (5% $= \frac{5}{100} = 0.05$).

■ 0.5% written as a decimal is 0.005 (0.5% $= \frac{0.5}{100} = \frac{5}{1000} = 0.005$).

 REMEMBER ● Move the decimal 2 places to the *left* and drop the percent sign.

◨ Converting a Decimal to a Percentage

◉◄◄◄◄◄◄◄RULE To change a decimal to a percentage, move the decimal point 2 places to the *right*, and add the percent sign.

EXAMPLES ■ 0.1 is a decimal. To make it a percentage, move the decimal point 2 places to the *right* and add the percent sign. Therefore 0.1 $= \frac{1}{10} = \frac{10}{100} = 10\%$.

■ Thus 0.001 $= \frac{1}{1000} = \frac{0.1}{100} = 0.1\%$.

---

*See page ●●● for division of fractions.

ANSWERS ON PAGE 318

WORKSHEET 1S

Percentages, Decimals, and Fractions

Fill in the following blanks with the appropriate equivalents:

	FRACTION	DECIMAL	PERCENTAGE
1.	$\frac{1}{2}$		
2.			$66\frac{2}{3}\%$
3.			6.5%
4.	$\frac{1}{12}$		
5.	$\frac{3}{1000}$		
6.		0.10	
7.			250%
8.		0.35	
9.	$\frac{4}{5}$		
10.			78%

◼ Finding the Percentage

STEPS Change the percentage to a decimal or common fraction.

Multiply the number by this decimal.

EXAMPLES 23% of 64 = 64 × 0.23 = 14.72
5% of 10 = 10 × 0.05 = 0.5

ANSWERS ON PAGE 319

WORKSHEET

1T **Finding the Percentage**

1. 114% of 240 =

2. 2% of 1500 =

3. $\frac{1}{2}$% of 9328 =

4. $\frac{1}{3}$% of 930 =

5. 28% of 50 =

6. 9% of 200 =

7. 120% of 400 =

8. 5% of 105.80 =

9. 10% of 520 =

10. 3% of 40.80 =

ANSWERS ON PAGE 320

WORKSHEET
1U Multiple-Choice Practice

Solve the following problems and select the correct answer. Estimate the correct answer before working the problem:

1. $\frac{41}{7}$ can be converted to which whole and mixed number:

   a. $7\frac{1}{4}$ **c.** $9\frac{1}{8}$

   b. $5\frac{6}{7}$ **d.** $6\frac{6}{8}$

2. Select the *improper fraction* equivalent for $3\frac{5}{6}$:

   a. $\frac{15}{6}$ **c.** $4\frac{1}{6}$

   b. $\frac{23}{6}$ **d.** $\frac{8}{6}$

3. $\frac{7}{8}$ and $\frac{3}{5}$ have which lowest common denominator:

   a. 8   **c.** 13

   b. 10   **d.** 40

4. $5\frac{1}{8} + 1\frac{1}{4} + = 4\frac{1}{2} =$

   a. $10\frac{7}{8}$ **c.** $12\frac{1}{2}$

   b. $9\frac{1}{6}$ **d.** $10\frac{3}{4}$

5. $6\frac{3}{4} - 5\frac{1}{3} =$

   a. $\frac{1}{2}$ **c.** $1\frac{5}{12}$

   b. $1\frac{1}{2}$ **d.** $1\frac{5}{8}$

6. $\frac{5}{6} \times \frac{2}{8} =$

   a. $\frac{1}{12}$ **c.** $\frac{7}{14}$

   b. $\frac{5}{24}$ **d.** $\frac{10}{44}$

7. Divide the following fraction and reduce the lowest term: $\frac{1}{6} \div \frac{1}{2}$

   a. $\frac{2}{12}$ **c.** $\frac{1}{6}$

   b. $\frac{1}{3}$ **d.** $\frac{1}{12}$

8. Divide the following fraction and reduce the *lowest* term: $\frac{5}{6} \div \frac{1}{3}$

   a. $\frac{1}{6}$ **c.** $1\frac{1}{6}$

   b. $\frac{5}{18}$ **d.** $2\frac{1}{2}$

9. Two and seventeen thousandths can be written in decimal form as:

   a. 2.017   **c.** 2.17

   b. 2.07   **d.** 2.170

10. $0.41 - 0.2538 =$

   a. 0.1562   **c.** 0.4138

   b. 0.2503   **d.** 0.6638

11. $5 \times 0.7 =$

   a. 5.7   **c.** 3.5

   b. 12.5   **d.** 35

12. $79.4 \div 0.87 =$

   a. 12.024   **c.** 80.276

   b. 21.084   **d.** 91.264

13. Change $8\frac{1}{6}$ to a decimal and round the answer to the *nearest* hundredth:

   a. 8.02   **c.** 8.166

   b. 8.0625   **d.** 8.17

14. 30% of 550 =

   a. 15   **c.** 50

   b. 165   **d.** 185

15. $6\frac{1}{4}\%$ of 9328 =

   a. 0.56   **c.** 583

   b. 540   **d.** 5596

16. Change 0.285 to a fraction:

   a. $\frac{285}{1000}$ **c.** $\frac{285}{100}$

   b. $\frac{28}{100}$ **d.** $\frac{29}{1000}$

17. Change $\frac{2}{5}$ to a decimal to the *nearest* tenth:

   a. 0.4   **c.** 0.04

   b. 0.25   **d.** 0.025

18. Change $\frac{1}{6}$ to a decimal to the *nearest hundredth:*

   a. 0.1   **c.** 0.17

   b. 0.2   **d.** 0.18

19. Round 58.007 to the *nearest tenth:*

   a. 58   **c.** 58.1

   b. 58.07   **d.** 58.7

20. Change 4% to a decimal:

   a. 0.4   **c.** 0.25

   b. 0.04   **d.** 0.2

 Refer to the Mathematics Review, Fractions, Decimals, and Percents sections of the enclosed CD-ROM for additional practice problems.

ANSWERS ON PAGE 320

CHAPTER **1** **FINAL**

Change to whole or mixed numbers:

1. $\frac{48}{7}$

2. $\frac{34}{6}$

Change to improper fractions:

3. $13\frac{3}{5}$

4. $3\frac{5}{6}$

Find the lowest common denominator in the following pairs of fractions:

5. $\frac{17}{20}$ and $\frac{4}{5}$

6. $\frac{7}{8}$ and $\frac{3}{5}$

Add the following:

7. $\frac{1}{18} + \frac{1}{4} + \frac{2}{9}$

8. $5\frac{1}{8} + 1\frac{1}{4} + 4\frac{1}{2}$

Subtract the following:

9. $\frac{7}{8} - \frac{2}{3}$

10. $6\frac{2}{4} - 5\frac{1}{2}$

Multiply the following:

11. $\frac{1}{5} \times \frac{1}{3}$

12. $\frac{5}{6} \times \frac{2}{8}$

Divide the following:

13. $\frac{3}{4} \div \frac{1}{8}$

14. $3\frac{3}{8} \div 4\frac{1}{2}$

Reduce the following fractions to lowest terms (numbers):

15. $\frac{2}{500}$

16. $\frac{9}{27}$

Write the following as decimals:

17. Thirty-six hundredths

18. Two and seventeen thousandths

Add the following:

19. $5.01 + 2.999$

20. $36.87 + 8.26 + 15.84$

Subtract the following:

21. $4 - 0.176$

22. $0.41 - 0.2538$

Multiply the following:

23. 0.0005×0.02

24. 5×0.7

Divide the following and carry to the third decimal place:

25. $158.4 \div 48$

26. $79.4 \div 0.87$

Change the following to decimals:

27. $\frac{57}{48}$

28. $8\frac{1}{16}$

Find the following percentages:

29. 24% of 52

30. $6\frac{1}{4}\%$ of 9328

Change the following decimals to fractions:

31. 0.4

32. 0.285

Fill in the following blanks with the appropriate equivalents:

	FRACTION	DECIMAL TO NEAREST TENTH	DECIMAL TO NEAREST HUNDREDTH	PERCENTAGE
33.	$\frac{1}{3}$			
34.				4%
35.	$\frac{2}{5}$			
36.				22%
37.	$\frac{3}{8}$			
38.				10%
39.	$\frac{1}{12}$			
40.				$\frac{1}{2}$%
41.	$\frac{5}{16}$			
42.				15%
43.	$\frac{1}{4}$			
44.				12%
45.	$\frac{7}{9}$			
46.				80%
47.	$\frac{1}{6}$			
48.				33%
49.	$\frac{1}{250}$			
50.				75%

Ratio and Proportion

2

INTRODUCTION

Ratio and proportion is the easiest provable method of drug dose calculation for most students. The setup of problems is logical and systematic. Answers can be proven if the setup is correct.*

● RATIO

A ratio indicates the relationship of one quantity to another. It indicates *division* and may be expressed in fraction form.

EXAMPLE $\frac{1}{3}$ may be expressed as the ratio 1:3.

ANSWERS ON PAGE 321

WORKSHEET
2A   Ratio: Expressing Ratios as Fractions

Express the following ratios as fractions reduced to lowest terms:

1. 3:6   **2.** 6:8   **3.** 2:500

4. 6:1000   **5.** 43:86   **6.** 2:13

7. 7:49   **8.** 1:10   **9.** 1:150

10. 4:100

● PROPORTION

A proportion shows the relationship between two equal ratios. A proportion may be expressed as 3 : 5 :: 6 : 10 or 3 : 5 = 6 : 10.
To solve the ratio and proportion problems, do the following.

STEPS   Multiply the two inside numbers.

Multiply the two outside numbers.

Check to see that the answers are the same.

---

*Students who are familiar with dimensional analysis and prefer to use this method of solving problems are referred to Chapter 12.

EXAMPLE   3 : 5 :: 6 : 10 or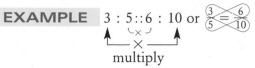

multiply

Multiply the two *inside* numbers: 5 × 6 = 30.
Multiply the two *outside* numbers: 3 × 10 = 30.

■ Solving Proportion Problems When One of the Numbers Is *Unknown,* or *x*

EXAMPLE   2 : 8 :: *x* : 24 or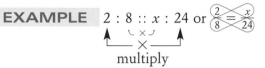

multiply

Multiply the two *inside* numbers (means).
$$8 \times x = 8x$$
Multiply the two *outside* numbers (extremes).
$$2 \times 24 = 48$$
Place the $8x$ on the **left** side of the equation. It will now look like this:
$$8x = 48$$

> **HINT ■ Placing the *x* product on the left side of the equation simplifies the work for many.**

Now you must get x to stand alone.

◉◀◀◀◀◀◀◀**RULES**   To get *x* alone, *divide* both sides of the equation by the number *next* to *x*. Those numbers will cancel each other. The result will be that *x* will stand alone.

What you do to one side of the equation, you must do to the other to keep the sides equal.

EXAMPLE
continued $\frac{\not{8}}{\not{8}}x = \frac{48}{8}$ This means 48 ÷ 8 or $8\overline{)48}$ $\begin{array}{r} 6 \\ \hline \end{array}$
$$\frac{48}{0}$$

$x = 6$
How do you know your answer is correct?

◉◀◀◀◀◀◀◀◀**RULE**   To check your answer, substitute the answer for the *x* in the problem, multiply the inside numbers together, and then multiply the outside numbers together. The products should be equal.

PROOF 8 × 6 = 48   (product of inside numbers, or means)
       2 × 24 = 48   (product of outside numbers, or extremes)

EXAMPLE $2 : 3 :: 6 : x$ $2 : 3 :: 6 : 9$

multiply

PROOF $2 \times 9 = 18$ (product of outside numbers)
$3 \times 6 = 18$ (product of inside numbers)

$2x = 18$

$\frac{\cancel{2}}{\cancel{2}}x = \frac{18}{2}$ $18 \div 2$ or $2\overline{)18} = 9$

$x = 9$

REMEMBER ● Divide both sides by the number next to x.

ANSWERS ON PAGE 322

WORKSHEET 2B

Solving Proportion Practice Problems for the Value of x

Multiply the two inside numbers, multiply the two outside numbers, and put _x_ on the _left_. Solve for _x_:

1. $9 : x :: 5 : 300$

2. $\frac{1}{2} : x :: 1 : 8$

3. $9 : 27 :: 300 : x$

4. $\frac{1}{4} : 500 :: x : 1000$

5. $36 : 12 :: \frac{1}{100} : x$

6. $6 : 24 :: 0.75 : x$

7. $x : 600 :: 4 : 120$

8. $0.7 : 70 :: x : 1000$

9. $\frac{1}{1000} : \frac{1}{100} :: x : 60$

10. $6 : 12 :: \frac{1}{4} : x$

ANSWERS ON PAGE 323

WORKSHEET 2C   Solving Proportion Practice Problems for the Value of x

Solve the following proportions for x, and prove your answers:

1. $15 : 30 :: x : 12$

2. $\frac{1}{200} : x :: 1 : 800$

3. $\frac{1}{1000} : \frac{1}{100} :: x : 30$

4. $6 : 12 :: 0.25 : x$

5. $300 : 5 :: x : \frac{1}{60}$

6. $\frac{1}{150} : \frac{1}{200} :: 2 : x$

7. $\frac{1}{2} : \frac{1}{6} :: \frac{1}{4} : x$

8. $7.5 : 12 :: x : 28$

9. $15 : x :: 1.5 : 10$

10. $10 : x :: 0.4 : 12$

ANSWERS ON PAGE 324

WORKSHEET 2D

Solving Proportion Practice Problems for the Value of *x*

Solve the following proportions for *x*, and prove your answers:

1. $9 : x :: 5 : 300$

2. $6 : 24 :: 0.75 : x$

3. $8 : 16 :: x : 24$

4. $x : 600 :: 4 : 120$

5. $5 : 3000 :: 15 : x$

6. $0.7 : 70 :: x : 1000$

7. $9 : 27 :: 300 : x$

8. $6 : 12 :: \frac{1}{4} : x$

9. $25 : x :: 75 : 3000$

10. $0.6 : 10 :: 0.5 : x$

● SETTING UP RATIOS AND PROPORTIONS

HINTS ■ To set up a ratio and proportion, you must always put on the *left*-hand side what you already *have*, or what you already *know*.
■ On the *right*-hand side, you will put your *x*, or what you *want* to know.
■ Each side of the equation is set up the *same way*.

EXAMPLE Apples : *Pears* :: Apples : *x Pears*

STEPS Multiply the two inside numbers. Multiply the two outside numbers.

Always put *x* on the left for your *final* multiplication.

Divide both sides by the number next to *x*.

Prove all answers and label them.

EXAMPLES ■ You wish to make a floral bouquet of 6 daffodils for every 4 roses. How many daffodils will you use for 30 roses?

Know   *Want to know*
6 daffodils : 4 roses :: *x* daffodils : 30 roses  **PROOF** $4 \times 45 = 180$
└──────── multiply ────────┘ $6 \times 30 = 180$

$\frac{\cancel{4}}{\cancel{4}}x = \frac{180}{4} = 180 \div 4 = 45$ daffodils

REMEMBER ● Place x on the left side of the equation to solve:

$$4x = 180$$
$$x = 45 \text{ daffodils}$$

■ Make a necklace that has 19 blue beads for every yellow bead. How many blue beads are needed if you have 8 yellow beads? (Prove your answer.)

Know   *Want to Know*

19 blue beads : 1 yellow bead :: x blue beads : 8 yellow beads

—————————— multiply ——————————

$x = 152$ blue beads needed

PROOF $19 \times 8 = 152$
                 $1 \times 152 = 152$

ANSWERS ON PAGE 325

WORKSHEET 2E

Setting Up Ratios and Proportions

Set up a proportion in each of the following problems, and label and prove your answers:

1. You have to make a fruit basket with 6 bananas for every 9 apples. How many bananas will there be for 72 apples?

2. You are making coffee, and 7 scoops make 8 cups. How many scoops make 40 cups?

3. You have a recipe for cocoa—4 scoops make 6 cups of cocoa. You want to make 18 cups for a party. How many scoops of cocoa are needed? Set up a proportion.

4. Ordered: 4 pills each day. The patient will be taking the medication for 21 days. How many pills will you give?

5. You wish to plant 8 bushes for every 2 trees in your yard. How many bushes will there be if there are 36 trees? (Estimate and prove.)

6. Ordered: 4 cups of bran every day. How many days would it take to consume 84 cups of bran? (Estimate and prove.)

7. It takes 4 cups of flour to make 3 loaves of bread. How many loaves of bread can be made from 24 cups of flour?

8. Your recipe for punch calls for 3 cups of soda for every $\frac{1}{2}$ cup of fruit juice. How many cups of soda will be needed for 2 cups of fruit juice?

9. You need 4 tbsp of sugar for every glass of lemonade you prepare. How many tablespoons of sugar will be needed for 6 glasses of lemonade?

10. Ordered: 4 capsules every day. How many capsules would be needed for 14 days?

ANSWERS ON PAGE 327

WORKSHEET

2F   Setting Up Ratios and Proportions

Use ratio and proportion to solve the following problems, and label and prove your answers:

1. The office needs 4000 envelopes. The boxes on hand contain 200 envelopes per box. How many boxes will you send?

2. Ordered are 300 computer disks. The packages on hand contain 10 disks per package. How many packages will you send?

3. If there is one computer allocated for every 18 students, how many computers will be needed for an enrollment of 1280 students?

4. Your doctor tells you to drink 3 glasses of water and eat 2 apples every day. How many apples will you have eaten when you have drunk 24 glasses of water?

5. If all the teachers were to receive 6 pens for every 8 pencils, how many pens would you give if the teachers have 72 pencils?

6. If the cook is making an omelet with $\frac{1}{2}$ tsp of salt for every 3 eggs, how many teaspoons of salt would be needed for 30 eggs?

7. If a coffeemaker makes 8 cups of coffee for every 7 scoops of coffee, how many scoops would be needed to make 24 cups of coffee?

8. The flower arrangements call for 5 carnations for each fern. How many carnations would be needed for 10 ferns?

9. If 2 tbsp of vinegar are needed for each cup of water, how many tablespoons would be needed for 10 cups of water?

10. If a recipe calls for $\frac{1}{2}$ cup of milk for every 3 cups of flour, how many cups of milk would be needed for 21 cups of flour?

ANSWERS ON PAGE 328

WORKSHEET

2G   Multiple-Choice Practice

Use ratio and proportion to solve the following problems, and label and prove your answers:

1. Ordered: 120 insulin syringes. They are delivered in units of 10 per package. How many packages will you receive?
   - **a.** 10 pkgs
   - **b.** 12 pkgs
   - **c.** 15 pkgs
   - **d.** 20 pkgs

2. You have to take 4 tsp of medicine every day. The bottle contains 80 tsp. How many days will the bottle last?
   - **a.** 2 days
   - **b.** 5 days
   - **c.** 10 days
   - **d.** 20 days

3. If you need 10 diapers a day, how many days will a package of 50 diapers last?
   - **a.** 5 days
   - **b.** 10 days
   - **c.** 15 days
   - **d.** 20 days

4. You have a vial with 30 mL of liquid. If the average dose given is 5 mL, how many doses are available?
   - **a.** 5 doses
   - **b.** 6 doses
   - **c.** 8 doses
   - **d.** 10 doses

5. Ordered: 3 pills per day. How many pills will the patient need for 21 days?
   - **a.** 12 pills
   - **b.** 20 pills
   - **c.** 31 pills
   - **d.** 63 pills

6. The hospital has allotted 120 days of inservice for 15 departments. How many days of inservice can each department use?
   - **a.** 4 days
   - **b.** 8 days
   - **c.** 12 days
   - **d.** 15 days

7. The hospital staffs every 8 patients with one RN. How many RNs will be needed when the census is 240?
   - **a.** 30 RNs
   - **b.** 60 RNs
   - **c.** 90 RNs
   - **d.** 120 RNs

8. The directions state that for every $\frac{1}{2}$ cup portion of baby cereal you will need 4 oz of milk. How many ounces of milk will you need to prepare 20 portions?
   - **a.** 20 oz
   - **b.** 40 oz
   - **c.** 80 oz
   - **d.** 100 oz

9. If you receive $15 an hour overtime, how many hours would you need to work overtime to receive $450 in overtime earnings?
   - **a.** 3 hrs
   - **b.** 15 hrs
   - **c.** 30 hrs
   - **d.** 45 hrs

10. There is one nurse assistant employed for every 20 beds. How many nurse assistants are employed for a 360-bed hospital?
    - **a.** 18 assistants
    - **b.** 20 assistants
    - **c.** 25 assistants
    - **d.** 30 assistants

 Refer to the Mathematics Review, Ratio and Proportion sections of the enclosed CD-ROM for additional practice problems.

ANSWERS ON PAGE 329

CHAPTER 2 FINAL

Use ratio and proportion to solve the following problems, and label and prove your answers:

1. If the patient is discharged with a 1-week supply of pills and is to take 4 pills per day, how many pills will the patient need?

2. Ordered: 2 tablets, 3 times daily. How many days will a bottle of 60 tablets last?

3. The patient is to drink 4 oz of water every $\frac{1}{2}$ hour. How much water will the patient have consumed in 8 hours?

4. The budget permits 96 inservice days per year. There are 12 units. How many inservice days could each unit receive?

5. A multidose vial contains 20 mL. If each dose is 2.5 ml, how many doses are in the vial?

6. If the average adult weight is 150 lb and the elevator can hold 1800 lb, how many people, on average, can ride the elevator?

7. If the patient has to take 1 pill every 6 hours, how many pills will he need for 3 days?

8. If each orientation for an RN costs approximately $3000, how many RNs can the hospital plan to hire with an annual orientation budget of $96,000?

9. If a guest speaker is paid a $50 honorarium, how many guest speakers can you have with a budget of $600?

10. If a patient needs a 30-day supply of tablets and takes 2 tablets four times a day, how many tablets will the patient need at discharge?

Patient Safety: Errors, Orders, Labels, and Records

3

OBJECTIVES

- List knowledge and skills needed for safe administration of medications.
- Describe safe nursing practices to reduce medication errors.
- Interpret medication labels.
- Identify equipment for oral medication administration.
- Identify oral and liquid forms of medications.
- Identify key characteristics of medication administration records (MARs).
- Convert time to military hours.
- Explain the need for incident reports.
- Analyze medication errors using critical thinking.

INTRODUCTION

Patient safety in medication administration involves more than accurate dose calculation. Knowledge of potential sources of error and commonly occurring errors, critical thinking in the nursing process, and attention to detail and patients' rights are required to protect each patient. Revisit this practical chapter throughout your clinical courses of study so that this knowledge can be applied whenever you are in the clinical setting.

● PATIENT SAFETY

Patient safety is a primary goal of patient care rendered by any provider: "First do no harm." Accurate dose calculation by the person who will administer the medication is one of many factors in the process of ensuring patient safety. To prevent errors, the health care provider also needs to have extensive knowledge of pharmacology and legal issues, as well as adequate clinical practice and supervision. In addition, the provider must integrate many skills and behaviors incorporating the patient's rights with the nursing process:

- Verifying and interpreting medication orders—the right order, a safe order
- Reading and understanding medication labels—the right drug
- Accurate dose calculation and drug preparation—the right dose
- Use of qualified resources when a question arises—patient safety
- Relevant patient assessment—readiness for and response to medications
- Accurate drug administration—the right route, the right time
- Relevant and prompt patient intervention and follow-up—patient protection
- Accurate, prompt, and complete documentation—patient protection

Several studies have shown that many medications are given in error, ranging from 2% to well over 10%, if underreporting and wrong time of administration factors are considered. Medication supplies, administration procedures, and related forms are constantly updated in an attempt to reduce errors. When errors occur, patient injury and lawsuits may follow. The errors may be made in the physician's prescription, in the pharmacy, by clerical employees, and by nurses. The nurse who is to administer the medication offers the last protection for the patient. Extensive nursing knowledge and skill are necessary to prevent errors. Everyone who administers medications has a responsibility to obtain adequate information and to request practice with supervision and assistance until safe independent practice is attained.

● HOW TO AVOID MEDICATION ERRORS

As you read through each of these safety suggestions, think about what kinds of injuries might be prevented.

The following current Internet references pertain to medication errors:

www.cc.nih.gov/phar
www.fda.gov/cder/drug/MedErrors
www.gov/oc/speeches/2002
www.ismp.org
www.medscape.com
www.pharmacyandyou.org

Physician's Orders

All medication-related forms in the hospital record must match exactly the provider's *original* orders (Figure 3-1).

GENERAL HOSPITAL
PHYSICIAN'S ORDERS

PROBLEMS:

DRUG ALLERGIES:

☐ IN ACCORDANCE WITH OUR FORMULARY SYSTEM THE USE OF
GENERIC EQUIVALENTS ACCEPTABLE UNLESS CHECKED.

▲▲ ADDRESSOGRAPH IMPRINT ▲▲

INSTRUCTIONS FOR USE

1. IMPRINT SET BEFORE PLACING IN CHART.
2. DETACH TOP CARBONLESS COPY AND SEND TO PHARMACY EACH TIME DOCTOR WRITES A SET OF ORDERS.
3. INDICATE CARBONLESS COPY REMOVED BY PLACING INITIALS IN COLUMN OPPOSITE PHYSICIAN'S SIGNATURE.

DATE	TIME	ORDERS AND SIGNATURE	CH'KD	NURSE
3/10	0940	Clindamycin 300 mg PO q6h		
		J R Doctor MD		

A

| 6/10 | 0700 | Digoxin 0.5 mg loading dose PO tab today | | |
| | | J Taylor MD | | |

B

FIGURE 3-1 A, Example of a legible handwritten order. It gives the name of the medication, strength, and route of administration. The nurse can initial the order and record the time the order was reviewed and sent to the pharmacy to be filled. The order is signed by the physician attending the patient. **B,** This order is written clearly with the date and time recorded, medication, dosage, route, and schedule. The order is signed by the physician caring for the patient.

Clarify any unclear orders with the provider (best source), pharmacy, or a knowledgeable supervisor, and then *document* the clarification on the patient record. Experience will dictate the best source for clarification. Orders may be improperly written, illegible, or inappropriate for a particular patient, or the patient may be allergic to a medication ordered.

Avoid verbal orders except in an emergency; if you must take a verbal order, read back the order to the person giving it. Spell the name of the drug. There are thousands of drugs, including many that have very similar names but very different actions. Also, the ear may not be able to distinguish sounds and consonants such as *Z* from *X*, *D* from *B*, and *T* from *D*.

The following are examples of drugs with similar names:

Cefzil	Keflin
clindamycin	clindamycin phosphate
glyburide	glipizide
penicillin G	penicillin V
Procardia	Procardia XL
Zantac	Xanax

On return from breaks and meals, always check for new orders and recheck the medication administration record. Do not rely on others to inform you of new orders or medications given in your absence.

◼ Preparation

1. Clean and clear the area. Focus on your task. Try to avoid distractions.
2. Note allergies cited on record, and reconfirm on medication administration record (MAR) when medication was last given.
3. If the patient is transfer or postoperative, check the operating room and recovery room notes to see what medications were given so that the patient does not receive a drug overdose or interaction with the new transfer orders.
4. Assess recent relevant laboratory results.
5. If dose will exceed the basic unit dose supplied (e.g., 1 tablet or capsule per package or 1 mL ampule), recheck the original order and a pharmacology reference. Remember that the basic unit dose applies only to the average adult and not to the elderly or children. If you have to prepare more than one pill or more than 1 mL in a syringe for an adult, RECHECK first. Do the same if you are preparing more than 1 tsp of an oral liquid.
6. Check for lack of sediment in liquids and intact seals on controlled substances.
7. Check the label again before returning or discarding medication from a multidose bottle. With single-dose medications, retain the container at least until the medication has been administered. Figures 3-2 and 3-3 show computerized and standard medication carts.

◼ Medication Packaging

- Unit dose (Figure 3-4)
- Multidose (Figures 3-5 and 3-6)

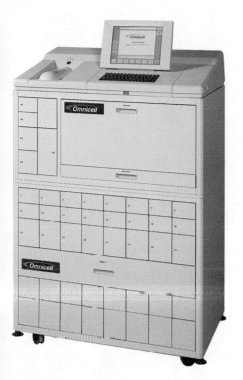

FIGURE 3-2 Sure-Med Unit Dose Center is an example of a computerized unit dose medication cart. Each dose is released individually, recorded automatically, and requires no counting when dispensed or at the end of a shift. It is used for monitoring controlled substances and high-use floor stock, supplies, and other charge items. *(From Omnicell, Inc., Palo Alto, CA.)*

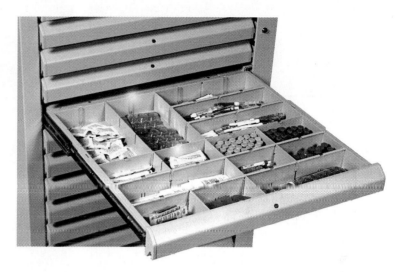

FIGURE 3-3 The Lighted Matrix Drawer is an example of a flexible medication and pharmacy supply drawer. *(From Omnicell, Inc., Palo Alto, CA.)*

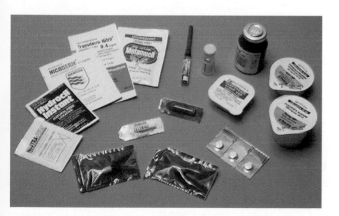

FIGURE 3-4 Unit dose packages. *(From Clayton BD, Stock YN: Basic pharmacology for nurses, ed 12, St Louis, 2001, Mosby. Courtesy of Chuck Dresner.)*

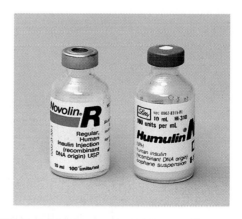

FIGURE 3-5 Multidose vials of Regular (Novolin R) and intermediate-acting (Humulin N) insulin. *(From Elkin M, Perry A, Potter P: Nursing interventions and clinical skills, ed 2, St Louis, 2000, Mosby.)*

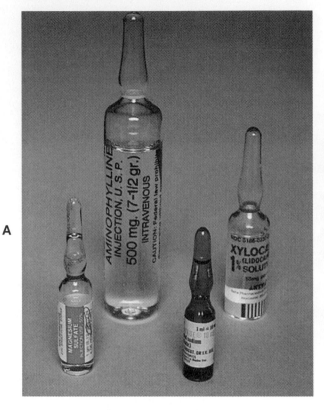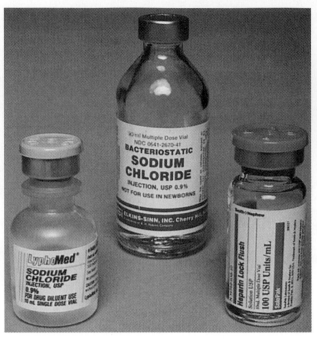

FIGURE 3-6 A, Medication in ampules. **B,** Medication in vials. *(From Potter P, Perry A: Basic nursing: essentials for practice, ed 5, St Louis, 2003, Mosby.)*

Labels

DRUG X
30 mg/tablet
100 tablets
Instructions: Take with full glass (8 oz) of warm water on empty stomach
Keep out of sunlight
Exp: 01/2007

- Check the complete label three times—before, during, and after preparation.*
- Focus on the order and label comparison.
- Clarify label questions with the pharmacy.

Calculations

- Learn to do your dose calculations accurately. Do not rely on peers.
- Check with the physician or pharmacy if you have a question about the dose. Document the verification on the medical record.
- Know the difference between a unit dose and total dose in a multidose container (refer to p. 53).
- Know the correct average and usual dose for the weight and age of your patient.
- Have a pharmacology and medication preparation reference on hand to verify usual dilution and administration timing techniques and the appropriate or usual dose for your patient.
- Read the package insert.

---

*Refer to p. 52 for label interpretation.

Administration

1. Identify the patient by asking his or her name. For a child, check the wristband and verify the name with a parent or other nurse.
2. Identify *all* patients by placing the ID that you are using to accompany the medication next to the patient's wristband. If you are distracted or rushed, a visual side-by-side comparison will make discrepancies more noticeable. Some agencies use bar code IDs to reduce errors.
3. Tell the patient the drug, the dose, and a brief understandable purpose. If the patient raises questions about the medication or refuses it, obtain more information, recheck the orders, and report to a supervisor. Then document the reason for refusal. The physician may need to be informed.
4. Reconfirm the patient's allergies with the patient and/or a family member. Sometimes the admission data provided are incomplete as a result of anxiety or the illness.
5. Place the medication on the patient's table, not on any other fixture in a room with two or more beds.
6. Make appropriate assessments—mental status, vital signs, skin integrity, ability to swallow, injection sites that should be avoided. Inquire about side effects and past problems with medications.
7. Be prepared to document the assessment findings on the chart and report them to appropriate personnel. Withhold the medication if there is a question about whether it can be safely given.
8. Show the medication and the label on the container to the physician if a *verbal order is being carried out at the bedside (e.g., in an emergency).*
9. Always incorporate and document teaching when you give medications to patient and family. Most patients are discharged shortly after admission. Remember that for effective two-way communication, you also need feedback from the patient or a family member to ensure understanding. Make full use of your time at the bedside.

Reporting and Documenting

1. After administration, document per policy and add relevant assessment and patient teaching data to the records according to agency policy.

REPORTING AND DOCUMENTING

Nurse's Notes
0800 *Refused Digoxin. Pulse A/R 82. Complains of nausea and halos around eyes.*
Dr. Cruz notified. Dig level drawn by lab. Instructed to take sips and chips.
Joe Mack, RN
0900 *Pulse A/R 66. States halos continue. Denies nausea. Dig levels pending.*
Taking sips and chips.
Joe Mack, RN

MEDICATION REFUSAL

2. Assess and evaluate the patient for consequences if an error was made. Document errors on record and on incident report after reporting to the provider and supervisor.

◉ Interventions

When a medication-related problem arises, take appropriate action using the nursing process. This includes the following steps:
- Identify the possible problem.
- Assess the patient.
- Report, plan, and intervene with the assistance of the appropriate physician or supervisor.
- Document errors and problem in the patient's record and on an incident report if necessary.
- Evaluate.
- Reassess the situation.

◉ Evaluation

Evaluate the patient for medication effects and side effects, and reassess at appropriate intervals for any problem noted and the action and duration of the medication given.

◉ INTERPRETING MEDICATION LABELS

Medication labels can be confusing because of the vast amount of information they contain and the small print. Some labels are prepared in-house by pharmacists or pharmacy technicians. The most important information is as follows:
- Name—generic (the first letter is usually lowercase) and proprietary, brand, or trade name (the first letter is usually capitalized)
- Route
- *Unit dose* per milliliter, per tablet, or per capsule
- *Total* amount in the container
- Instructions for preparation, if applicable
- Instructions for storage
- Expiration date (stamped by firm or pharmacist after manufacture)

EXAMPLE

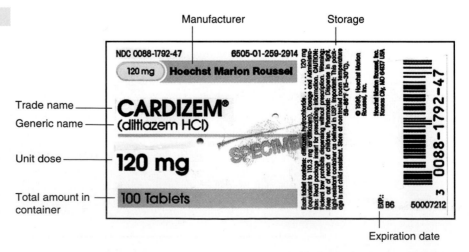

Cardizem is the proprietary, or trade, name for this Hoechst Marion Roussel product. Diltiazem is the generic name used by all companies that produce this drug. There are 100 tablets total in the container; each tablet contains 120 mg (unit dose). Tablets are usually given by mouth. The route is not specified, but the storage directions are given and there is space provided for an expiration date. When calculating a dose, place the 120 mg : 1 tab on the left side of your ratio and proportion.

EXAMPLE

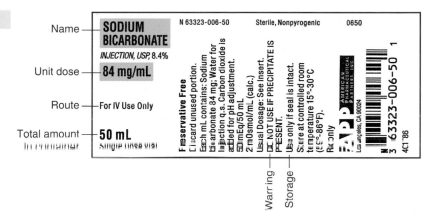

This vial of sodium bicarbonate contains 50 mL of 84 mg/mL intravenous injection fluid. It is a single-dose vial. The directions state that the unused portion should be discarded. A multidose vial may be kept for a specified period and used for more than one patient or on more than one occasion. When calculating a dose, place the 84 mg : 1 mL on the left side of your ratio and proportion as your "have."

EXAMPLE

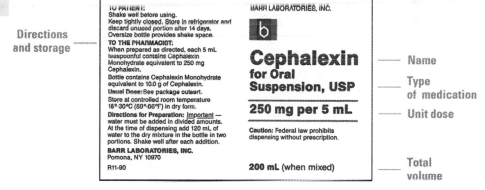

This multidose preparation, cephalexin, is an aqueous suspension (solid particles suspended in liquid). Whether it is dispensed for hospital or home use, it is obvious that the directions for preparation, storage, and use are very important for

CLINICAL ALERT!

A lethal error can be made if the *total dose* in a multidose container is mistaken for the *unit* dose or an IM preparation is given intravenously because the administrator failed to check the route.

distributing the medication properly throughout the suspension, for dispensing the correct strength, and for maintaining the strength of the drug during storage (in the refrigerator). When calculating a dose, use 250 mg:5 mL for the left side of your ratio and proportion. Note that 200 mL would contain 40 doses of 250 mg each. Any dose other than 250 mg will require some metric mathematical skills!

EXAMPLE

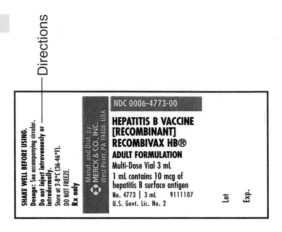

Directions

NDC 0006-4773-00

HEPATITIS B VACCINE [RECOMBINANT] RECOMBIVAX HB® **ADULT FORMULATION** Multi-Dose Vial 3 mL 1 mL contains 10 mcg of hepatitis B surface antigen No. 4773 | 3 mL   9111107 U.S. Govt. Lic. No. 2

SHAKE WELL BEFORE USING. Dosage: See accompanying circular. Do not inject intravenously or intradermally. Store at 2-8°C (36-46°F). DO NOT FREEZE. Rx only

Manuf. and Dist. by: MERCK & CO., INC. West Point, PA 19486, USA

Lot

Exp.

This hepatitis B vaccine label emphasizes that it is for adult use. The routes to be avoided are also emphasized. You would have to read the accompanying literature to determine whether it is to be given po or IM. (It is to be administered IM.) Also note the dose: 10 μg (mcg):1 mL. The nurse must be very aware of the difference between micrograms (μg) and milligrams (mg). This vaccine, like many medications, is also issued in other strengths. It is important to note that this is a *multidose* 3-mL vial, *not* a unit dose vial.

◼ Oral Drug Forms: Solids and Liquids

◼ Solids (Figure 3-7)

- Plain tablets (Figure 3-7, *A*): compressed powdered drugs
- Scored tablets (Figure 3-7, *B*): tablets with indentation; the only kind of tablet that may be broken
- Enteric-coated tablets (Figure 3-7, *C*): tablets with coating for delayed dissolution; should not be crushed or chewed
- Capsules (caps) (Figure 3-7, *D*): soluble case, usually gelatin, that holds liquid or dry particles of drug
- Extended-release capsules (S-R, slow-release) (Figure 3-7, *E*): capsules that contain beaded particles of drug for delayed absorption
- Powders/granules (Figure 3-7, *F*): loose or molded drug substance; usually to be dissolved in liquid or food

◼ Liquids (Figure 3-8)

- Aqueous suspensions: solid particles suspended in liquid that must be mixed well before administration
- Elixirs: sweetened alcohol and water solution
- Emulsions: fats or oils suspended in liquid with an emulsifier

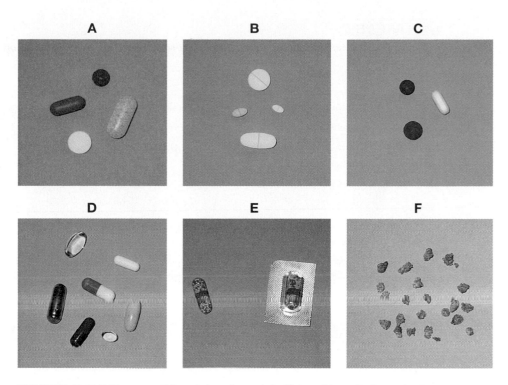

FIGURE 3-7 Different solid oral drug forms. **A,** Plain tablets. **B,** Scored tablets. **C,** Enteric-coated tablets. **D,** Capsules. **E,** Extended-release capsules. **F,** Granules. *(Courtesy of Amanda Politte, St Louis, MO.)*

- Extract: syrup or derived form of an active drug
- Fluid extracts: concentrated alcoholic liquid extract of plants or vegetables

Liquids are administered in medicine cups, with medicine droppers, and sometimes with syringes. When pouring medicines into a cup, pour to the meniscus at your eye level. Note the equivalent household amounts for the metric system: Tbsp, oz, mL.

FIGURE 3-8
A, Liquid medication in single-dose package. **B,** Liquid measured in medicine cup. **C,** Oral liquid medicine in syringe. *(From Potter P, Perry A: Basic nursing: essentials for practice, ed 5, St Louis, 2003, Mosby.)*

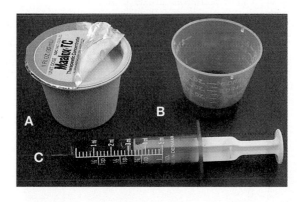

CLINICAL ALERT!

Do not substitute one ordered form of a drug for another. Do not substitute household utensils such as spoons, cups, and droppers for measuring medications. Medication utensils are calibrated for exact dosages according to the metric system of measurement.

EXAMPLES

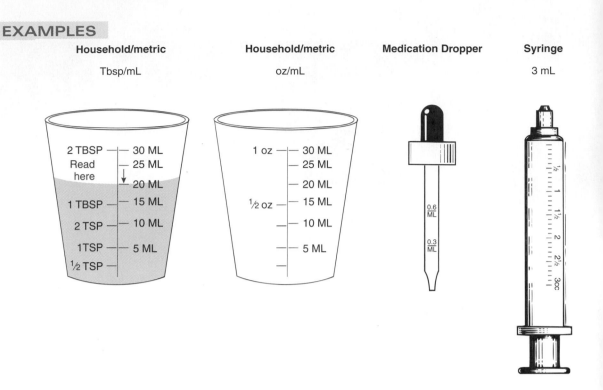

Household/metric	Household/metric	Medication Dropper	Syringe
Tbsp/mL	oz/mL		3 mL

ANSWERS ON PAGE 329

WORKSHEET
3A   Interpreting Medication Labels

Examine the label and fill in the requested information. Check your answers in the Answer Key before moving on to the next problem.

What you have or know (unit dose), 100 mg:1 tab or 50 mg:1 mL, is determined from the label and is inserted on the left side of your ratio and proportion.

1.

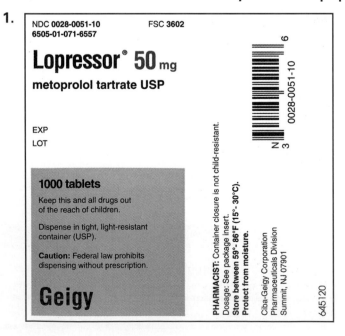

NDC 0028-0051-10   FSC 3602
6505-01-071-6557

Lopressor® 50 mg

metoprolol tartrate USP

EXP
LOT

1000 tablets

Keep this and all drugs out of the reach of children.

Dispense in tight, light-resistant container (USP).

Caution: Federal law prohibits dispensing without prescription.

Geigy

PHARMACIST: Container closure is not child-resistant.
Dosage: See package insert.
Store between 59°- 86°F (15°- 30°C).
Protect from moisture.

Ciba-Geigy Corporation
Pharmaceuticals Division
Summit, NJ 07901

645120

N 3 0028-0051-10 6

a. Trade name (registered patent or brand name, capital first letter)
b. Generic name (common name, *usually* lowercase and in parentheses)
c. Unit dose and form (tab/cap/mL)
d. Total amount in container
e. Ratio for "what you have or know" (left side of your proportion)

ANSWERS ON PAGE 329

WORKSHEET

3A   Interpreting Medication Labels—cont'd

2.

NDC 0068-0510-30

150 | mg   MARION MERRELL DOW INC.

RIFADIN®
(rifampin capsules)

NEW CAPSULE SIZE

150 mg

30 Capsules

Each capsule contains: rifampin...............................150 mg

Usual Dose: See accompanying product information.

CAUTION: Federal law prohibits dispensing without prescription. Keep tightly closed. **Store in a dry place**. Avoid excessive heat. Dispense in tight, light-resistant container with child-resistant closure.

©1992 Marion Merrell Dow Inc.   54134

Merrell Dow Pharmaceuticals Inc.
Subsidiary of Marion Merrell Dow Inc.
Kansas City, MO 64114

a. Trade (brand) name
b. Generic (common) name
c. Unit dose and form
d. Total amount in container
e. Ratio for "what you have or know"

3.

AMOXIL®
125mg/5mL

125mg/5mL
NDC 0029-6008-23

AMOXIL®
AMOXICILLIN
FOR ORAL SUSPENSION

Directions for mixing: Tap bottle until all powder flows freely. Add approximately 1/3 total amount of water for reconstitution (total=78 mL), shake vigorously to wet powder. Add remaining water; again shake vigorously. Each 5 mL (1 teaspoonful) will contain amoxicillin trihydrate equivalent to 125 mg amoxicillin. **Usual Adult Dosage:** 250 to 500 mg every 8 hours. **Usual Child Dosage:** 20 to 40 mg/kg/day in divided doses every 8 hours, depending on age, weight and infection severity. See accompanying prescribing information.

100mL
(when reconstituted)

Keep tightly closed.
Shake well before using.
Refrigeration preferable but not required.
Discard suspension after 14 days.

SB SmithKline Beecham

NSN 6505-01-153-3662
Net contents: Equivalent to 2.5 grams amoxicillin. Store dry powder at room temperature.
Caution: Federal law prohibits dispensing without prescription.
SmithKline Beecham Pharmaceuticals
Philadelphia, PA 19101

3 0029-6008-23 1

LOT
EXP.
9405793-E

a. Trade name
b. Total amount (mL) of sterile water to add for reconstitution
c. Unit dose
d. Total amount (mL) in container after reconstitution
e. Ratio for "what you have"
f. Length of time permitted for storage

CLINICAL ALERT!

The unit dose is usually the average dose ordered for adults (*not* children or elderly). If your calculations call for more than one or two times the unit dose (more than 1-2 tab or 1-2 mL), double check the order and your math, and research the reason. This commonsense approach has saved many lives.

ANSWERS ON PAGE 329

4.

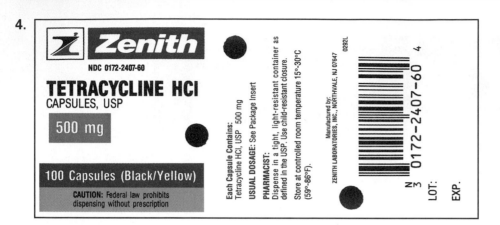

a. Generic name
b. Unit dose
c. Total amount in container
d. Ratio for "what you have"

5.

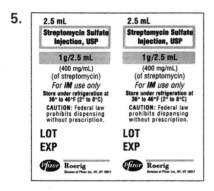

a. Generic name
b. Route
c. Unit dose (mg per mL)
d. Total amount in container
e. Storage directions
f. Route

● THE 24-HOUR CLOCK: 0000-2400 HOURS

Most facilities use a 24-hour computer-compatible clock, also known as *military time* or *international time* (Figure 3-9). At 2400, midnight (12 AM), the clock *changes* to 0000 for counting purposes. Thus 0001 is 1 minute after midnight. The sequential numbering system helps to avoid AM/PM time confusion and potential errors.

The AM clock begins at midnight, 0000, and ends at noon, 1200 hours.

The PM clock begins at noon, 1200, and ends at 2400 hours, midnight.

Thus midnight is noted *two* ways. It is most frequently written as 2400, but each minute *after* midnight is written as if midnight were 0000.

All times are expressed with 4 digits from 0001 to 2400 without colons and without AM and PM labels.

The afternoon hours begin at noon (12 PM) when the PM side of the clock is accessed and the major difference in numbering from traditional time is noted at 1300 (1 PM).

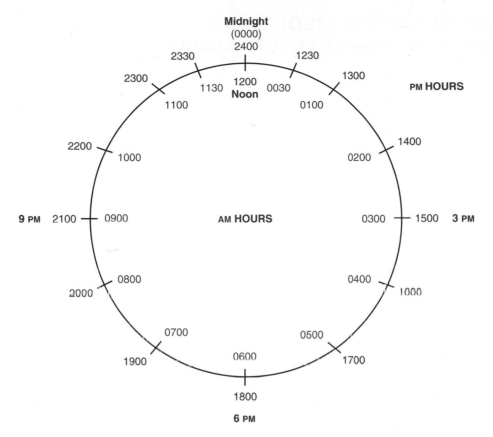

FIGURE 3-9 The 24-hour clock, 0000 hours to 2400 hours.

◉◀◀◀◀◀◀◀◀◀RULE   To convert traditional PM time to the 24-hour clock, begin at 1:00 PM and add 1200 to the time. Delete colons and AM/PM notation.

EXAMPLES   1:00 PM + 1200 = 1300   or   1 + 12 = 13 and add 2 zeroes
3:00 PM + 1200 = 1500   or   3 + 12 = 15 and add 2 zeroes

PM Hours   **AM Hours**
1200 = Noon (12 PM)   2400 = Midnight (12 AM) (0000)
1230 = Half past 12 noon   0030 = 1 half hour after midnight
1300 = 1 PM   0100 = 1 AM

Learning the key times 0100 and 1300 to 2400 is helpful.

1159 = 1 minute before noon   2359 = 1 minute before midnight
1201 = 1 minute after noon   0001 = 1 minute after midnight

It is also helpful to study some key times in your daily schedule:

Your usual breakfast hour: _____
The time your shift begins: _____
The time your shift ends: _____
Your usual dinner hour: _____
Your usual bedtime hour: _____

● UNDERSTANDING MEDICATION ADMINISTRATION RECORDS (MARs)

Every nursing institution has its own MAR forms. Similar in content, most of these forms are self-explanatory. All contain places to record identifying patient data; allergies; medication orders with the dose, route, and frequency or time desired for administration; and full signature (with date) of the person administering the medication. Most MARs list suggested codes to use in filling out the form.

During orientation, a new employee needs to identify agency policies that are not stated on the form. These include how to add a new order, how to indicate discontinuance of a medication on the form, procedures for data entry and reporting medication errors, and additional documentation required to support the MAR. Examples of MARs are shown in Figures 3-10 to 3-11.

Entering the time on the wrong MAR, wrong date, or wrong shift may result in time-consuming frustration. To avoid entry errors on the MAR, it is recommended to use the following order when checking or entering data for a patient:

1. Patient ID
2. Correct date on MAR
3. Correct medication
4. Time that the medication was last given
5. Correct shift column

If the last dose of a scheduled medication was given late, it may be necessary to delay the next dose that you are preparing. This is done to protect the patient from a drug overload injury.

Many agencies have policies for charting by "exception," meaning entering a narrative explanation for data requiring more explanation than provided on a flow sheet.

If a medication is withheld, the time due is entered on the MAR, usually circled and initialed. According to hospital policy, this is sometimes noted on the MAR with a word such as "refused" or "ref" and circled and initialed with a brief narrative explanation in the nurse's notes section (see Figure 3-10).

Any time a nonscheduled medication is given, such as a stat or prn medication, it is necessary to document prompt follow-up assessments and the time. This can be recorded on the nurse's notes or flow sheet, according to hospital policy. For example, "1630 states nausea is relieved."

If an entry error is made, follow hospital policy for corrections; an example of a medication incident report is shown in Figure 3-12. The original data must all be legible. It is *illegal* to discard a record or to erase or obscure any entry on medical records.

As with all medical records, the MAR is considered confidential information, and permission must be obtained to make photocopies.

Some institutions preprint the *exact* times for administration on the MAR (refer to the MAR if the medication is administered at a *different* time; the time printed should be *circled*, and the correct time, written in next to it with the nurse's initials.

Legally it is impossible to give five different patients their medications at, for instance, 0900. Some institutions allow the nurse to initial the printed time if it is within 1 half hour. An experienced nurse knows which medications do not permit flexible administration times and *prioritizes* the medication administration order.

ANSWERS ON PAGE 330

WORKSHEET 3B   Interpreting the MAR

Using the MAR in Figure 3-10, answer the following questions:

1. Does the patient have a commonly seen surname? If so, why should the medication nurse take special note of this?   _____

2. Does the patient have any medication allergies? Is so, which?   _____

3. This MAR indicates how many days of medication administration?   _____

4. Which drug ordered was withheld or not given as scheduled?   _____

5. By what route is Clotrimazole 1% to be administered?   _____

6. Which order has expired?   _____

7. Which drug was given at 11 PM and in which location?   _____

8. When must the meperidine order be discontinued or reordered to continue administration?   _____

9. When is the next time Tylenol may be given according to the 24-hour clock; and traditional time?   _____

10. Why do you think this form requires both the initials and the signature of the person giving medications?   _____

● THE SIX RIGHTS OF DRUG ADMINISTRATION

THE SIX RIGHTS	SAFETY MEASURES
Right Patient	Always carry written patient/medication ID for each drug prepared and do a visual comparison with the wrist identification band. Ask the patient to state his or her name. Do not ask, "Are you Mr. Smith?"
Right Drug	Match the order to the drug three times during preparation. Verify complete spelling and form of drug. Refer to references for all unknown drugs. Be aware that many drugs have similar names but very different uses, schedules, and routes.
Right Dose	Always recheck if the dose is greater than the unit dose–1 to 2 pills, 1 to 2 mL. If the patient is a child or frail adult, a *fractional dose*, which is less than the average dose, is more likely to be ordered. Always recheck these orders. Recheck for decimals that may be absent, in the wrong place, or look like a "1"; a zero (0) added after decimal, but the decimal may not be noticed. Keep current on all abbreviations. Do not guess what abbreviations such as µg, gr, and mU mean. Do not rely on peers for correct calculations except to double-check your own. Know the difference between a unit dose and total dose in a multiple-dose vial or ampule.
Right Time	Prioritize emergency and *stat* drugs. Ask for help if your workload is too heavy. Always check to see when medication was last given.

Brown, John
ID# 45764304
Age: 50   Sex: M   Rm: 406A
Dr. Marin, Cruz

ALLERGIES: DRUGS: *IV iodine, Aspirin*
FOODS: Denies

RN Verification: *FD*

MAR Date: 05-07-03 0700 - 05-08-03 0659

MEDICATION: Dose Route Freq

Time of Administration, Site, and Initials

	START	**STOP**	**0700 TO 1459**	**1500 TO 2259**	**2300 TO 0659**
SCH	05-05-03 Digoxin 0.125 mg po Q AM	05-12-03	(0900) *JM* R		
SCH	05-05-03 Tylenol (acetaminophen) 500 mg po BID	05-12-03	0800 *JM*	2000	
SCH	05-05-03 Clotrimazole 1% CR TOP bid to affected area	05-12-03	0900 *JM* L	2100	

This is a pharmacy-generated MAR for a 24 hr period stated in military time beginning with the day shift, 5-7-03. The RN who signs the verification is verifying that the medication orders accurately match the provider orders and that the allergies have been noted. SCH means a regularly scheduled medication versus a PRN order. You must use the agency *code* for administration sites. A circled time denotes med NOT given. Additional documentation may need to be added elsewhere in the nurse's record. PRN meds and One time only meds have *separate* placeholders. You may add new orders by writing them in (refer to promethazine). This pharmacy prints instructions for diluting intravenous medications. The narcotic (meperidine) has an automatic 48 hr limit and then must have a written renewal order. This hospital policy calls for a yellow highlight to denote discontinued/expired orders. All discontinued orders, automatic or other must be renewed if it is necessary to continue them. On the SITE CODES note that if a medication is withheld other than for NPO or surgery, the reason must be documented on the patient record eg: "refused acetaminophen and states it "dosen't do anything for him". Dr. Marin notified."

ONE TIME ONLY AND PRN MEDS

	Start	**Stop**	**Time**	**Initials**	**Full Name/Title**

PRN	05-07-03 Meperidine
	  25 mg IV q6h PRN
	  Dilute in 5 mL NS and give over 5 min
		05-09-03
		0700
			2300
			C
				FD	*Florence Dane, RN*

	05-07-03 promethazine 25 mg IM STAT	*5/7/03*	*1900 J*	*TR*	*T Robbins, RN*

Sign: *Joe Mack*   Initials: *JM*   Sign: *T Robbins*   Initials: *TR*   Sign: *Florence Dane*   Initials: *FD*

SITE CODES   **GENERAL HOSPITAL**

A	Abdomen (L)	J	Gluteus (LUQ)
B	Abdomen (R)	K	Gluteus (RUQ)
C	Arm (L)	L	Thigh (L)
D	Arm (R)	M	Thigh (R)
E	Eyes (both) O.U.	N	Ventrogluteal (L)
F	Eyes (left) O.S.	O	Ventrogluteal (R)
G	Eyes (right) O.D.	P	NPO: Lab
H	Deltoid (mid L)	Q	NPO: Surgery
I	Deltoid (mid R)	R	Withheld/See nurses notes

Clinical Alert!   Verify pharmacy data on this sheet including dilution instructions. Remember this form is not a *copy* of the original orders. These data have been recopied into the computer.

FIGURE 3-10 Sample medication administration record (MAR).

Acct: Admitted: 10/05/02 1630 Att Phys: Diagnosis: Respiratory Allergies: Morphine/Beta-Adrenergic blocking agts			MR#: Age: 77Y Sex: F HT: 5'7.0" / 170.2cm WT: 224lbs / 101.606kg		M A R	MEDICATION AMINISTRATION RECORD
					Page:4 From:10/10/02 0731 Thru:10/11/02 0730	

Start Date/Time	Stop Date/Time	RN/ LPN	Medication	0731-1530	1531-2330	2331-0730
			** ****************** **PRN** ****************** **			
10/05 2143	11/04 2142		**Promethazine HCL (Phenergan Equiv) 25 mg=0.5 mL** IV **#020 Q6H PRN PRN N/V**			
			When administering IV: Must be diluted to a final concentration of 25mg/mL. IV administration to be at a rate not to exceed 25mg/minute.			
10/05 2100	11/10 2059		**Zolpidem Tartrate (Ambien) 10 mg=2 tablet** Oral **#016 HS PRN **Narcotic sign-out****			*DC*
10/05 2200	11/04 2159		**Alum-Mag Hydroxide-Simethicone (Maalox Plus/Mylanta Equiv) 30 mL=30mL** Oral **#022 Q4H PRN Stagger one hr from other meds**			

This is an example of a computer-generated MAR for PRN orders only. There are many similarities to the MAR in Figure 3-10 and also some differences noted: this MAR states the medication unit dose supplied; the medication nurse must enter the exact time the medication was given. In addition to dilution instructions, scheduling instructions are given with the last medication. The site code is different and the dose omission code is amplified. Even if no medication is given to a patient, the MAR must be signed by the nurse responsible for the patient each shift. Medications which are refused, withheld, or mischarted must be circled, timed, and initialed—a standard procedure which may require additional entries on the patient record if the code is not self-explanatory.

Order Date	RN INIT.	Date/Time To Be Given	One Time Orders and Pre-Operatives Medication-Dose-Route	Actual Time Given	Site Codes		Dose Omission Code
					Arm Deltoid Ventrogluteal Gluteal Abdomen Abdomen	LA RA LD RD LVG RVG LG RG LUQ RUQ LLQ RLQ	A = pt absent H = hold M = med absent N = NPO O = other R = refused U = unable to tolerate
					INIT	Signature	INIT Signature

60321 (8/98)A   CHART   **CONTINUED**

FIGURE 3-11 Computer-generated MAR sample for prn orders. *(From Scottsdale Healthcare, Scottsdale, AZ.)*

MEDICATION INCIDENT REPORT

Patient name: _____   Date of incident: _____
                                                          Time of incident: _____

Where incident occurred: Hospital: _____   Unit: _____

Admitting diagnosis: _____

Type of incident: _____   Wrong drug
                                     _____   Wrong time
                                     _____   Wrong dose
                                     _____   Wrong patient
                                     _____   Wrong route

Medication order: _____

Account of incident and intervention taken: _____
_____
_____
_____

Was the physician notified? _____   Time: _____

Why do you feel the incident occurred? _____
_____

What were possible consequences to the patient as a result of this incident? _____
_____
_____

What can you do to prevent this type of incident from occurring again? _____
_____
_____

Persons familiar with incident or involved: _____
_____

_____   _____
Provider signature   Date   Supervisor signature   Date

FIGURE 3-12 Example of medication incident report.

Right Route   Use the route ordered. If the patient cannot swallow, obtain a written order for a change of route. Read the fine print on the labels. Do not substitute NG for PO or IV for IM.

Right Documentation   Accurate and timely reporting to appropriate resources and documentation is an essential addition to patient rights.

There are additional rights with legal implications to keep in mind:
Right to confidentiality
Right to information about the medication being taken
Right to refuse medications
Right to competent care

ANSWERS ON PAGE 331

WORKSHEET
3C   Multiple-Choice Practice

1. When administering a medication at the bedside, which should be the *first* priority?
   a. Make appropriate assessments
   b. Identify the patient
   c. Document the administration of the medication
   d. Recheck the medication label

2. If a medication-related problem is identified, which should be the *first* measure the nurse takes:
   a. Assess the patient for side effects
   b. Notify the supervisor
   c. Call the physician
   d. Document the problem in detail on an incident report

3. Which is the *unit dose* for the medication shown below?
   a. 300 mg/mL
   b. 3 grams/10 mL
   c. 10 mL
   d. 250 mg

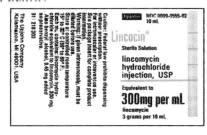

4. If a hand-written medication order is illegible or unclear, which would be the best nursing decision:
   a. Check with pharmacy
   b. Rewrite the order to make it more legible
   c. Give the usual unit dose and clarify
   d. Clarify with the physician who wrote it

5. The nurse gives a medication at 1 PM. The correct equivalent international or military time would be:
   a. 1000
   b. 1300
   c. 1500
   d. 0100

ANSWERS ON PAGE 331

WORKSHEET

3C   Multiple-Choice Practice—cont'd

6. Which of the following statements regarding medications is *true?*
   a. Each nurse needs to be able to perform accurate simple and complex medication calculations.
   b. The unit dose and the total dose in a vial are one and the same.
   c. It is wise to rely on experienced colleagues to calculate drug dosages.
   d. Medication errors rarely occur in the hospital setting.

7. Which of the following statements regarding potential medication errors is *false?*
   a. Medications to which the patient is allergic need to be documented on admission and verified each time a new medication is administered.
   b. Many drugs have similar sounding names.
   c. Verbal orders are best reserved for emergencies and have potential for error.
   d. Memorized calculation formulas are the most helpful measures to protect the nurse from making medication calculation errors with complex dosage calculations.

8. A tablet is ordered for a patient with a nasogastric feeding tube who is NPO. Which is the most appropriate action for the nurse to take?
   a. Crush the tablet, dilute with water, and administer via the tube.
   b. Consult with the charge nurse about the medication routine for NPO patients.
   c. Ask the patient if there have been any problems with swallowing the pill and then give it by mouth.
   d. Clarify the route with the physician who wrote the order.

9. An inexperienced nurse reads an order for Tylenol #2 stat for John L. Green. She asks his name, checks the patient name band against the label she has made for the medication, and gives two (2) plain Tylenol tablets stat to John L. Green and charts "Tylenol #2 given" and signs her name. Which patient right was NOT violated?
   a. The right drug
   b. The right dose
   c. The right documentation
   d. The right patient

10. An order for meperidine 50 mg IM q4h prn for pain expired after 48 hours, during the last shift. The patient continues to complain of postoperative pain and requests another pain injection. Which action is an *inappropriate* nursing action?
    a. Attempt alternative measures for pain relief such as repositioning and other comfort measures.
    b. Administer the medication, since the patient has had no untoward side effects from any of the prior doses.
    c. Assess the patient for unexplained sources of continued pain.
    d. Explain that the medication order has expired but that you will call for a renewed order.

Refer to the **How to Read a Drug Label** section on the enclosed CD-ROM for additional Practice Problems.

■ CRITICAL THINKING EXERCISES

Analyze the following examples of medication errors with your peers and/or instructor and discuss the issues suggested in the left-side guidelines using this chapter and pharmacology references. As you study the error, consider which patient rights on pp. 64 and 65 have been violated. What suggestions might you have for procedural changes at the institution to prevent this from happening again? Include those that might involve pharmacy staff, providers, nurses, and patients.

1. **Order:**   Tylenol # 2, stat

   On Hand: Tylenol in patient medication drawer and Tylenol #2 (in locked cabinet)

   Given: Two Tylenol tablets

   Error: The wrong medication was given. Two tablets of plain Tylenol were given instead of one tablet of Tylenol #2, which has a narcotic added. (If an incident report must be filed, this is the way the incident should be described in the space provided for a description of the incident.)

   Nursing Actions: Obtain orders to give additional pain medication.
   Report to supervisor and provider.
   Document on medical record and file incident report per hospital policy.
   Assess patient periodically for side effects and document the results.

   Potential Injuries: Lack of comfort and its physiologic and emotional effects; lack of security; need for an alternative medication, perhaps to avoid acetaminophen (Tylenol) overdose.

   Preventive Measures: Familiarize self with the medications ordered and commonly used in the unit, as well as all controlled medications supplied including emergency.

If this common medication was known to the giver and a lack of attention or focus was a contributing cause, then techniques to avoid distractions need to be addressed. If this medication was not known to the giver, a pharmacology review of more commonly used medications is in order. Nurses should always look up unfamiliar medications in current pharmacology references or check with the pharmacy before administration. Nursing students need to check with an instructor or supervisor after the reference check if they are unfamiliar with a medication. It is also wise to inform the patient at the bedside exactly which medications are to be given, because the patient may question the order. An informed patient presents the last line of defense in error prevention.

2. **Order:**   Aspirin 650 mg, two tablets at bedtime

   Supplied: Aspirin 325 mg per tablet

   Given: Aspirin 650 mg, two tablets by one nurse; aspirin 325 mg, two tablets by another nurse

   Error:

   Nursing Actions:

   Potential Injuries:

   Preventive Actions:

3. **Order:** Narcotic for pain q3h prn, last noted on record as given by recovery room nurse at 1445 (2:45 PM).

   Given: Narcotic for pain at 1545 (3:30 PM) by nurse who just started evening shift and admitted patient to unit.

   Error:

   Nursing Actions:

   Potential Injuries:

   Preventive Actions:

4. **Order:** Prednisone 10 mg qod
   Given: Prednisone 10 mg qid
   Error:

   Nursing Actions:

   Potential Injuries:

   Preventative Measures:

5. **Order:** Percocet (automatic discontinuation 8/10)
   Given: 8/11 Percodan recorded on the medical record, patient allergic to aspirin

   Error:

   Nursing Actions:

   Potential Injuries:

   Preventive Measures:

Metric System Calculations

4

OBJECTIVES

- Convert milligrams, micrograms, grams, and kilograms.
- Memorize milliliter and liter conversions.
- Calculate gram and milligram conversion problems.
- Round medication doses to the nearest measurable amount.
- Identify metric and household liquid equivalents.
- Identify one- and two-step metric conversion problems.
- Distinguish unit and milliequivalent labels.
- Calculate one- and two-step oral and parenteral metric conversion problems by the ratio-proportion method.
- Distinguish metric, household, and apothecary terms.
- Analyze medication errors using critical thinking.

INTRODUCTION

Medications are ordered and supplied primarily in the metric system of measurement. This chapter teaches the application of basic mathematics, ratio and proportion, nursing process and critical thinking used in safe medication preparation. Mastery of this chapter will provide the reader with an excellent foundation for all drug dose calculations.

● METRIC SYSTEM

The International System of Units (SI), which is commonly known as *the metric system*, is now being used exclusively in the United States Pharmacopeia. SI is the abbreviation for the French *Système International d'Unités*. The metric system is becoming the preferred system for weights, volume, and lengths and is used in computers. Soon it will be the only system used in medication administration.

It is a decimal system based on the number 10 and all the math involved is done by moving decimals. The basic units are multiplied and divided by a multiple of 10 to form the entire system. There are a few equivalents used frequently in medicine. These should be memorized and are as follows:

MEMORIZE   **WEIGHT**

1 mg (milligram)	= 1000 μg or mcg (micrograms)
1 g (gram)	= 1000 mg or mgm (milligrams)
1 kg (kilogram)	= 1000 g or Gm (grams) = 2.2 lb

VOLUME

1 L (liter) = 1000 mL (milliliters) or 1000 cc (cubic centimeters)

A milliliter (mL) is equivalent to a cubic centimeter (cc), and for all practical purposes these units may be used interchangeably. However, the use of milliliter is preferable. Hence:

$$1 \text{ L (liter)} = 1000 \text{ cc}$$
$$1 \text{ L (liter)} = 1000 \text{ mL}$$

 REMEMBER ● The symbol (such as g or mg) always *follows* the amount in the metric system.

EXAMPLES   1000 mg
1 g

CLINICAL ALERT!

Some physicians and nurses may use the symbol mgm for mg (milligram), mcg for μg (microgram), gm for g (gram), and lowercase l for liter. These abbreviations are obsolete and are not part of the standard system of metric abbreviations that was adopted in 1960. However, mgm and mcg may be easier to read correctly than mg and μg.

Table 4-1 Metric Measurements, Prefixes, and Their Values

Prefix	Numerical Value	Power of Base 10	Meaning	Examples	Meaning
deci (d)	.1	10^{-1}	Tenth, part of	deciliter	one tenth of a liter
centi (c)	.01	10^{-2}	Hundredth, part of	centimeter	one hundredth of a meter
milli (m)	.001	10^{-3}	Thousandth, part of	milliliter	one thousandth of a liter
micro (μ)	.000001	10^{-6}	Millionth, part of	microgram	one millionth of a gram
nano (n)	.000000001	10^{-9}	Billionth, part of	nanogram	one billionth of a gram
deka (da)	10	10	10 times	dekagram	ten grams
hecto (h)	100	10^{2}	100 times	hectogram	one hundred grams
kilo (k)	1000	10^{3}	1000 times	kilogram	one thousand grams
mega (M)	1000000	10^{6}	1,000,000 times	Megabyte	one million bytes
giga (G)	1000000000	10^{9}	1,000,000,000 times	Gigabyte	one billion bytes

These prefixes can be combined with liters and grams. They can be seen in medication prescriptions and/or laboratory reports.

EXAMPLES

WEIGHT	VOLUME	LENGTH
decigram (dg)	deciliter (dL)	kilometer (km)
kilogram (kg)	kiloliter (kL)	meter (m)
milligram (mg)	milliliter (mL)	centimeter (cm)

● METRIC CONVERSIONS BY MOVING DECIMALS

The metric system is a *decimal system.*

 REMEMBER ● 1000 mg = 1 g
1000 μg = 1 mg

◀◀◀◀◀◀◀◀◀**RULE**   To convert grams (large) to milligrams (small), multiply by 1000 or move the decimal point 3 places to the *right*.

EXAMPLES   5 g   = 5.000. mg = 5000 mg

0.2 g = 0.200. mg = 200 mg

0.04 g = 0.040. mg = 40 mg

◀◀◀◀◀◀◀◀◀**RULE**   To convert milligrams (small) to grams (large), divide by 1000 or move the decimal point 3 places to the *left*.

EXAMPLES   250 mg = 0.250. g = 0.25 g

20 mg = 0.020. g = 0.02 g

5 mg   = 0.005. g = 0.005 g

◀◀◀◀◀◀◀◀◀**RULE**   To convert milligrams (large) to micrograms (small), multiply by 1000 or move the decimal point 3 places to the *right*.

EXAMPLES   5 mg   = 5.000. μg = 5000 μg

0.8 mg = 0.800. μg = 800 μg

0.05 mg = 0.050. μg = 50 μg

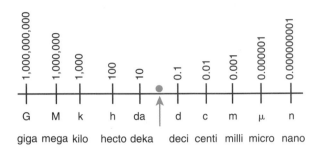

⊙ ◄◄◄◄◄◄◄◄◄RULE   To convert micrograms (small) to milligrams (large), divide by 1000 or move the decimal point 3 places to the *left.*

EXAMPLES   2500 μg = 2.500. mg = 2.5 mg

400 μg = 0.400. mg = 0.4 mg

10 μg = 0.010. mg = 0.01 mg

FIGURE 4-1
Metric units number line.

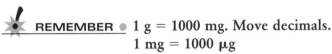

ANSWERS ON PAGE 332

WORKSHEET
4A
Metric Conversions by Moving Decimals

Make the following conversions by moving the decimals.

REMEMBER ● **1 g = 1000 mg. Move decimals.**
1 mg = 1000 μg

1. 1 g = _____ mg
2. 2 g = _____ mg
3. 1.5 g = _____ mg
4. 0.5 g = _____ mg
5. 0.05 mg = _____ μg
6. 0.25 g = _____ mg
7. 0.05 g = _____ mg
8. 0.1 g = _____ mg
9. 1.1 g = _____ mg
10. 0.3 g = _____ mg
11. 25 mg = _____ g
12. 5 mg = _____ μg
13. 3000 mg = _____ g
14. 1500 mg = _____ g
15. 15,000 mg = _____ g
16. 10 mg = _____ g
17. 100 μg = _____ mg
18. 0.5 mg = _____ g
19. 7.5 mg = _____ g
20. 20.15 mg = _____ g

CLINICAL ALERT!

The *microgram, milligram,* and *gram* are the most commonly used units of measurement in medication administration.

Medication tablets and capsules are most often supplied in milligrams. Antibiotics can be supplied in grams, milligrams, or units (abbreviation U).* Micrograms are used in pediatrics and critical care cases for small dosages and/or for powerful drugs, and the need to convert is frequent. You *must* be skilled in the measurement and conversion of all three units.

*Refer to p. 77 for more explanation.

● ROUNDING MEDICATION DOSES

When the medication supplied is *not* the same strength as the *ordered dose*, recheck your order and calculations and check with the pharmacy to see if there is another strength available.

EXAMPLE   You have to give 750 mg, and on hand is 300 mg. Call the pharmacy.

You have to give 50 mg, and on hand is 10 mg. Recheck the order, the usual dose, your calculations, and then call the pharmacy and request a different strength. Pediatric forms of medications are often available in lower strengths than the adult form, and the adult form may have been sent.

 REMEMBER ● Seldom should a patient receive more than one or two multiples of the unit dose supplied.

◐◀◀◀◀◀◀◀◀**RULE**   Always round your answers to the nearest *measurable dose after* you verify that the dose is correct for that patient.

EXAMPLE   **Tablets:** *scored*   Round to the nearest $\frac{1}{2}$ tablet
   1.8 tabs   Give 2 tablets
   1.5 tabs   Give 1.5 tablets
   1.4 tabs   Give 1.5 tablets
   1.2 tabs   Give 1 tablet

Tablets: *unscored*   Do not break unscored tablets. Verify order. Recheck if the dose is more than 1 or 2 tablets.

■ Rounding Milliliters

Examine the equipment you plan to use. On a syringe, markings might be tenths or hundredths of a milliliter. On a larger syringe, markings might be in 0.2-mL increments. On an IV electronic infusion device, you would most likely use the nearest whole number in milliliters.

■ Rounding to the Nearest Tenth

◐◀◀◀◀◀◀◀◀**RULE**   To round to the **nearest tenth,** examine the *hundredths* column. If it is 0.05 or greater, round up to the next tenth. If it is 0.04 or less, the tenths column remains the same.

EXAMPLE   1.5**5** mL or 1.5**7** mL: Round to 1.6 mL
   1.5**3** mL or 1.5**4** mL: Round to 1.5 mL

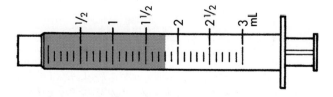

Ordered 1.7**5** mL. The 3-mL syringe shown above, the most commonly used syringe, is shaded to 1.**8** mL, the nearest tenth, the nearest measurable dose.

◼ Rounding to the Nearest Hundredth

◉◄◄◄◄◄◄◄◄RULE To round to the **nearest hundredth,** examine the thousandths column. If it is 0.005 or greater, round up to the next hundredth.

EXAMPLE 0.756 : Round to 0.76
0.754 : Round to 0.75

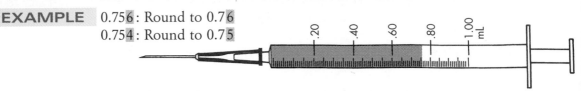

The 1-mL syringe is shaded to 0.75 mL, because the 1-mL syringe is calibrated in hundredths and permits more exact measurement of small doses.*

◼ Rounding Drops

Drops are so small that it is impossible to divide them into parts.
Any remainder of 0.5 or above is given the next higher number

EXAMPLES 31.4 drops per minute for a gravity IV: Infuse at 31 drops per minute.
31.7 drops per minute for a gravity IV: Infuse at 32 drops per minute
If a specially calibrated dropper is provided to give drops of liquid medicines, you must use that calibrated dropper and measure exactly.

If an oral medication is to be administered, use the calibrated special spoon, prefilled syringe, or dropper provided (Figures 4-2 and 4-3) or draw it up in an appropriate syringe (without the needle) to the exact or nearest measurable amount (Figure 4-4). Then transfer it to a medication cup promptly.

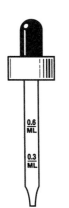

FIGURE 4-2
Medicine dropper.

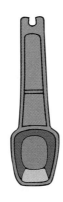

FIGURE 4-3
Measuring teaspoon.
(From Clayton BD, Stock YN: Basic pharmacology for nurses, ed 12, St Louis, 2001, Mosby.)

FIGURE 4-4
Withdrawing medicine from a cup with a syringe. *(From Clayton BD, Stock YN: Basic pharmacology for nurses, ed 12, St Louis, 2001, Mosby.)*

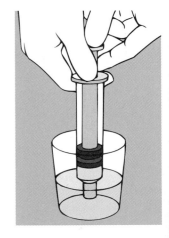

◉◄◄◄◄◄◄◄◄RULE Always round to the *nearest measurable calibration* on the equipment you are using.

CLINICAL ALERT!

To avoid overdosing the patient, never round up liquid medications to the nearest whole number. If the answer is 1.7 mL, DO NOT round up to 2 mL. Use a syringe with the appropriate calibrations to measure an exact dose.

*For further discussion of syringe calibrations, refer to Figure 4-5.

● ONE-STEP METRIC RATIO AND PROPORTION CALCULATIONS

You learned how to move decimals 3 places to the left or right to calculate metric equivalents on pp. 71 and 72. Ratio and proportion is a provable method of solving medication calculation problems. They can be used to calculate metric equivalents and medication doses with accuracy and logic. There are two types of metric one-step calculations: metric equivalent problems and metric dose problems.

EXAMPLE   40 mg = ? g (metric equivalent problem)

◀◀◀◀◀◀◀◀RULE   Place the known metric equivalents from the metric tables on the **left**. Be sure to select the equivalents with the same terms as your problem (e.g., mg to g), and place the unknown on the **right** side of the equation in the same order as shown below.

Follow the same procedures as in Chapter 2 for ratio and proportion. Label all terms and prove your answer.

Know	*Want to Know*	**PROOF**	**ANSWER**
1000 mg : 1 g :: 40 mg : x g		$1000 \times 0.04 = 40$	40 mg = 0.04 g
(mg : g :: mg : g)		$1 \times 40 = 40$	

$\frac{\cancel{1000}}{\cancel{1000}} x \frac{\cancel{40}}{1000}$ or $100\overline{)4}$

$x = 0.04$ g (Always label problems and answers.)

EXAMPLE   **Ordered:** 50 mg **Unit dose on label:** 25 mg/tab (medication dose problem)

The second example of common metric one-step ratio and proportion problems is this: *Ordered: 50 mg. Label for the medicine: 25 mg/tab.* Since *both* the order and the label are in the same terms—milligrams—this only involves a *one-step* calculation.

◀◀◀◀◀◀◀◀RULE   Place what you have on hand or what you know (the label unit dose) on the **left** and what is ordered (want to have or know) on the right. Follow through with your math as in Chapter 2.

Know	*Want to Know*	**PROOF**	**ANSWER**
25 mg : 1 tab :: 50 mg : x tab		$25 \times 2 = 50$	Give 2 tabs
		$1 \times 50 = 50$	

$\frac{\cancel{25}}{\cancel{25}} x = \frac{50}{25} = 2$

$x = 2$ tab

▰ CLINICAL ALERT!

Some of these problems can be easily solved without being written. However, it is safer to establish a routine using the **provable** ratio and proportion method, (e.g., *Ordered: 0.3 mg—Label: 0.5 mg/2 mL*) so that you can solve more complex medication problems with ease when the need arises.

ANSWERS ON PAGE 332

WORKSHEET
4B   **One-Step Metric Equivalents**

Use ratio and proportion to solve the following one-step metric equivalent problems. Prove and label all answers.

REMEMBER ● 1000 μg = 1 mg
1000 mg = 1 g
1000 g   = 1 kg (2.2 lb)
1000 mL = 1 L (liter)

Change milligrams to grams:

1. 200 mg   **2.** 4 mg   **3.** 0.3 mg

4. 25 mg   **5.** 15 mg

Change grams to milligrams:

6. 0.01 g   **7.** 4.6 g   **8.** 0.03 g

9. 0.5 g   **10.** 2.5 g

Change micrograms to milligrams:

11. 150 μg   **12.** 3000 μg   **13.** 50 μg

14. 2500 μg   **15.** 500 μg

Change milligrams to micrograms:

16. 20 mg   **17.** 200 mg   **18.** 5 mg

19. 0.1 mg   **20.** 0.04 mg

Change kilograms to grams (these measurements are both used for infant weights):

21. 5.5 kg   **22.** 12 kg   **23.** 3 kg

24. 1.3 kg   **25.** 0.5 kg

Change liters to milliliters:

26. 0.5 L   **27.** 1.3 L   **28.** 1.5 L

29. 3 L   **30.** 2.8 L

ANSWERS ON PAGE 335

WORKSHEET 4C

Understanding Units and Milliequivalents in Medication Dosages

Measurements in addition to micrograms, milligrams, and grams may be seen in medication orders. They may also be seen in laboratory values.

TERM	ABBREVIATION	MEANING
unit	U, u	A quantity that represents a laboratory standard of measurement; often used as unit of measure for products that have some or all animal or plant contents (e.g., heparin, insulin, antibiotics).
milliunit	mU	Equals 1/1000 of a unit. Pitocin is an example of a medication ordered this way.
Milliequivalent	mEq	Represents the number of grams of solute dissolved in a milliliter of solution. Electrolytes are commonly dissolved in solution and measured in milliequivalents (e.g., sodium, potassium, chlorides).
mEq/L		Equals one thousandth of 1 g of a specific substance dissolved in a liter of a solution. Electrolytes are frequently supplied in milliequivalents per liter for intravenous infusion (e.g., KCl 40 mEq/L).
mEq/mL		Equals one thousandth of 1 g of a specific substance dissolved in 1 mL. (The 1 is implied when a number is absent in front of mL.) 2 mEq/mL would equal two thousandths of a gram dissolved in 1 mL.

Continued

CLINICAL ALERT!

It is preferred that "unit" be written out to avoid confusion with the number "0".

ANSWERS ON PAGE 335

WORKSHEET 4C

Understanding Units and Milliequivalents in Medication Dosages—cont'd

Examine the following labels for unit and total dose in the containers and fill in the blanks as noted in problem 1. The unit dose is the individual dose supplied. Notice the similarities and differences in terms.

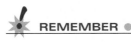 **REMEMBER** • Distinguish u for unit and μg for microgram (one thousandth of a gram). They look similar but are different symbols with different meanings.

1. a. Unit dose <u>300 mg</u>   **b.** Total amount in container <u>30 capsules</u>

NDC 0068-0508-30
300 mg   MARION MERRELL DOW INC.
RIFADIN®
(rifampin capsules)
300 mg
30 Capsules

Each capsule contains: rifampin..........................300 mg
Usual Dose: See accompanying product information.
CAUTION: Federal law prohibits dispensing without prescription.
Keep tightly closed. Store in a dry place. Avoid excessive heat.
Dispense in tight, light-resistant container with child-resistant closure.

© 1993 Marion Merrell Dow Inc.
Merrell Dow Pharmaceuticals Inc.
Subsidiary of Marion Merrell Dow Inc.
Kansas City, MO 64114   H 3 6 4 C

2. a. Unit dose _____   **b.** Alternative unit dose measurement _____

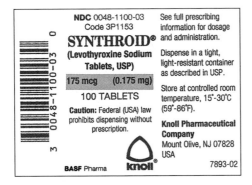

NDC 0048-1100-03
Code 3P1153
SYNTHROID®
(Levothyroxine Sodium Tablets, USP)
175 mcg   (0.175 mg)
100 TABLETS
Caution: Federal (USA) law prohibits dispensing without prescription.
BASF Pharma   knoll®

See full prescribing information for dosage and administration.
Dispense in a tight, light-resistant container as described in USP.
Store at controlled room temperature, 15°-30°C (59°-86°F).
Knoll Pharmaceutical Company
Mount Olive, NJ 07828 USA
7893-02

3. a. Unit dose _____   **b.** Total volume in container _____

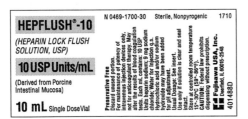

HEPFLUSH®-10
(HEPARIN LOCK FLUSH SOLUTION, USP)
10 USP Units/mL
(Derived from Porcine Intestinal Mucosa)
10 mL Single Dose Vial

N 0469-1700-30   Sterile, Nonpyrogenic   1710

4. Unit dose if 10.2 mL diluent is added: **a.** _____

   b. Usual dose _____   **c.** Total dose in container _____

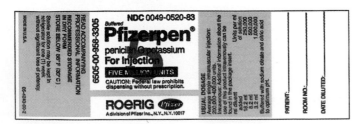

NDC 0049-0520-83
Buffered
Pfizerpen®
penicillin G potassium
For Injection
FIVE MILLION UNITS
CAUTION: Federal law prohibits dispensing without prescription.
ROERIG Pfizer
A division of Pfizer Inc., N.Y., N.Y. 10017

ANSWERS ON PAGE 335

WORKSHEET
4C

Understanding Units and Milliequivalents in Medication Dosages—cont'd

5. a. Unit dose _____   **b.** Total dose/total volume in container _____

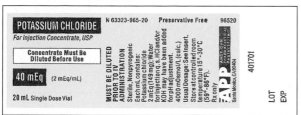

6. a. Unit dose _____   **b.** Total volume in vial _____

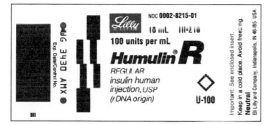

7. a. Unit dose _____   **b.** Alternative unit dose measurement _____

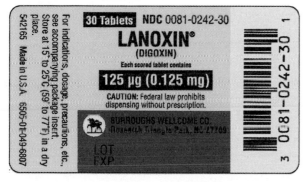

Questions 8-10 pertain to the lactated Ringer's injection USP * IV contents label

8. Total volume in milliliters in IV _____ mL

9. Milliequivalents per liter of potassium in container _____ mEq/L

10. Milligrams of potassium in container _____ mg

LOT   EXP

⊙   ⊙   2B2324
                              NDC 0338-0117-04
                              DIN 00061085   **1**

Lactated Ringer's Injection USP   **2**

3

1000 mL
EACH 100 mL CONTAINS   600 mg SODIUM CHLORIDE USP
310 mg SODIUM LACTATE   30 mg POTASSIUM CHLORIDE USP   **4**
20 mg CALCIUM CHLORIDE USP   pH 6.5 (6.0 TO 7.5)   mEq/L
SODIUM 130 POTASSIUM 4 CALCIUM 2.7 CHLORIDE 109
LACTATE 28   OSMOLARITY 273 mOsmol/L (CALC)   STERILE
NONPYROGENIC SINGLE DOSE CONTAINER   **NOT FOR USE IN THE**
TREATMENT OF LACTIC ACIDOSIS   ADDITIVES MAY BE   **5**
INCOMPATIBLE CONSULT WITH PHARMACIST IF AVAILABLE WHEN
INTRODUCING ADDITIVES USE ASEPTIC TECHNIQUE   MIX
THOROUGHLY DO NOT STORE DOSAGE INTRAVENOUSLY AS
DIRECTED BY A PHYSICIAN SEE DIRECTIONS CAUTIONS   **6**
SQUEEZE AND INSPECT INNER BAG WHICH MAINTAINS PRODUCT
STERILITY DISCARD IF LEAKS ARE FOUND MUST NOT BE USED IN
SERIES CONNECTIONS DO NOT ADMINISTER SIMULTANEOUSLY
WITH BLOOD DO NOT USE UNLESS SOLUTION IS CLEAR FEDERAL
(USA) LAW PROHIBITS DISPENSING WITHOUT PRESCRIPTION
STORE UNIT IN MOISTURE BARRIER OVERWRAP AT ROOM   **7**
TEMPERATURE (25°C/77°F) UNTIL READY TO USE AVOID
EXCESSIVE HEAT SEE INSERT

Baxter   **8**
BAXTER HEALTHCARE CORPORATION
DEERFIELD IL 60015 USA

MADE IN USA   Viaflex® CONTAINER
DISTRIBUTED IN CANADA BY   PL 146® PLASTIC
BAXTER CORPORATION   FOR PRODUCT INFORMATION
TORONTO ONTARIO CANADA   CALL 1-800-933-0303   **9**

⊙   ⊙

_____
*USP refers to the United States Pharmacopoeia, a national listing of drugs.

ANSWERS ON PAGE 335

WORKSHEET
4D One-Step Oral Medication Problems

Use ratio and proportion and metric conversions to solve the following problems, and prove all work:

1. Ordered: Lanoxin (digoxin) 0.2 mg cap qd po. How many *capsules* will you give?

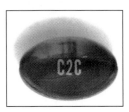

Lanoxin Capsule 0.2mg

2. Ordered: Erythromycin ethylsuccinate suspension 300 mg po. How many milliliters will you administer? How will you prepare the dose?

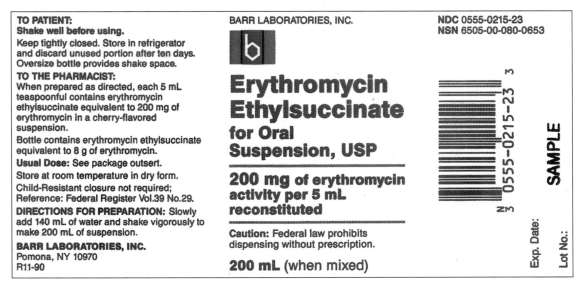

TO PATIENT:
Shake well before using.
Keep tightly closed. Store in refrigerator and discard unused portion after ten days. Oversize bottle provides shake space.
TO THE PHARMACIST:
When prepared as directed, each 5 mL teaspoonful contains erythromycin ethylsuccinate equivalent to 200 mg of erythromycin in a cherry-flavored suspension.
Bottle contains erythromycin ethylsuccinate equivalent to 8 g of erythromycin.
Usual Dose: See package outsert.
Store at room temperature in dry form.
Child-Resistant closure not required; Reference: Federal Register Vol.39 No.29.
DIRECTIONS FOR PREPARATION: Slowly add 140 mL of water and shake vigorously to make 200 mL of suspension.
BARR LABORATORIES, INC.
Pomona, NY 10970
R11-90

BARR LABORATORIES, INC.

Erythromycin Ethylsuccinate
for Oral Suspension, USP

200 mg of erythromycin activity per 5 mL reconstituted

Caution: Federal law prohibits dispensing without prescription.

200 mL (when mixed)

NDC 0555-0215-23
NSN 6505-00-080-0653

0555-0215-23   SAMPLE

Exp. Date: Lot No.:

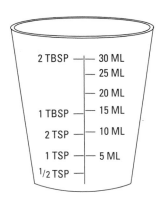

2 TBSP —— 30 ML
—— 25 ML
—— 20 ML
1 TBSP —— 15 ML
2 TSP —— 10 ML
1 TSP —— 5 ML
1/2 TSP ——

ANSWERS ON PAGE 335

WORKSHEET

4D

One-Step Oral Medication Problems—cont'd

3. Ordered: Lanoxin 0.0625 mg qd po. How many *tablets* will you give?

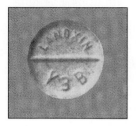

Lanoxin Tablet 0.125 mg

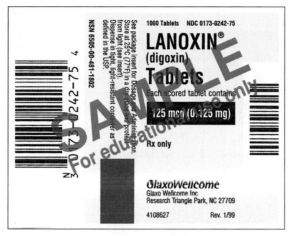

Reproduced with permission of Glaxo Wellcome, Inc.

> **HINT** ■ If a tablet is "scored," that is, has a line cut across it to denote a breaking point, you may break it. Unscored tablets may not be broken because they will not break evenly and because the medication is not distributed evenly in the tablet.

4. Ordered: Synthroid (levothyroxine sodium) 350 μg qd po. How many *tablets* will you give?

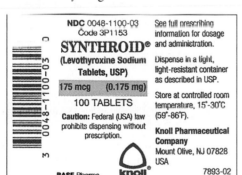

Continued

ANSWERS ON PAGE 335

5. Ordered: Infants' Tylenol (acetaminophen) Concentrated Drops 40 mg q4h po prn for pain/restlessness. How many milliliters will you give?

ASPIRIN FREE
ALCOHOL FREE
IBUPROFEN FREE

Directions:
1. Shake well before using.
2. Find right dose on chart below. If possible, use weight to dose; otherwise, use age.
3. Only use enclosed dropper; fill to prescribed level and dispense liquid slowly into child's mouth toward inner cheek.
4. Replace dropper tightly to maintain child resistance.
5. If needed, repeat dose every 4 hours.
6. Do not use more than 5 times a day.

WEIGHT (lb)	AGE (yr)	DOSE
Under 24	Under 2	Consult Doctor
24-35	2-3	2 Dropperfuls (2 x 0.8 mL)

Attention:
This product has been specifically designed for use only with enclosed dropper. Do not use any other dosing device with this product.

● Tylenol® products are the first choice of Pediatricians.

● Infants' Tylenol® Drops are more concentrated than Children's Tylenol® Liquids. For accurate dosing, follow the dosing instructions on this label.

● Only use enclosed dropper to dose.

● Never use spoons, droppers or cups that come with other medicines.

Infants' TYLENOL®
Acetaminophen

CONCENTRATED DROPS
Fever Reducer - Pain Reliever

Pediatricians' First Choice

NEW !

SAFE-TY-LOCK™ Bottle
Unique Safety Barrier

TYLENOL Stage One INFANTS

Grape Flavor

1/2 FL OZ (15 mL) 80 mg per 0.8 mL

CLINICAL ALERT!

Read your liquid labels carefully to determine the unit dose and to see whether the liquid must be diluted, rolled, shaken, or mixed before administration.

WORKSHEET
4E

Metric Oral One-Step
Practice Problems

Use ratio and proportion and metric conversion to solve the following problems, and prove all work:

1. Ordered: Phenobarbital 30 mg. Label: 15 mg/tab. How many tablet(s) will you give?

2. Ordered: Lanoxin 0.25 mg. Label: 0.125 mg/tab. How many tablet(s) will you give?

3. Ordered: Theo-Dur 450 mg. Label: 300 mg scored tablets. How many tablet(s) will you give?

4. Ordered: Digitoxin 0.2 mg. Label: 0.1 mg tablets. How many tablet(s) will you give?

5. Ordered: KCl 20 mEq. Label: 8 mEq/5 mL. How many milliliters will you give?

6. Ordered: Synthroid 0.02 mg. Label: 0.01 mg tablets. How many tablet(s) will you give?

7. Ordered: Desyrel 75 mg. Label: Desyrel 50 mg scored tablets. How many tablet(s) will you give?

8. Ordered: Diazepam 5 mg. Label: Diazepam 10 mg scored tablets. How many tablet(s) will you give?

9. Ordered: Clinoril 800 mg. Label: Clinoril 400 mg tablets. How many tablet(s) will you give?

10. Ordered: Voltaren 450 mg. Label: Voltaren 150 mg tablets. How many tablet(s) will you give?

● TWO-STEP METRIC RATIO AND PROPORTION CALCULATIONS

When a medication is ordered that is not in the same terms of measurement as the label–for example, grams ordered and milligrams on label, or micrograms ordered and milligrams on label–a two-step calculation must be completed.

EXAMPLE   Ordered: 100 **mg.** You have 0.05 **g** tablets on hand. How many tablets will you give?

Step 1   Select the correct equivalents.
Have grams on hand. Need to change **mg** to the equivalent **g** on hand.

Equivalency tables: $1000 \ \mu g \ = 1 \ mg$
                                    1000 mg = 1 g

Know   *Want to Know*
$1000 \ mg : 1 \ g :: 100 \ mg : x \ g$
         $(mg : g :: mg : g)$

$\frac{\cancel{1000}}{\cancel{1000}}x = \frac{\cancel{100}}{\cancel{1000}} = 0.1$

$x = 0.1 \ g$

PROOF
$1000 \times 0.1 = 100$
$1 \times 100 = 100$

Step 2   Insert the equivalent measure from Step 1 into your ratio and proportion now that all terms of measurement are the same.

Have   *Want to Have*
$0.05 \ g : 1 \ tab :: 0.1 \ g : x \ tab$

$\frac{\cancel{0.05}}{\cancel{0.05}}x = \frac{0.1}{0.05}$ or $0.05\overline{)0.1}$

$x = 2 \ tabs$

PROOF
$0.05 \times 2 = 0.1$
$1 \times 0.1 = 0.1$

How to Avoid Errors

1. Analyze your problem. Is it a one-step or two-step calculation? (Are the terms the same or different?)
2. Always place a zero in front of a decimal when the number is less than one. It reminds you that the next figure is a decimal, not a number 1 (0.4).
3. Eliminate zeros at the end of a decimal (0.75̶0̶).
4. Write neatly; estimate and prove each step. Ask yourself whether this is a reasonable amount of medication. (Close to unit dose?)
5. If you doubt your math, recalculate without looking at your original work. If still in doubt, check reliable sources.

ANSWERS ON PAGE 337

WORKSHEET
4F   Metric Oral Two-Step Problems

Use ratio and proportion and metric equivalents to change the order to what is on hand for the first step, then use ratio and proportion to determine the correct dose for the second step. Prove all work. Remember to estimate your answer when you set up the second step. Refer to the metric equivalency table, page 71, and the two-step explanation, page 84.

1. Ordered: Procanbid (procainamide HCl) 0.5 g. How many tablets will you give?

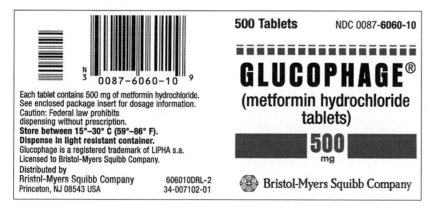

2. Ordered: Rifadin (rifampin) 0.3 g. How many capsules will you give?

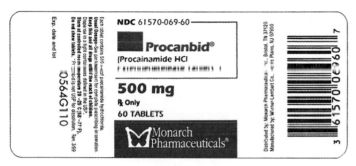

Step 1   **Step 2**

3. Ordered: Glucophage (metformin) 1 g. How many tablets will you give?

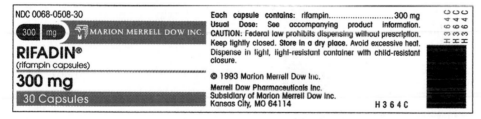

Step 1   **Step 2**   *Continued*

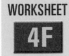
4. Ordered: Dilantin (extended phenytoin sodium) capsules 0.3 g. How many capsules will you give?

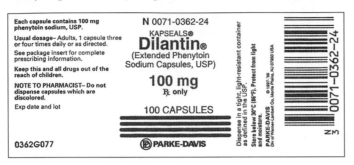

Each capsule contains 100 mg phenytoin sodium, USP.

Usual dosage– Adults, 1 capsule three or four times daily or as directed.

See package insert for complete prescribing information.

Keep this and all drugs out of the reach of children.

NOTE TO PHARMACIST– Do not dispense capsules which are discolored.

Exp date and lot

0362G077

N 0071-0362-24
KAPSEALS®
Dilantin®
(Extended Phenytoin Sodium Capsules, USP)

100 mg
℞ only

100 CAPSULES

ⓟ **PARKE-DAVIS**

Dispense in a tight, light-resistant container as defined in the USP.

Store below 30°C (86°F). Protect from light and moisture.

© 1997-98

PARKE-DAVIS
Div of Warner-Lambert Co, Morris Plains, NJ 07950 USA

0071-0362-24

Step 1   **Step 2**

5. Ordered: Lopid (gemfibrozil) 0.6 g. How many tablets will you give?

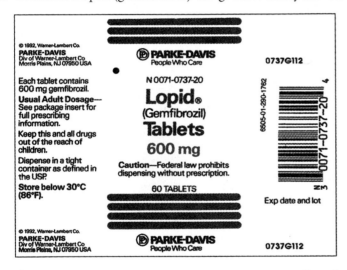

© 1992, Warner-Lambert Co.
PARKE-DAVIS
Div of Warner-Lambert Co
Morris Plains, NJ 07950 USA

Each tablet contains 600 mg gemfibrozil.

Usual Adult Dosage— See package insert for full prescribing information.

Keep this and all drugs out of the reach of children.

Dispense in a tight container as defined in the USP.

Store below 30°C (86°F).

© 1992, Warner-Lambert Co.
PARKE-DAVIS
Div of Warner-Lambert Co
Morris Plains, NJ 07950 USA

ⓟ **PARKE-DAVIS**
People Who Care

0737G112

N 0071-0737-20
Lopid®
(Gemfibrozil)
Tablets
600 mg

Caution—Federal law prohibits dispensing without prescription.

60 TABLETS

ⓟ **PARKE-DAVIS**
People Who Care

0737G112

6505-01-290-1782

0071-0737-20

Exp date and lot

Step 1   **Step 2**

ANSWERS ON PAGE 338

WORKSHEET 4G

More Practice in Metric Oral Two-Step Problems

Solve the following two-step problems using ratio and proportion. First convert the order to the equivalent on hand; then calculate the amount of medication. Prove all work.

1. Ordered: Lanoxin (digoxin) 0.25 mg qod po for congestive heart failure.
Label: 125 µg tablets. How many tablets will you give?

Step 1   **Step 2**

2. Ordered: Valium (diazepam) 0.01 g bid po for a patient with anxiety.
Label: 5 mg tablets. How many tablets will you give?

Step 1   **Step 2**

3. Ordered: Dilantin (phenytoin) 0.2 g bid po for a patient with seizures.
Label: 100 mg capsules. How many capsules will you give?

Step 1   **Step 2**

4. Ordered: Diuril (chlorothiazide) 0.05 g po qd for a patient with
hypertension. Label: 25 mg tablets. How many tablets will you give?

Step 1   **Step 2**

5. Ordered: Halcion (triazolam) 125 µg HS po for a patient with insomnia.
Label: 0.125 mg tablets. How many tablets will you give?

Step 1   **Step 2**

CLINICAL ALERT!

qd, qod, and qid orders have been misread resulting in serious errors. The risk of error is especially high when the order is written with "periods" between the letters, for example, "q.d." because the period can be misread as an "i."

ANSWERS ON PAGE 339

WORKSHEET 4H More Practice in Metric Oral Two-Step Problems

1. Ordered: Naproxen 0.5 g bid po for a patient with arthritis. Label: 250 mg tablets. How many tablets will you give?

Step 1   **Step 2**

2. Ordered: Atenolol 0.025 g qd po for a patient with hypertension. Label: 50 mg scored tablets. How many tablets will you give?

Step 1   **Step 2**

3. Ordered: Tetracycline 250 mg qid po for a patient with Type B gastritis. Label: 0.25 g tablets. How many tablets will you give?

Step 1   **Step 2**

4. Ordered: Cimetidine 0.45 g qid for a patient with esophageal reflux. Label: 150 mg tablets. How many tablets will you give?

Step 1   **Step 2**

5. Ordered: Glipizide 5000 μg daily with breakfast. Label: 2.5 mg tablets. How many tablets will you give?

Step 1   **Step 2**

CLINICAL ALERT!

Each of the medications ordered on this worksheet has a potential for adverse effects in the elderly for physiologic reasons.

These effects include high risk for injury due to confusion, sedation, anorexia, hypotension, urinary incontinence, potassium imbalances, dehydration, elevated and toxic serum levels of the medication, and medication interactions, to name a *few*. Many other medications are also dangerous for the elderly. If the patient experiences a *new* problem after admission (e.g., confusion, constipation, diarrhea, or others from the above named list), review the medication orders and drug serum levels if applicable and available, and you may discover the source of the problem.

● MEASURING AND READING AMOUNTS IN A SYRINGE

The best way to learn to read the measurements on a syringe is to examine some unfilled syringes while you read this (Figure 4-5). Then examine some filled syringes, and verify the amounts with your instructor or lab partner.

| **STEPS** | Examine the *total amount* the syringe contains. The 3 mL hypodermic syringe is most commonly used for intramuscular injections and also for subcutaneous injections. The 1 mL tuberculin syringe is used mainly for skin tests. |

Locate the *1 mL* markings on each syringe.

Examine the calibrations in 1 mL, 0.2 mL, 0.1 mL, or 0.01 mL, depending on the size of the syringe. The larger the syringe, the larger the calibration.

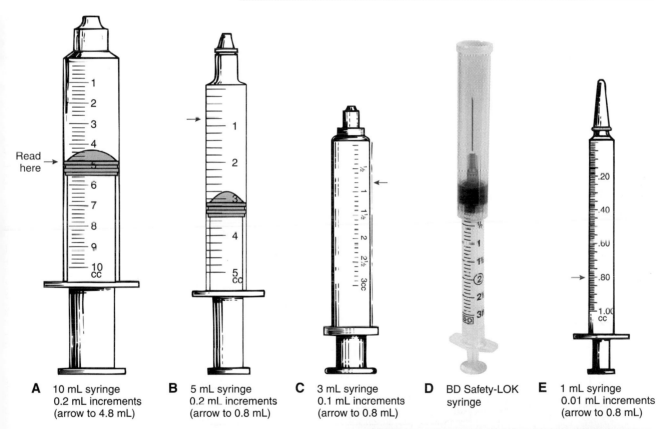

A 10 mL syringe	**B** 5 mL syringe	**C** 3 mL syringe	**D** BD Safety-LOK	**E** 1 mL syringe
0.2 mL increments	0.2 mL increments	0.1 mL increments	syringe	0.01 mL increments
(arrow to 4.8 mL)	(arrow to 0.8 mL)	(arrow to 0.8 mL)		(arrow to 0.8 mL)

FIGURE 4-5

Comparison of syringe sizes and calibrations. Note where the dose is measured. There are two black rings on the plunger and a rounded or pointed tip. Ignore the rounded/pointed tip and read the uppermost ring as shown on **A**. The rings are not shown in **C** and **E** so the dose and calibrations can be better visualized. **E**, Tubex Blunt Pointe sterile cartridge unit. (*D, Courtesy Becton Dickinson and Company, Franklin Lakes, NJ. E, Courtesy ESI Lederle, Division of American Home Products Corporation, St. Davids, PA; F, From Potter P, Perry A:* Basic nursing: essentials for practice, *ed 5, St Louis, 2003, Mosby.*)

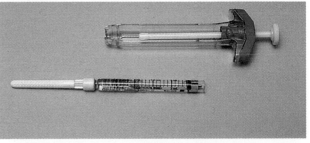

F   Carpuject syringe and prefilled sterile cartridge with needle.

ANSWERS ON PAGE 341

WORKSHEET

41   **Syringe Volume Practice**

Examine the following syringes. Note the total capacity and the 1 mL and 0.5 mL markings. Fill in the blanks and shade the syringe to the volume requested. If possible, practice with real syringes.

1. Total capacity: _____ mL. Calibrated in tenths or hundredths of a milliliter? (Circle one) Indicate 1.6 mL:

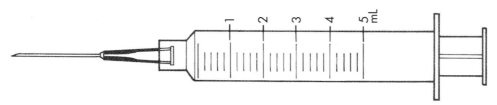

2. Total capacity: _____ mL. Calibrated in 0.1, 0.2, or 0.01 mL increments? (Circle one) Indicate 4.6 mL:

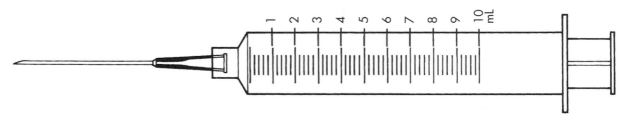

3. Total capacity: _____ mL. Calibrated in 0.1, 0.2, or 0.01 mL increments? (Circle one) Indicate 3.4 mL:

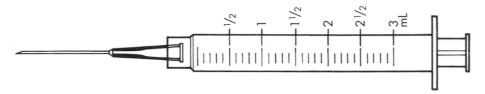

4. Total capacity: _____ mL. Calibrated in tenths or hundredths of a milliliter? (Circle one) Indicate 2.5 mL:

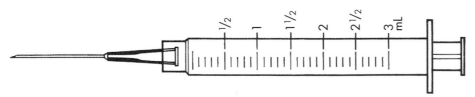

5. Total capacity: _____ mL. Calibrated in tenths or hundredths of a milliliter? (Circle one) Indicate 0.75 mL:

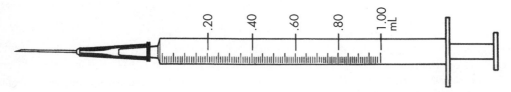

ANSWERS ON PAGE 342

WORKSHEET
4J   Metric Parenteral Mixes

Combinations of the following narcotics and antiemetics, antihistamines, or anticholinergics are commonly ordered.

Calculate the amount to be given in milliliters *to the nearest tenth* for each of the two drugs ordered using the labels provided. Then *add* the results to find the total volume to be combined and administered in one syringe.* Estimate your answer. Round to the nearest tenth of a milliliter. Prove all work. Does your estimate match your answer? Shade in the total amount to be drawn on the 3 mL syringe illustration.

1. Ordered: Meperidine HCl 25 mg and Vistaril (hydroxyzine HCl) 25 mg IM q4h prn for pain.

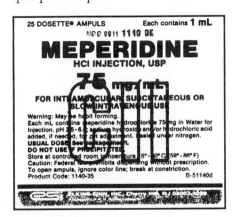

a. How many mg/mL of meperidine are available? (label)

b. How many milliliters of meperidine will you prepare?

c. How many mg/mL of hydroxyzine are available? (label)

d. How many milliliters of hydroxyzine will you prepare?

e. Total volume in syringe? (to nearest tenth) (Shade in syringe below.)

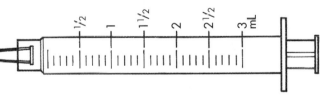

Continued

CLINICAL ALERT!

Always consult a current, reliable compatibility reference before mixing parenteral medications. Consult a pharmacist if a reference is unavailable.

---

*Orders for mixes are usually bracketed in the medication administration record (MAR).

ANSWERS ON PAGE 342

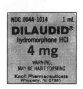

WORKSHEET 4J   **Metric Parenteral Mixes—cont'd**

2. Ordered: Dilaudid (hydromorphone HCl) 3 mg and prochlorperazine 2.5 mg IM stat for pain and nausea.

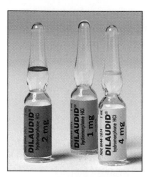

a. How many mg/mL of hydromorphone are available? (label)

b. How many milliliters of hydromorphone will you prepare?

c. How many mg/mL of Compazine will you prepare?

d. Total volume in syringe? (Shade in syringe below.)

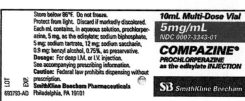

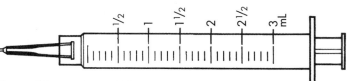

3. Ordered: Meperidine HCl 50 mg and atropine sulfate 0.6 mg IM preoperatively on call from OR.

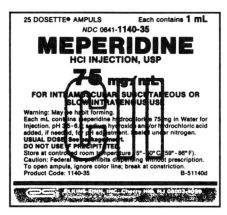

a. How many mg/mL of meperidine are available? (label)

b. How many milliliters of meperidine will you prepare?

c. How many mg/mL of atropine are available? (label)

d. How many milliliters of atropine will you prepare?

e. Total volume in syringe? (Shade in syringe.)

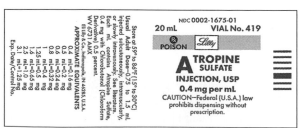

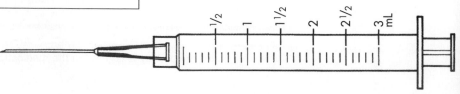

ANSWERS ON PAGE 342

WORKSHEET 4J   Metric Parenteral Mixes—cont'd

4. Ordered: Dilaudid (hydromorphone HCl) 2 mg and Vistaril (hydroxyzine HCl) 35 mg IM q4-6h prn for pain.

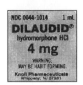

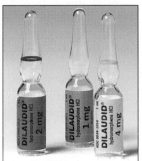

a. How many milliliters of hydromorphone will you prepare?

b. How many milliliters of hydroxyzine will you prepare?

c. Total volume in syringe? (Shade in syringe below.)

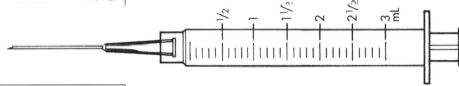

 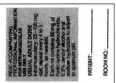

Continued

CLINICAL ALERT!

To prepare the correct total volume, it is safer to prepare and verify the total for *each* medication separately and then combine the two.

Beginning practitioners who prepare a mix using only one syringe risk withdrawing an improper amount for the second syringe.

ANSWERS ON PAGE 342

WORKSHEET 4J Metric Parenteral Mixes—cont'd

5. Ordered: Morphine sulfate 8 mg and Vistaril 25 mg IM postoperatively.

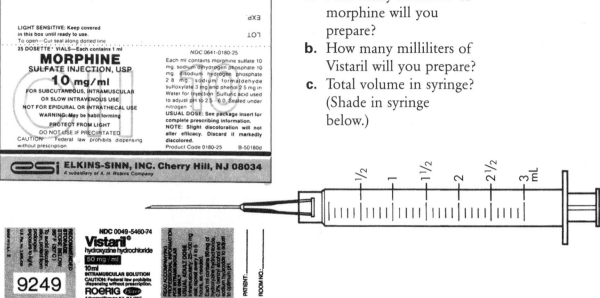

a. How many milliliters of morphine will you prepare?

b. How many milliliters of Vistaril will you prepare?

c. Total volume in syringe? (Shade in syringe below.)

ANSWERS ON PAGE 344

WORKSHEET 4K Metric One-Step and Two-Step Oral and Parenteral Problems

Examine the orders and labels below. Is the problem *one-step* or *two-step?* Before you perform the *final calculation,* determine whether you will give *more* or *less* of what you have on hand. Calculate the dose (to the nearest tenth of a milliliter if applicable). Prove your answers.

1. Ordered: Cleocin phosphate 0.2 g IM stat. (One-step or two-step?)

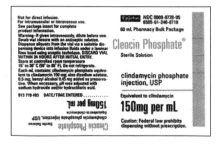

2. Ordered: Xanax 500 µg po HS. (One-step or two-step?)

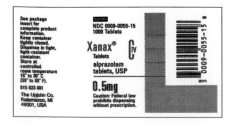

ANSWERS ON PAGE 344

WORKSHEET 4K   Metric One-Step and Two-Step Oral and Parenteral Problems—cont'd

3. Ordered: Solu-Cortef 0.2 g IM. (One-step or two-step?)

Single-Dose Vial   For IV or IM use
Contains Benzyl Alcohol as a Preservative
See package insert for complete
product information.
Per 2 mL (when mixed):
* hydrocortisone sodium succinate equiv.
to hydrocortisone, 250 mg. Protect
solution from light. Discard after 3 days.
814 070 205   Reconstituted . . . .
The Upjohn Company
Kalamazoo, MI 49001, USA

2 mL Act-O-Vial®   NDC 0009-0909-08
Solu-Cortef®   Sterile Powder
hydrocortisone sodium succinate
for injection, USP
250 mg*

4. Ordered: Solu-Medrol 75 mg IM. (One-step or two-step?)

Single-Dose Vial   For IM or IV use
Contains Benzyl Alcohol as a Preservative.
See package insert for complete
product information.
Each 2 mL (when mixed) contains:
* methylprednisolone sodium succinate
equiv. to methylprednisolone, 125 mg
lyophilized in ampoules
812 893 406
The Upjohn Company
Kalamazoo, MI 49001, USA

NDC 0009-0190-09   2 mL Act-O-Vial
Solu-Medrol®   Sterile Powd
methylprednisolone sodium
succinate for injection, USP
125 mg*

5. Ordered: Medrol 32 mg po. (One-step or two-step?)

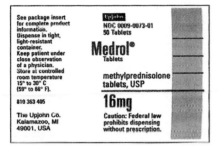

See package insert
for complete product
information.
Dispense in tight,
light-resistant
container.
Keep patient under
close observation
of a physician.
Store at controlled
room temperature
15° to 30° C
(59° to 86° F).

810 363 405

The Upjohn Co.
Kalamazoo, MI
49001, USA

Upjohn
NDC 0009-0073-01
50 Tablets
Medrol®
Tablets
methylprednisolone
tablets, USP
16mg
Caution: Federal law
prohibits dispensing
without prescription.

6. Ordered: Motrin 0.8 g po. (One-step or two-step?)

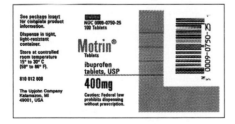

See package insert
for complete product
information.
Dispense in tight,
light-resistant
container.
Store at controlled
room temperature
15° to 30° C
(59° to 86° F).

810 012 808

The Upjohn Company
Kalamazoo, MI
49001, USA

Upjohn
NDC 0009-0750-25
100 Tablets
Motrin®
Tablets
ibuprofen
tablets, USP
400mg
Caution: Federal law
prohibits dispensing
without prescription.

7. Ordered: Lincocin 250 mg IM. (One-step or two-step?)

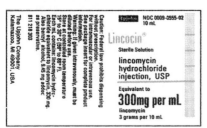

The Upjohn Company
Kalamazoo, MI 49001, USA
811 218 303

Caution: Federal law prohibits dispensing
without prescription.
For intramuscular or intravenous use.
See package insert for complete product
information.
Warning: If given intravenously, must be
diluted before use.
Store at controlled room temperature
15° to 30° C (59° to 86° F).
Each mL contains: lincomycin hydrochloride equivalent to lincomycin, 300 mg.
Also benzyl alcohol, 9.45 mg added
as preservative.

Upjohn   NDC 0009-0555-02
10 mL
Lincocin®
Sterile Solution
lincomycin
hydrochloride
injection, USP
Equivalent to
300mg per mL
lincomycin
3 grams per 10 mL

Continued

WORKSHEET 4K Metric One-Step and Two-Step Oral and Parenteral Problems—cont'd

8. Ordered: Depo-Provera 0.3 g IM. (One-step or two-step?)

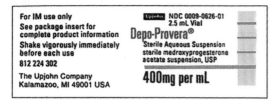

For IM use only
See package insert for complete product information
Shake vigorously immediately before each use
812 224 302

The Upjohn Company
Kalamazoo, MI 49001 USA

Upjohn NDC 0009-0626-01
2.5 mL Vial
Depo-Provera®
Sterile Aqueous Suspension
sterile medroxyprogesterone
acetate suspension, USP
400mg per mL

9. Ordered: Halcion 125 µg HS po. (One-step or two-step?)

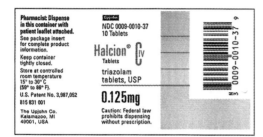

Pharmacist: Dispense in this container with patient leaflet attached.
See package insert for complete product information.
Keep container tightly closed.
Store at controlled room temperature 15° to 30° C (59° to 86° F).
U.S. Patent No. 3,987,052
815 831 001
The Upjohn Co.
Kalamazoo, MI 49001, USA

Upjohn
NDC 0009-0010-37
10 Tablets
Halcion® C IV
Tablets
triazolam tablets, USP
0.125mg
Caution: Federal law prohibits dispensing without prescription.

10. Ordered: Synthroid 350 µg po daily. (One-step or two-step?)

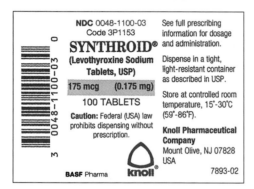

NDC 0048-1100-03
Code 3P1153
SYNTHROID®
(Levothyroxine Sodium Tablets, USP)
175 mcg (0.175 mg)
100 TABLETS
Caution: Federal (USA) law prohibits dispensing without prescription.

See full prescribing information for dosage and administration.
Dispense in a tight, light-resistant container as described in USP.
Store at controlled room temperature, 15°-30°C (59°-86°F).
Knoll Pharmaceutical Company
Mount Olive, NJ 07828 USA
7893-02
BASF Pharma knoll®

ANSWERS ON PAGE 346

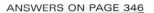

WORKSHEET 4L   Comparing Metric, Household, and Apothecary Measurements

As stated earlier, the metric system is the preferred system for measurement of medications. Household measures have become increasingly important with the trend toward home health care. The apothecary system is an imprecise, old, English system of measurement that is not very often seen today. As you will see from the equivalents, the nurse must be aware of the differences and the nomenclature, particularly the difference between *mg, g (gm),* and *gr.*

You have learned that the metric system is written with Arabic numerals and decimals. The apothecary system is written in Roman numerals and whole numbers and fractions.

ARABIC NUMERALS: 1, 2, 3, 4, 5, 6, 7, 8, 9, 10
ROMAN NUMERALS: I, II, III, IV, V, VI, VII, VIII, IX, X

The metric medication system uses the terms, *milligrams* and *grams* and *milliliters* and *liters.* The apothecary system uses grains *(gr)** for solids and *ounces (oz)* (℥) for liquids. The apothecary terms for other liquid measures, dram and minim, are now obsolete. You are already familiar with the household designations of cup, pint, and quart.

Table 4-2 Approximate Equivalents of Metric, Apothecary, and Household Measures

Metric	Household	Apothecary
5 mL (or cc)*	1 teaspoon (tsp)	1 teaspoon (tsp)
15 mL	1 tablespoon (tbs)	
30 mL	2 tablespoons (tbs)	1 ounce (℥)
240 mL	1 measuring cup	8 ounces
500 mL	1 pint	16 ounces
1000 mL	1 quart	32 ounces

*The abbreviations *mL* and *cc* are used interchangeably; however, *mL* should be used for liquids, *cc* for solids and gases, and *g* for solids.

Table 4-3 Volume Equivalents and Weight Equivalents

Volume	Weight
4000 milliliters (mL) = 1 gallon (gal) = 4 quarts (qt)	1000 mg = 1 g = gr XV (15)
1000 milliliters (mL) = 1 liter (L) = 1 quart (qt) = 2 pints (pt) = 32 oz (℥)	500 mg = 0.5 g = gr Viiss
1 mL = 1 cubic centimeter (cc)	60–67 mg = gr i
500 mL = 1 pint (pt) = 16 oz (℥)	gr ss = gr $\frac{1}{2}$
30 mL = 1 ounce (℥) or 8 drams (ℨ) = 6 tsp	0.6 mg = gr $\frac{1}{100}$
5 mL = 1 dram = 1 tsp = 4 or 5 mL	0.4 mg = gr $\frac{1}{150}$
	0.3 mg = gr $\frac{1}{200}$
	0.2 mg = gr $\frac{1}{300}$

*The grain measurement for weight was originally derived from a grain of wheat.

Continued

ANSWERS ON PAGE 346

WORKSHEET
4L

Comparing Metric, Household, and Apothecary Measurements—cont'd

The apothecary system does not convert exactly to metric, and neither the apothecary nor the metric system converts exactly to the household system. The patient at home must use special equipment for teaspoons and droppers if provided.

Discharge teaching must be scrupulous in explaining correct measurement to the patient and the family, taking into account that the equipment may not be provided and that the patient does not know that all droppers and teaspoons are not equal.

A good way to compare is to use the conversion clock (Figure 4-6). As you can see, a grain is 60 times larger than a milligram.

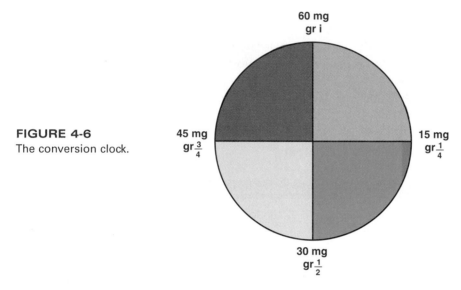

FIGURE 4-6
The conversion clock.

The apothecary system has been mostly phased out of use, but these medication labels still provide the metric/apothecary equivalent in case someone writes an order using the apothecary system.

Examine the following labels and fill in the *unit dose* metric and apothecary equivalents in the spaces provided:

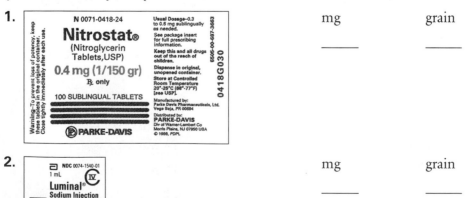

1.   mg   grain
      ——   ——

2.   mg   grain
      ——   ——

ANSWERS ON PAGE 346

WORKSHEET 4L Comparing Metric, Household, and Apothecary Measurements—cont'd

3.

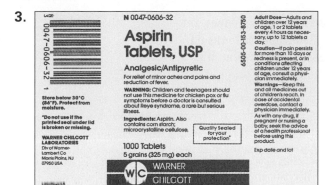

N 0047-0606-32

Aspirin Tablets, USP

Analgesic/Antipyretic

For relief of minor aches and pains and reduction of fever.

WARNING: Children and teenagers should not use this medicine for chicken pox or flu symptoms before a doctor is consulted about Reye syndrome, a rare but serious illness.

Ingredients: Aspirin. Also contains corn starch; microcrystalline cellulose.

Quality Sealed for your protection*

Store below 30°C (86°F). Protect from moisture.

*Do not use if the printed seal under lid is broken or missing.

WARNER CHILCOTT LABORATORIES
Div of Warner-Lambert Co
Morris Plains, NJ
07950 USA

1000 Tablets
5 grains (325 mg) each

WC WARNER CHILCOTT

6505-00-153-8750

Adult Dose—Adults and children over 12 years of age, 1 or 2 tablets every 4 hours as necessary, up to 12 tablets a day.

Caution—if pain persists for more than 10 days or redness is present, or in conditions affecting children under 12 years of age, consult a physician immediately.

Warnings—Keep this and all medicines out of children's reach. In case of accidental overdose, contact a physician immediately.

As with any drug, if pregnant or nursing a baby, seek the advice of a health professional before using this product.

Exp date and lot

mg _____   grain _____

4.

NDC 0002-0313-02
100 TABLETS No. 1571

Lilly

FERROUS SULFATE TABLETS USP

5 grs (324 mg)

For Iron Deficiency in Hypochromic Anemias.

Usual Adult Dose—One or two tablets 3 times a day after meals, or as directed by the physician.

WARNINGS: Keep all medications out of the reach of children. As with any drug, if you are pregnant or nursing a baby, seek the advice of a health professional before using this product.

Do not purchase if Lilly band around cap is missing or broken. After purchasing, do not use initially if red Lilly seal under cap is missing or broken. Tampering may have occurred.

Each Tablet equivalent to 65 mg elemental iron. Also contains cellulose, FD&C Blue No. 1, D&C Red No. 40, FD&C Yellow No. 6, lactose, magnesium stearate, silicon dioxide, sodium lauryl sulfate, talc, titanium dioxide and other inactive ingredients.

Keep Tightly Closed
Store at 59° to 86°F
Eli Lilly & Co., Indianapolis, IN 46285, U.S.A.
YA-8009 AMX
Expiration Date/Control No.

mg _____   grain _____

5.

20
15
10
5

APPROXIMATE VOLUME SCALE

NDC 0002-1636-01
20 ml VIAL No. 335

POISON *Lilly* C II

CODEINE PHOSPHATE 30

INJECTION, USP

30 mg (1/2 gr) per ml

Multiple Dose

YA 9725 AMX
Eli Lilly & Co., Indianapolis, IN 46206, U.S.A.

APPROXIMATE EQUIVALENTS
0.5 ml=15 mg (1/4 gr)
1 ml=30 mg (1/2 gr)
2 ml=60 mg (1 gr)

Usual Adult Dose—0.5 to 2 ml subcutaneously every 4 hours. Each ml contains Codeine Phosphate 30 mg (1/2 gr), Chlorobutanol (Chloroderivative) 5%, and more than 0.1% sodium bisulfite.

Store at Controlled Room Temperature 59° to 86°F (15° to 30°C).
Protect from light.

Exp. Date/Control No.

mg _____   grain _____

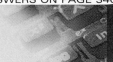

CLINICAL ALERT!

Never confuse g or g*m* with gr. Some writers' *r*'s and *m*'s are very similar in appearance. If an order is written in grains, the label will have the metric nearest equivalent as noted in the above labels.

Refer to the Introducing Drug Measures, section of the enclosed CD-ROM for additional practice problems.

ANSWERS ON PAGE 346

WORKSHEET

4M Multiple-Choice Practice

Solve the following problems and circle the correct answer. Use scrap paper, set up your ratio and proportion neatly, and *prove* your work. Remember to focus on whether the calculation is one-step or two-step and *estimate* your answer. If it does not seem right, recalculate the problem without looking at your original work.

1. Ordered: Demerol (meperidine HCl) 35 mg IM stat preoperatively. Label: 50 mg/mL. How many milliliters will you give?
   a. 0.5   **b.** 0.6   **c.** 0.7   **d.** 1.0

2. Ordered: Compazine (prochlorperazine maleate) 25 mg q4h IM prn for nausea. Label: 10 mg/mL. How many milliliters will you give?
   a. 0.5   **b.** 2.0   **c.** 2.5   **d.** 2.9

3. Ordered: Potassium chloride elixir 20 mEq bid po for a patient with potassium deficiency. Label: 8 mEq/5 mL. How many milliliters will you give?
   a. 12.5   **b.** 15   **c.** 32   **d.** 40

4. Ordered: Atropine 0.4 mg IM stat. Label: 0.3 mg/0.5 mL. How many milliliters will you give?
   a. 0.1   **b.** 0.5   **c.** 0.6   **d.** 0.7

5. Ordered: Quinidine sulfate 0.3 g bid po for a patient with an arrhythmia. Label: 150 mg tablets. How many tablets will you give?
   a. 0.5   **b.** 1   **c.** 2   **d.** 3

6. Ordered: L-Dopa (levodopa) 2 g bid po for a patient with Parkinson's disease. Label: 500 mg tablets. How many tablets will you give?
   a. 2   **b.** 3   **c.** 4   **d.** 5

7. Ordered: Vitamin B_{12} 1000 μg deep IM once a month for a patient who has had a gastrectomy. Label: 0.5 mg/mL. How many milliliters will you give?
   a. 1   **b.** 1.5   **c.** 2   **d.** 2.5

8. Ordered: AZT (zidovudine) 0.2 g q4h po for symptomatic HIV infection. Label: 100 mg tablets. How many tablets will you give?
   a. 0.5   **b.** 1   **c.** 1.5   **d.** 2

9. Ordered: Lanoxin 0.25 mg qd po for a patient with CHF. Label: 0.125 mg tablets. How many tablets will you give?
   a. 0.5   **b.** 1   **c.** 1.5   **d.** 2

10. Ordered: Nembutal 0.1 g HS po for sleep prn. Label: 50 mg capsules. How many capsules will you give?
    a. 1   **b.** 2   **c.** 3   **d.** 4

Refer to the Calculating Dosages Introduction, Systems of Measurement section of the enclosed CD-ROM for additional practice problems.

CRITICAL THINKING EXERCISES

Analyze this anecdote.

Mr. R. is an alert, anxious-appearing, frail gentleman, 76 years old, weighing 65 kilograms. He had been admitted two days before with complaints of chest pain. His medication orders included Lanoxin 0.125 mg daily every morning. This was the only medication ordered for the morning. On hand was digoxin 0.25 mg/tablet.

After you provided care for him on the evening shift, he mentioned that his doctor must have changed his orders because for two days he had been taking only a half of a tablet in the morning, and yesterday and today, his new nurse had given him two tablets each day. His wife agreed. He wanted to know if this meant that his heart problem was getting worse.

Order:

Given:

Error/s:

Potential Injury:

Nursing Actions:

Preventive measures: How could this have been avoided? If you were on a hospital committee to study incidents, what sort of recommendations would you make for this specific incident and the nurse involved and the pharmacy department, keeping in mind that you would not want to discourage the reporting of medication errors?

ANSWERS ON PAGE 346

CHAPTER 4 FINAL

Use ratio and proportion and your knowledge of conversion tables to solve these problems. Focus on whether you should use a one-step or a two-step calculation. *Estimate* and *prove* all work. Label your answers.

1. Ordered: Promethazine HCl tablets 0.05 g po q6h prn nausea for a postoperative patient. How many tablets will you give?

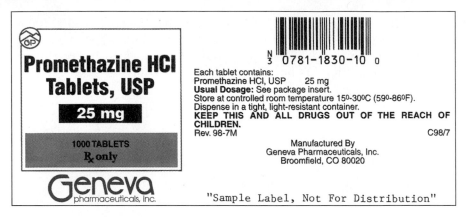

2. Ordered: Voltaren (diclofenac sodium) 0.05 g bid po for a patient with arthritis. How many tablets will you give?

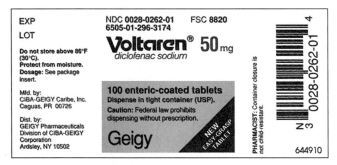

3. Ordered: Cimetidine 0.8 g bid po for a patient with an ulcer. How many tablets will you give?

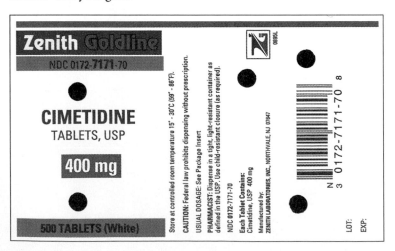

4. Ordered: Minoxidil 0.04 g once a day for hypertension. How many tablets will you give?

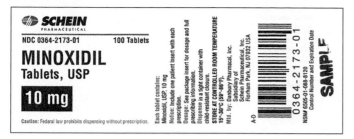

5. Ordered: Meperidine HCl 50 mg and atropine sulfate 0.3 IM preoperatively. How many milliliters (to the nearest tenth) will you prepare each of meperidine and atropine, and how many milliliters in the combined dose (to the nearest tenth)?

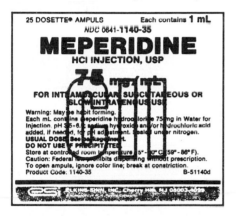

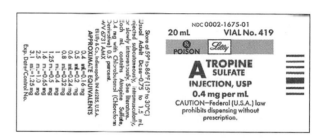

6. Ordered: Amoxil oral suspension 500 mg q6h for an elderly woman with influenza. How many milliliters will you prepare? Shade in the correct dose on the medication cup.

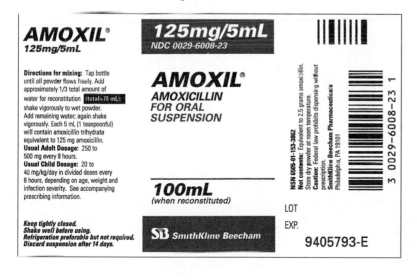

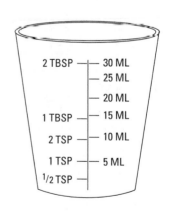

7. Ordered: Dilantin (phenytoin sodium) 0.2 g po qd for a patient with seizures. How many capsules will you give?

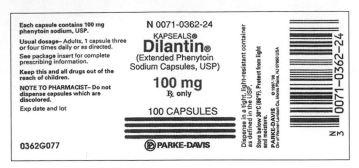

8. Ordered: Lanoxin (digoxin) 125 μg IM qd.
   a. How many milliliters will you give?
   b. SDR is 0.125-0.5 mg daily for adults. Is the order safe?

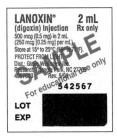

9. Ordered: Isoniazid 0.3 g qd po as preventive therapy for a patient at high risk for tuberculosis. How many tablets will you give?

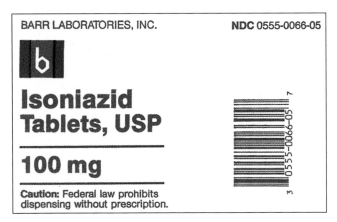

10. Ordered: Dexamethasone 3000 μg po stat for a patient with a severe allergic reaction. How many tablets will you give?

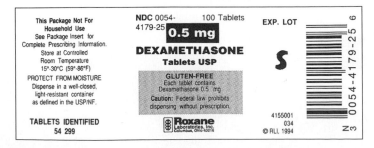

Medications from Powders and Crystals

5

- Read reconstitution labels to determine specific doses, conditions for storage, and expiration dates.
- Understand the importance of initialing and writing the date and time of reconstitution on the medication vial or bottle.
- Determine the best dilution strength to use for multiple dosage strength vials.
- Calculate the dosage in milligrams, grams, and milliliters for oral and parenteral routes.
- Reconstitute and measure liquid medications.
- Reconstitute medications from powders and crystals.

INTRODUCTION

Preparation of reconstituted medications from powders and crystals, mostly antibiotics, is usually the nurse's responsibility. The medications are reconstituted by adding a diluent (liquid) recommended by the manufacturer as the means for administration. The shelf life of reconstituted medications is usually shorter; therefore careful consideration must be given to how they are stored, the date and time of reconstitution (initialed by the nurse), the expiration date, and the route of administration. This chapter teaches the steps to safely prepare medications from powders and crystals. The measurement of units will be spelled out in the physician's orders, but the symbol U will be used in the problem setup.

● MEASURING LIQUID MEDICATIONS

When measuring a liquid medication, hold the transparent measuring device at eye level. The liquid curve in the center is called *the meniscus* (Figure 5-1). All liquid medication is measured at the meniscus level.

Medications can be measured in a medicine cup and transferred to an oral syringe for ease in administration and accuracy (Figure 5-2).

Liquid medications can be measured more accurately in a syringe than in a medicine cup (Figure 5-3).

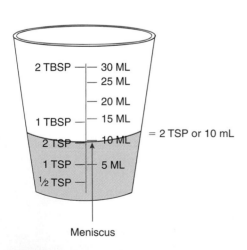

FIGURE 5-1 Measuring cup showing meniscus.

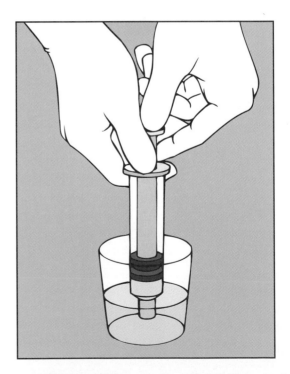

FIGURE 5-2 Filling a syringe directly from medicine cup. (*From Clayton BD, Stock YN: Basic pharmacology for nurses, ed 12, St Louis, 2001, Mosby.*)

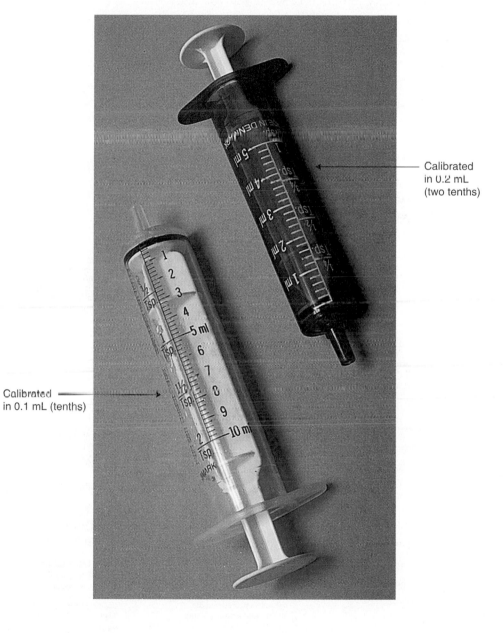

FIGURE 5-3 Oral syringes. *(From Clayton BD, Stock YN:* Basic pharmacology for nurses, *ed 12, St Louis, 2001, Mosby. Courtesy Chuck Dresner.)*

Calibrated in 0.2 mL (two tenths)

Calibrated in 0.1 mL (tenths)

ANSWERS ON PAGE 347

WORKSHEET
5A

Practice in Reconstituting, Administering, and Measuring Liquid Medications

Show your calculations and proofs in the following problems. Shade in the correct dose on the medicine cup.

1. Augmentin suspension 200 mg po q8h.
   a. How many milliliters of water will you add?
   b. How many total milliliters are in the bottle?
   c. How many milliliters of Augmentin will you administer?

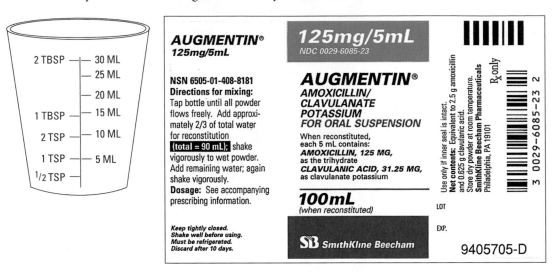

2. Ordered: Erythromycin ethylsuccinate suspension 0.3 g po for intestinal amebiasis.
   a. How many milliliters of water will you add?
   b. How many total grams are in the 200 mL bottle?
   c. How many milliliters will you administer?

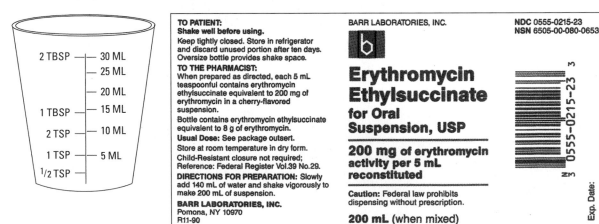

ANSWERS ON PAGE 347

WORKSHEET 5A

Practice in Reconstituting, Administering, and Measuring Liquid Medications—cont'd

3. Ordered: Amoxil (amoxicillin) 500 mg po q8h for endocarditis prophylaxis.

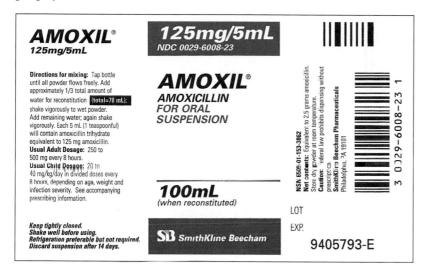

AMOXIL®
125mg/5mL

125mg/5mL
NDC 0029-6008-23

Directions for mixing: Tap bottle until all powder flows freely. Add approximately 1/3 total amount of water for reconstitution (total=78 mL); shake vigorously to wet powder. Add remaining water; again shake vigorously. Each 5 mL (1 teaspoonful) will contain amoxicillin trihydrate equivalent to 125 mg amoxicillin.
Usual Adult Dosage: 250 to 500 mg every 8 hours.
Usual Child Dosage: 20 to 40 mg/kg/day in divided doses every 8 hours, depending on age, weight and infection severity. See accompanying prescribing information.

Keep tightly closed.
Shake well before using.
Refrigeration preferable but not required.
Discard suspension after 14 days.

AMOXIL®
AMOXICILLIN
FOR ORAL SUSPENSION

100mL
(when reconstituted)

SB SmithKline Beecham

NSN 6505-01-153-3862
Net contents: Equivalent to 2.5 grams amoxicillin.
Store dry powder at room temperature.
Caution: Federal law prohibits dispensing without prescription.
SmithKline Beecham Pharmaceuticals
Philadelphia, PA 19101

3 0029-6008-23 1

LOT
EXP.
9405793-E

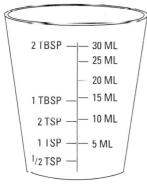

2 TBSP — 30 ML
— 25 ML
— 20 ML
1 TBSP — 15 ML
2 TSP — 10 ML
1 TSP — 5 ML
1/2 TSP —

a. How many milliliters of diluent will you add?
b. How many total milligrams are in the bottle?
c. How many milliliters will you administer per dose?
d. How many doses are in the bottle?

Continued

CLINICAL ALERT!

For accuracy, read the medication at the meniscus level.

ANSWERS ON PAGE 347

WORKSHEET

5A

Practice in Reconstituting, Administering, and Measuring Liquid Medications—cont'd

4. Ordered: Lorabid 150 mg po bid.

Follow mixing directions on the label.

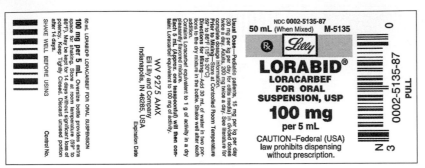

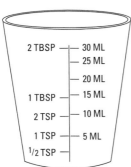

a. How many total milliliters of water are needed?

b. How many total milliliters of Lorabid are in the bottle?

c. How many milliliters will provide 150 mg of Lorabid?

d. How many doses are in the bottle?

5. Ordered: Vancocin HCl 300 mg po bid for colitis.

Follow mixing directions on the label.

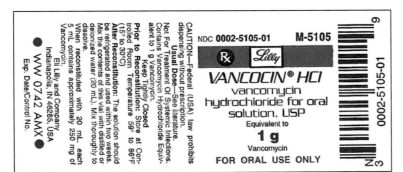

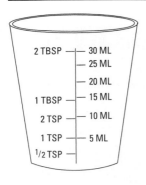

a. How many milliliters of distilled water are needed?

b. How many total milligrams of Vancocin are in the bottle?

c. How many milliliters of Vancocin HCl will provide 300 mg?

ANSWERS ON PAGE 347

WORKSHEET 5A   Practice in Reconstituting, Administering, and Measuring Liquid Medications—cont'd

6. Ordered: Lorabid 200 mg po q12h 1 hour ac for bacterial bronchitis.

Follow mixing directions on the label.

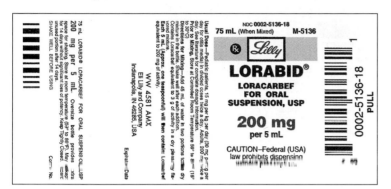

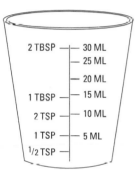

a. How many total milliliters of water are needed?

b. How many total milliliters of Lorabid are in the bottle?

c. How many milliliters will the patient receive per dose?

d. How many doses are in the bottle?

e. For how many days will the reconstituted medicine be effective?

7. Ordered: Lorabid 400 mg po q12h × 14 days 1 hour ac for pneumonia.

Follow mixing directions on the label.

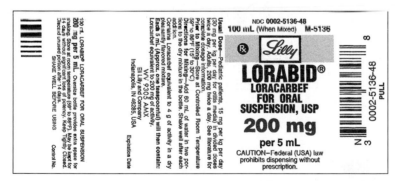

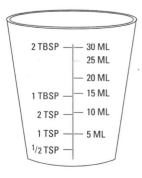

a. How many total milliliters of water are needed?

b. How many total milliliters of Lorabid are in the bottle?

c. How many milliliters will provide 400 mg?

d. How many doses are in the bottle?

Continued

ANSWERS ON PAGE 347

> **WORKSHEET**
> **5A**

Practice in Reconstituting, Administering, and Measuring Liquid Medications—cont'd

8. Ordered: 500 mg of Vancocin suspension bid po.

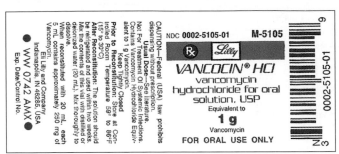

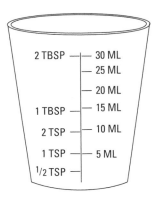

a. How many milligrams are in the bottle?
b. How many milliliters will you administer?

9. Ordered: 400 mg of Augmentin suspension po tid.

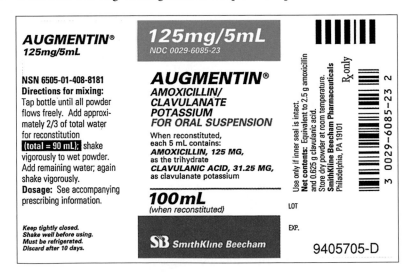

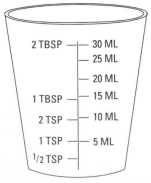

a. How many milliliters will you administer per dose?

ANSWERS ON PAGE 347

10. Ordered: Erythromycin suspension 500 mg po bid.

TO PATIENT:
Shake well before using.
Keep tightly closed. Store in refrigerator and discard unused portion after ten days. Oversize bottle provides shake space.

TO THE PHARMACIST:
When prepared as directed, each 5 mL teaspoonful contains erythromycin ethylsuccinate equivalent to 200 mg of erythromycin in a cherry-flavored suspension.
Bottle contains erythromycin ethylsuccinate equivalent to 8 g of erythromycin.
Usual Dose: See package outsert.
Store at room temperature in dry form.
Child-resistant closure not required; Reference: Federal Register Vol.39 No.29.
DIRECTIONS FOR PREPARATION: Slowly add 140 mL of water and shake vigorously to make 200 mL of suspension.
BARR LABORATORIES, INC.
Pomona, NY 10970
R11-90

BARR LABORATORIES, INC.

Erythromycin Ethylsuccinate
for Oral Suspension, USP

200 mg of erythromycin activity per 5 mL reconstituted

Caution: Federal law prohibits dispensing without prescription.

200 mL (when mixed)

NDC 0555-0215-23
NSN 6505-00-080-0653

N 3 0555-0215-23 3

SAMPLE

Exp. Date: Lot No.:

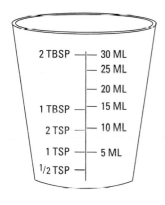

2 TBSP ——— 30 ML
—— 25 ML
—— 20 ML
1 TBSP —— 15 ML
2 TSP —— 10 ML
1 TSP —— 5 ML
1/2 TSP ——

a. How many milliliters will you administer?

● RECONSTITUTING MEDICATIONS

Reconstituting medications is much like making a cup of soup out of dried soup mix from a package or using freeze-dried coffee crystals to make a cup of coffee. The concept is the same. When a lot of liquid, or diluent as it is referred to when mixing medications, is used, the soup or coffee becomes weaker. The less liquid or diluent that is used makes the soup or coffee stronger. Some medications that must be reconstituted have different amounts of diluent or liquid that can be added to produce various strengths of the medicine. As an example, if you add 16 oz or 1 quart of water to 1 tbsp of instant coffee, you will have very weak coffee. If you add 8 oz of water to 1 tbsp of instant coffee, you will have stronger coffee, in less total volume. The main point is that the amount of instant coffee remains constant; only the amount of liquid (diluent) changes to make stronger or weaker coffee. Reconstituting medications works in the same manner. There is always a certain amount of powder or crystals in the container before the diluent is added. The drug manufacturer will tell you what the displacement factor is. This amount is added to the amount of diluent to give the total number of milliliters. The label on the medication vial will state strength (amount) of medication in the vial. That amount never changes. The only thing that can change is the amount of diluent (liquid) that is added.

Most reconstituted medications come in single-dose vials rather than multiple-dose vials, which have different amounts of diluent that can be added to make varying strengths of medication.

■ Types of Diluents

It is important to use the type of diluent described in the directions for reconstitution. The diluents used to reconstitute powders vary based on the chemical properties of the powder. For example, erythromycin must be reconstituted with sterile water. If normal saline (NS) is used, the powder clumps and will not go into solution. The Bacteriostatic agent used in bacteriostatic water is benzyl alcohol. If sterile water is used instead of bacteriostatic water, it may cause some products to clump instead of going into solution. The choice of diluent is based on the pH and the physical properties of the product (medication).

Dibasic sodium is added to some powders to correct the final pH of the product.

Lidocaine is added to ease pain during IM administration. The amount of lidocaine added to the medication would not affect vasoconstriction.

DILUTING POWDERS OR CRYSTALS IN VIALS

Directions for dissolving medications in vials can be found in the accompanying literature. What will be given is the volume of the powder after it is dissolved in the diluent. For instance, the directions may read: *Add 1.4 mL NS to make 2 mL of reconstituted solution.* These directions tell the user that the powder takes up to 0.6 mL of space.

$$1.4 \text{ mL} + 0.6 \text{ mL} = 2 \text{ mL of medication}$$

EXAMPLE   Read the medication label to find out how many units, grams, milligrams, or micrograms are in each milliliter of the reconstituted drug.

Begin by adding 2.7 mL of air to the sterile water for injection (diluent) vial, and then invert the vial to withdraw the 2.7 mL of diluent. Add the 2.7 mL of diluent to the oxacillin sodium vial to make 500 mg of medication in 3 mL (Figure 5-4).

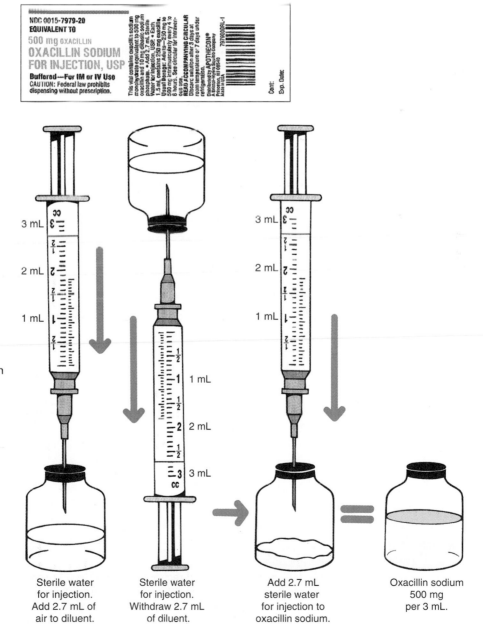

FIGURE 5-4
Diluting oxacillin sodium in sterile water for injection.

Sterile water for injection. Add 2.7 mL of air to diluent.

Sterile water for injection. Withdraw 2.7 mL of diluent.

Add 2.7 mL sterile water for injection to oxacillin sodium.

Oxacillin sodium 500 mg per 3 mL.

Ordered: 250 mg oxacillin sodium IM q6h.

Know   *Want to Know*

3 mL : 500 mg :: x mL : 250 mg

$500x = 3 \times 250 = 750$

$\quad x = 1.5$ mL

PROOF

$500 \times 1.5 = 750$

$3 \times 250 = 750$

Give 1.5 mL of reconstituted solution for each 250 mg.

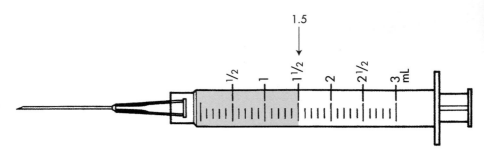

CLINICAL ALERT!

When giving intramuscular injections, always aspirate before injecting.

Medications for reconstitution with attached diluent ensures sterility and accuracy of reconstituted powder (Figure 5-5). Some medications are reconstituted by the manufacturer and are delivered in prefilled cartridges or syringes (Figure 5-6).

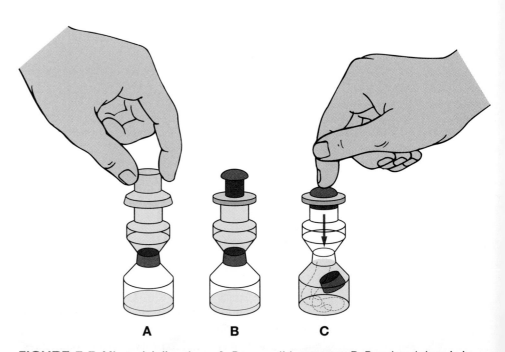

FIGURE 5-5 Mix-o-vial directions. **A,** Remove lid protector. **B,** Powdered drug is in lower half; diluent is in upper half. **C,** Push firmly on the diaphragm-plunger. Downward pressure dislodges the divider between the two chambers. *(From Clayton BD, Stock YN: Basic pharmacology for nurses, ed 12, St Louis, 2001, Mosby.)*

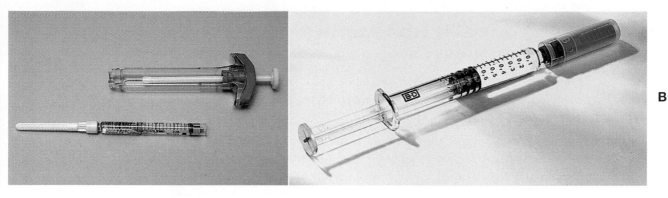

FIGURE 5-6 A, Carpuject syringe and pre-filled sterile cartridge with needle. *(From Potter P, Perry A: Basic nursing: essentials for practice, ed 5, St Louis, 2003, Mosby.)* **B,** BD-Hypak Pre-filled Syringe. *(From Bectin Dickinson Division, Franklin Lakes, N.J.)*

RECONSTITUTION: MEDICATION LABELS

Medication labels for reconstitution contain information about the amount of diluent to use and the resulting concentration. The important information is as follows:

- Strength-reconstitution directions
- Usual dose
- Route
- Name–generic and proprietary
- Expiration date
- Storage conditions/shelf life

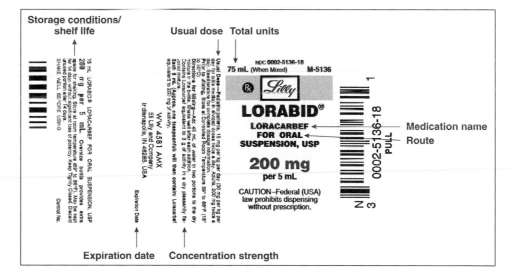

CLINICAL ALERT!

If the vial is a multiple-dose vial, the nurse must put the date, time, amount of diluent used, and his or her initials on the label.

Many solutions are unstable after being reconstituted. Read labels carefully for directions on storing the solution in the refrigerator or in a dark place. There is usually a time limit or expiration date on the vial. It is important to date, label, and initial all reconstituted medications.

WORKSHEET 5B Practice in Reconstituting Parenteral Dosages

Show your calculations and proofs in the following problems. Shade in the correct doses on the syringes.

1. Ordered: Oxacillin sodium 500 mg IV q6h. Available: A multidose vial that reads *Oxacillin sodium; add 5.7 mL sterile water for injection.* Each 1.5 mL of solution contains 0.25 g. How many milliliters will you administer?

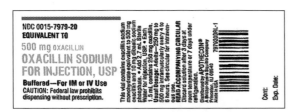

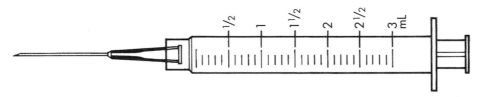

2. Ordered: Penicillin G potassium 300,000 U IM q4h. Available: A multidose vial containing one million units and the following directions:

ADD DILUENT	CONCENTRATION OF SOLUTION
9.6 mL	100,000 U/mL
4.6 mL	200,000 U/mL
1.6 mL	500,000 U/mL

Select the most appropriate dilution for the ordered dose. Work out all concentrations to determine the appropriate dosage for the patient.

a. Which dilution will you make and label?

b. What amount will you administer?

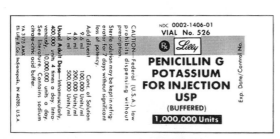

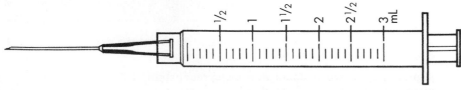

ANSWERS ON PAGE 350

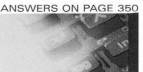

WORKSHEET 5B

Practice in Reconstituting Parenteral Dosages—cont'd

3. Ordered: 100 mg ampicillin IM q12h.
   a. How many milliliters of diluent will be added?
   b. What is the shelf life after reconstitution?
   c. What is the total amount of medication in the vial?
   d. How many milliliters of ampicillin will you administer?

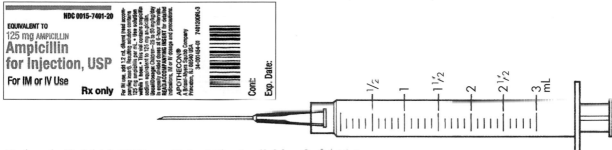

4. Ordered: Cefobid 1000 mg IM q12h. Available: Cefobid 1 g. Reconstitute IM doses with 2.2 mL of bacteriostatic water for injection (taken from insert). The powder displaces 0.4 mL. How many milliliters will be administered?

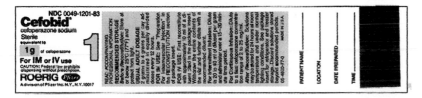

5. Ordered: Tazicef 250 mg IM q8h.
   Available: Tazicef 1 g for IM or IV use.
   Follow insert directions for reconstitution directions.
   a. How many mL of diluent will be added to the powder?
   b. How many mg/mL will this make?
   c. How many mL will you give IM?

RECONSTITUTION

Single Dose Vials:
For I.M. injection, I.V. direct (bolus) injection, or I.V. infusion, reconstitute with Sterile Water for injection according to the following table. The vacuum may assist entry of the diluent. SHAKE WELL.

Table 5

Vial Size	Diluent to Be Added	Approx. Avail. Volume	Approx. Avg. Concentration
Intramuscular or Intravenous Direct (bolus) Injection			
1 gram	3.0 ml.	3.6 ml.	280 mg./ml.
Intravenous Infusion			
1 gram	10 ml.	10.6 ml.	95 mg./ml.
2 gram	10 ml.	11.2 ml.	180 mg./ml.

Withdraw the total volume of solution into the syringe (the pressure in the vial may aid withdrawal). The withdrawn solution may contain some bubbles of carbon dioxide.

NOTE: As with the administration of all parenteral products, accumulated gases should be expressed from the syringe immediately before injection of 'Tazicef'.

These solutions of 'Tazicef' are stable for 18 hours at room temperature or seven days if refrigerated (5°C.). Slight yellowing does not affect potency.

For I.V. infusion, dilute reconstituted solution in 50 to 100 ml. of one of the parenteral fluids listed under COMPATIBILITY AND STABILITY.

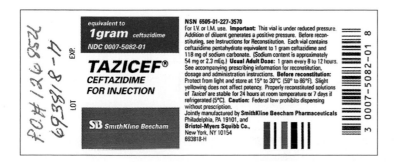

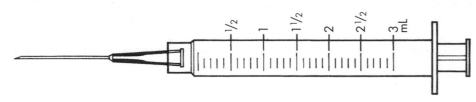

Continued

ANSWERS ON PAGE 350

WORKSHEET 5B

Practice in Reconstituting Parenteral Dosages—cont'd

6. Ordered: Cefobid 2 g IM q12h. Available: Cefobid 2 g vial. Reconstitution for IM use is found on the package insert. Directions read: Add 3.4 mL of sterile water for injection. The Cefobid powder displaces 0.6 mL. Administer the entire dose.
   a. How many milliliters will you give for the first dose?
   b. How many injections will you administer?
   c. What sites will you select?

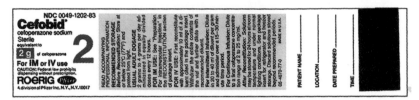

7. Ordered: Pfizerpen (penicillin G potassium) 300,000 U IM bid. Available: One million U. Directions read:

mL DILUENT ADDED	UNITS PER mL OF SOLUTION
20.0	50,000
10.0	100,000
4.0	250,000
1.8	500,000

Calculate the strength closest to the ordered amount.
   a. How many milliliters of diluent will you add?
   b. How many milliliters will you give?
   c. How many doses are in the multidose vial?

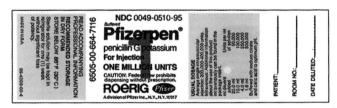

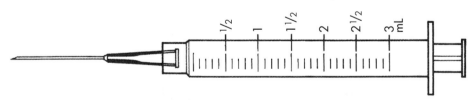

CLINICAL ALERT!

The maximum single injection for adults is 3 to 4 mL. Not all patients can tolerate a 3 mL injection. Assess patient for muscle mass at the site of injection to ensure ability to tolerate medication amount.

ANSWERS ON PAGE 350

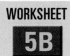

WORKSHEET 5B Practice in Reconstituting Parenteral Dosages—cont'd

8. Ordered: Ampicillin 1000 mg q6h. Available: Ampicillin 1 g. Directions read: *Add 3.5 mL diluent. Each mL = 250 mg.*
   a. How many milliliters will you administer?
   b. How many milliliters will you give in each site?

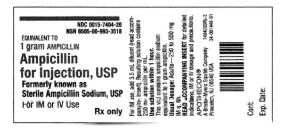

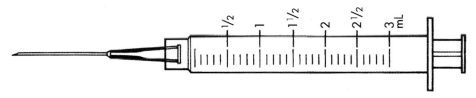

9. Ordered: Cefadyl 700 mg IM q6h. Available: Cefadyl 1 g. Directions read: *For IM use, add 2 mL sterile or bacteriostatic water for injection. USP. Each 1.2 mL contains 500 mg of cephapirin.*
   a. How many milliliters will you administer per injection?
   b. How many milligrams will the patient receive in 24 hours?
   c. How many vials will you need for a 24-hour period?

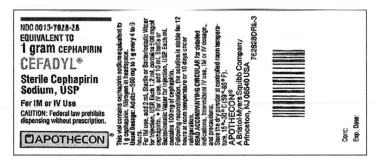

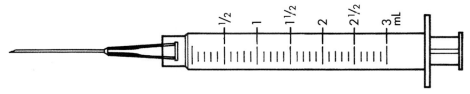

Continued

CLINICAL ALERT!

Do not confuse Units of medication with milligrams.

ANSWERS ON PAGE 350

WORKSHEET 5B

Practice in Reconstituting Parenteral Dosages—cont'd

10. Ordered: Pfizerpen (penicillin G potassium) 400,000 U IM q12h.
Available: one million U. Directions read:

mL DILUENT ADDED	UNITS PER mL OF SOLUTION
20.0	50,000
10.0	100,000
4.0	250,000
1.5	500,000

Select the most appropriate dilution for the ordered dose.
a. How many milliliters of diluent will you add?
b. How many milliliters will you administer?
c. How many doses are in the vial?

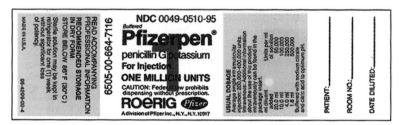

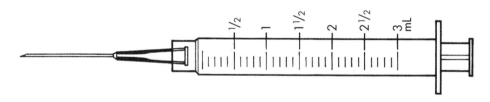

Doe, John
ID# 45764304
Age: 50 Sex: M Rm: 406A
Dr. Marin, Cruz

ALLERGIES: DRUGS: ___Codeine___
FOODS: ___none___

RN Verification: ___*Mary Smith*___

Date: *11-09-02* **(Beg)**
      11-13-02 **(End)**

MEDICATION: Dose Route Freq   Time of Administration, Site, and Initials

START	STOP	0700 TO 1459	1500 TO 2259	2300 TO 0659
SCH *11-09-02 Kefzol*	*11-13-02*	*0700*	*1500*	*2300*
300 mg IM q8h		*N MS*	*O IB*	*N JB*

This is a pharmacy generated MAR for 24 hours stated in military time for 8-hour shifts beginning at 0700. At the top, the orders must be signed by an RN indicating that the original order has been verified and is correct and allergies have been noted. SCH is a regularly scheduled medication. The start and stop dates are printed. PRN orders and One Time Only Meds are written in a separate space. Narcotic orders must be rewritten q48h. Discontinued orders are highlighted according to hospital policy and must be renewed if it is necessary to continue them. Site codes are in alpha order. Withheld meds use the code R circled with a nurse's note on the chart. The nurses giving the meds must initial each dose and sign the bottom of the MAR to identify their initials.

ONE TIME ONLY AND PRN MEDS

Start	Stop	Time	Initials	Full name/title
Lasix 11-16-02		*2000*	*IB*	*Irene Butler, RN*
40 mg IV STAT				

Sign: *Mary Smith*   Initials: *MS*   Sign: *Irene Butler*   Initials: *IB*   Sign: *Jill Book*   Initials: *JB*

SITE CODES   **GENERAL HOSPITAL**

A	Abdomen (L)	J	Gluteus (LUQ)
B	Abdomen (R)	K	Gluteus (RUQ)
C	Arm (L)	L	Thigh (L)
D	Arm (R)	M	Thigh (R)
E	Eyes (both) O.U.	N	Ventrogluteal (L)
F	Eyes (left) O.S.	O	Ventrogluteal (R)
G	Eyes (right) O.D.	P	NPO: Lab
H	Deltoid (mid L)	Q	NPO: Surgery
I	Deltoid (mid R)	R	Withheld/see nurse's notes

FIGURE 5-7 Medication administration record (MAR).

ANSWERS ON PAGE 354

WORKSHEET

5C Reconstituted Parenteral Dosages

Answer the questions in the following problems. Show your calculations and proofs; then shade in the correct dose on the syringes.

1. Ordered: Cefadyl 500 mg IM q4h for osteomyelitis. Follow directions on the label.
   a. How many milliliters of sterile water will be added?
   b. How many milliliters will be administered per dose?
   c. How many vials will be needed in 24 hours?

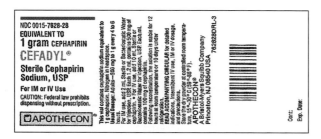

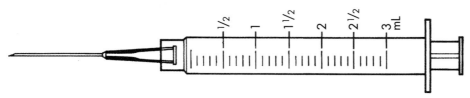

2. Ordered: Oxacillin sodium 450 mg IM q6h.
   a. How many milliliters of sterile water for injection will be used?
   b. How many mg/mL will it make?
   c. What is the shelf life of the medication after reconstitution?
   d. What is the total amount of medication in the vial?
   e. How many milliliters will you administer?

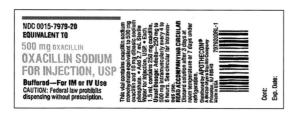

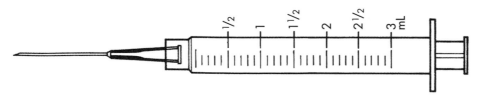

ANSWERS ON PAGE 354

WORKSHEET
5C

Reconstituted Parenteral Dosages—cont'd

3. Ordered: Ampicillin 500 mg IM q6h.
   a. How many milliliters of diluent are needed to reconstitute?
   b. How many mg/mL will it make?
   c. What is the shelf life of the medication?
   d. How many milliliters will you administer?

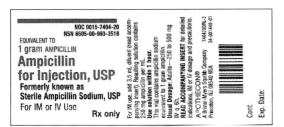

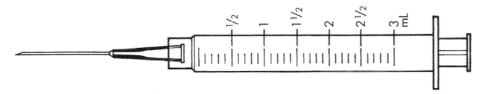

4. Ordered: Oxacillin sodium 300 mg IM q4h.
   a. How many milliliters of diluent should be used to reconstitute?
   b. How many mg/mL will it make?
   c. What is the shelf life of the medication?
   d. How many milliliters will you administer?

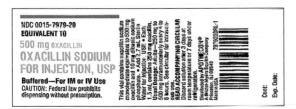

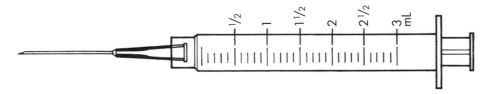

Continued

CLINICAL ALERT!

Check medication history for drug sensitivity before administration of antiin-fectives. Keep epinephrine, an antihistamine, and resuscitation equipment nearby in the event of an anaphylactic shock reaction.

ANSWERS ON PAGE 354

WORKSHEET
5C

Reconstituted Parenteral Dosages—cont'd

5. Ordered: Rocephin 500 mg IM bid

Directions: For IM use, add sterile water for injection according to directions. Withdraw entire contents to yield 500 mg. Give deep in a large muscle. Aspirate before giving. Calculate both dosages to determine which amount is appropriate for your patient.

VIAL DOSAGE SIZE	AMOUNT OF DILUENT TO BE ADDED
	1.8 mL ――― 250 mg/mL
500 mg	1.0 mL ――― 350 mg/mL

Which concentration did you choose? Measure it on the syringe.

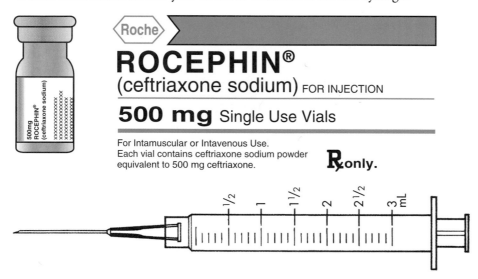

6. Ordered: Penicillin G potassium 750,000 U IM q8h. Select the most appropriate dilution for the ordered dose. The directions read: *Sterile solution may be kept in refrigerator for 7 days without significant loss of potency. Add diluent 9.6 mL for 100,000 units/mL for concentration of solution; add diluent 4.6 mL for 200,000 units/mL; add diluent 1.6 mL for 500,000 units/mL.*

a. Which strength will you use?

b. How many milliliters of diluent will be used?

c. How many milliliters of medication will you administer?

d. What is the shelf life of the medication after reconstitution?

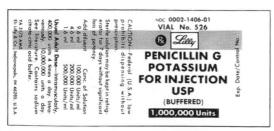

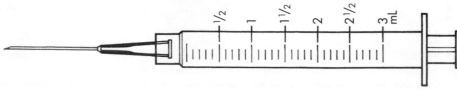

ANSWERS ON PAGE 354

WORKSHEET
5C

Reconstituted Parenteral Dosages—cont'd

7. Ordered: Ticar 750 mg IM q8h.
   a. How many milliliters of diluent will be added?
   b. 2.6 mL of Ticar contains how many grams?
   c. What is the shelf life of the medication?
   d. What is the total amount of medication in the vial?
   e. How many milliliters will you administer?

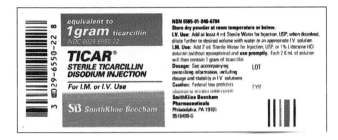

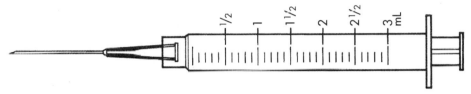

8. Ordered: Pfizerpen 400,000 U IM q12h.
   a. Calculate all 3 strengths to decide the best dosage amount for your patient based on a normal adult male.
   b. Fill in the amount you will administer on the syringe.

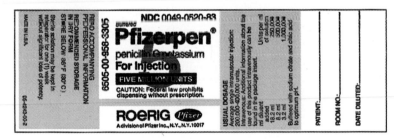

3 strengths to determine dosage
18.2 mL =   250,000 U/mL
 8.2 mL =   500,000 U/mL
 3.2 mL = 1,000,000 U/mL

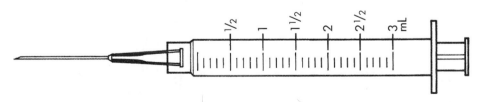

Continued

ANSWERS ON PAGE 354

9. Ordered: 400,000 U Pfizerpen IM q6h.
   Available: Pfizerpen one million U with mixing options.
   Choose between adding 4 mL and adding 1.5 mL of diluent.
   a. How many U/mL will you administer if you use 4 mL of diluent?
   Mark the syringe.
   b. How many U/mL will you administer if you use 1.5 mL of diluent?
   Mark the syringe.

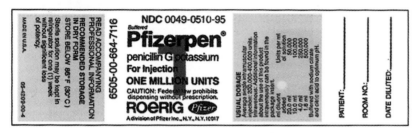

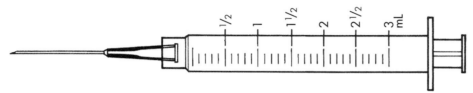

10. Ordered: Cefadyl (cephapirin) 500 mg IM q6h.
    a. How many milliliters of sterile water will you add?
    b. How many mg/mL will you have?
    c. How many milliliters will you administer?

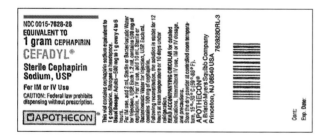

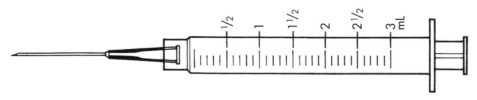

CLINICAL ALERT!

Always make sure that the patient's body mass is adequate for the amount of medication, which will be given intramuscularly.

ANSWERS ON PAGE 357

WORKSHEET

5D   Multiple-Choice Practice

1. Ordered: Ticar 500 mg IM tid.

Available: Ticar 1 gram.

Directions read: Add 2 mL of sterile water for injection.

How many milliliters will you administer?
- **a.** 2.6 mL
- **b.** 2 mL
- **c.** 1.3 mL
- **d.** 3.0 mL

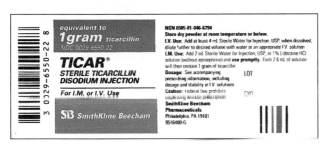

2. Refer to question 1.

How many vials of Ticar will be needed in 24 hours?
- **a.** 3 vials
- **b.** 4 vials
- **c.** 2 vials
- **d.** 5 vials

3. Ordered: Oxacillin sodium 500 mg IM q6h.

Available: Oxacillin 1 gram

How many milliliters of sterile water will you add?
- **a.** 3.7 mL
- **b.** 5 mL
- **c.** 3.1 mL
- **d.** 5.7 mL

How many milliliters will you give?
- **a.** 1.5 mL
- **b.** 3 mL
- **c.** 2.5 mL
- **d.** 2 mL

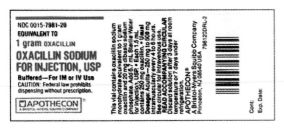

4. Ordered: Pfizerpen 400,000 U IM bid.

Available: Pfizerpen (penicillin G potassium) one million U.

How many milliliters of diluent will you add?
- **a.** 5.0 mL
- **b.** 10 mL
- **c.** 1.5 mL
- **d.** 20 mL

How many milliliters will you give?
- **a.** 2.0 mL
- **b.** 2.5 mL
- **c.** 1.6 mL
- **d.** 0.8 mL

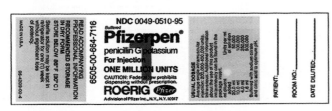

Continued

ANSWERS ON PAGE 357

WORKSHEET 5D — Multiple-Choice Practice—cont'd

5. Ordered: Streptomycin 500 mg IM bid.

   Available: Streptomycin sulfate 5.0 g.

   What is the concentration after dilution?
   a. 500 mg/mL   **b.** 1.0 g/mL   **c.** 400 mg/mL   **d.** 0.5 g/mL

   How many milliliters will you give?
   a. 1.3 mL   **b.** 1.0 mL   **c.** 2.2 mL   **d.** 1.8 mL

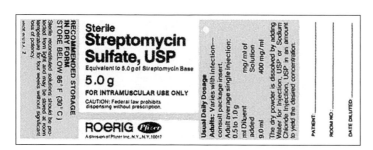

6. Ordered: Cefobid 1g IM q12h.

   Available: Cefobid 2 g vial.

   Directions for IM use read: Add 3.4 mL of sterile water for injection.
   Each 4 mL yields 2 g.

   How many milliliters will you give?
   a. 3.5 mL   **b.** 4 mL   **c.** 2 mL   **d.** 2.5 mL

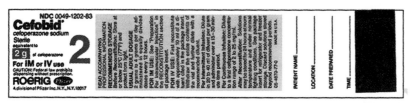

7. Ordered: Ampicillin 250 mg IM q12h.

   Available: Ampicillin 125 mg.

   How many milliliters of diluent will you add?
   a. 2 mL   **b.** 1.2 mL   **c.** 3 mL   **d.** 1.5 mL

   How many vials will you need in 24 hours?
   a. 1 vial   **b.** 2 vials   **c.** 3 vials   **d.** 4 vials

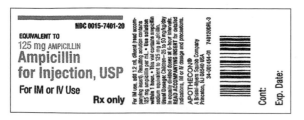

ANSWERS ON PAGE 357

WORKSHEET
5D   Multiple-Choice Practice—cont'd

8. Ordered: Cefobid 1.5 g IM q12h.

   Available: Cefobid 1 g vial.

   Directions read: Add 1.4 mL of sterile water for injection. Each 2 mL yields 1 g.

   How many milliliters will you give?
   a. 2.5 mL   **b.** 3 mL   **c.** 2 mL   **d.** 1.5 mL

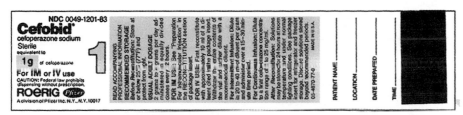

9. Ordered: Lorabid 200 mg po bid.

   Available: Lorabid 100 mg for oral use.

   How many milliliters of water will you add?
   a. 60 mL   **b.** 30 mL   **c.** 50 mL   **d.** 100 mL

   How many milliliters of medication will you give?
   a. 20 mL   **b.** 10 mL   **c.** 5 mL   **d.** 15 mL

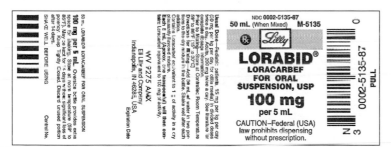

Continued

ANSWERS ON PAGE 357

WORKSHEET
5D
Multiple-Choice Practice—cont'd

10. Ordered: Erythromycin 200 mg po q12h.

Available: Erythromycin ethylsuccinate for oral suspension 200 mg/5 mL.

How many total milligrams of medication are in the 200 mL of erythromycin suspension?

a. 80,000 mg   **b.** 40,000 mg   **c.** 4,000 mg   **d.** 8,000 mg

How many milliliters will you give per dose?

a. 10 mL   **b.** 15 mL   **c.** 5 mL   **d.** 20 mL

TO PATIENT: **Shake well before using.** Keep tightly closed. Store in refrigerator and discard unused portion after ten days. Oversize bottle provides shake space. **TO THE PHARMACIST:** When prepared as directed, each 5 mL teaspoonful contains erythromycin ethylsuccinate equivalent to 200 mg of erythromycin in a cherry-flavored suspension. Bottle contains erythromycin ethylsuccinate equivalent to 8 g of erythromycin. **Usual Dose:** See package outsert. Store at room temperature in dry form. Child-Resistant closure not required; Reference: Federal Register Vol.39 No.29. **DIRECTIONS FOR PREPARATION:** Slowly add 140 mL of water and shake vigorously to make 200 mL of suspension. **BARR LABORATORIES, INC.** Pomona, NY 10970 R11-90	BARR LABORATORIES, INC. **Erythromycin Ethylsuccinate** **for Oral Suspension, USP** **200 mg of erythromycin activity per 5 mL reconstituted** **Caution:** Federal law prohibits dispensing without prescription. **200 mL** (when mixed)	NDC 0555-0215-23 NSN 6505-00-080-0653 0555-0215-23 3 **SAMPLE** Exp. Date: Lot No.:

 Refer to the Calculating Dosages, Oral Dosages, and Parenteral Dosages sections of the enclosed CD-ROM for additional practice problems.

CRITICAL THINKING EXERCISES

Penicillin G potassium has these directions for reconstitution:

ADD DILUENT	CONCENTRATION OF SOLUTION
9.6 mL	100,000 U/mL
4.6 mL	200,000 U/mL
1.6 mL	500,000 U/mL

The medication was reconstituted with 1.6 mL of diluent.

Order: Penicillin G potassium 200,000 IM q6h
Given: Penicillin G potassium 1 mL IM q6h
Error:
Preventive measures:
Potential injury:

Discussion

Which concentation would have been better to use?

Could the nurse use the 500,000 U/mL concentration and give the ordered dose of penicillin? How many milliliters should the nurse have given?

ANSWERS ON PAGE 359

CHAPTER **5** **FINAL**

1. Ordered: Penicillin G potassium 100,000 U IM q4h for pneumonia. The directions read: *Sterile solution may be kept in refrigerator for 7 days without significant loss of potency. Add diluent 9.6 mL for 100,000 units/mL concentration of solution; add diluent 4.6 mL for 200,000 units/mL; add diluent 1.6 mL for 500,000 units/mL.*
   a. Which dilution will you use? Why?
   b. How many milliliters will you administer? Shade in the amount on the syringe.

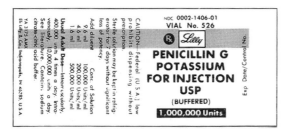

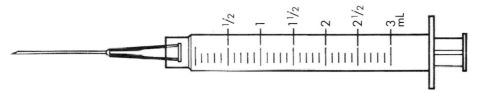

2. Ordered: Oxacillin sodium 250 mg IM q4h for a urinary tract infection (UTI).
   a. How many milliliters of diluent will you add?
   b. How many milliliters of oxacillin sodium will you administer? Shade in the amount on the syringe.

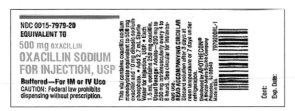

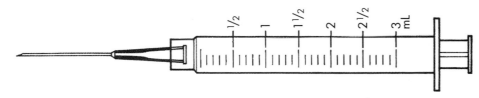

3. Ordered: Pfizerpen 300,000 U IM q12h.
Available: Pfizerpen five million U.
If you add 18.2 mL of diluent to the Pfizerpen:
   a. How many units/mL will this yield?
   b. How many milliliters will you give?
   c. How many doses are in the multidose vial?

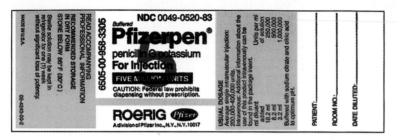

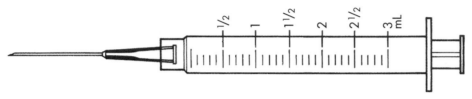

4. Ordered: Ticar 0.5 g IM q6h for salpingitis.
   a. How much diluent will you add?
   b. How many milliliters will you administer? Shade in the amount on the syringe.

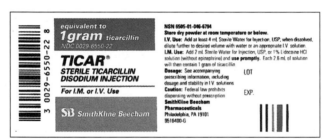

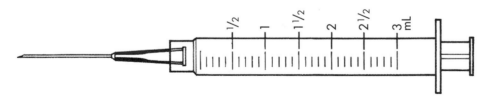

5. Ordered: Ampicillin 250 mg IM q4h for endocarditis prophylaxis.
   a. How much diluent will you add?
   b. How many milliliters will you administer? Shade in the amount on the syringe.

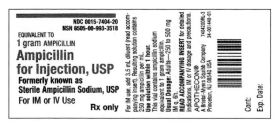

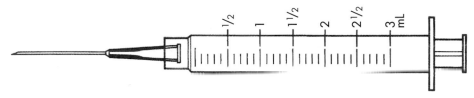

6. Ordered: Penicillin G 300,000 U IM q4h. Available: Penicillin G 3 million U in dry crystal form. Dilute with 4.2 mL normal saline to make 5 mL. How many milliliters will you administer?

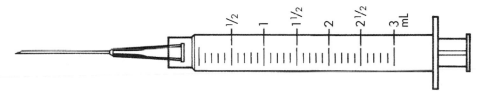

7. Ordered: Keflin 0.5 g IM q6h. Available: a vial of sodium cephalothin (Keflin) 1 g in powder form. Directions read: *Add 4 mL sterile water to make two 0.5 g doses of 2.2 mL each.* How many milliliters will you administer?

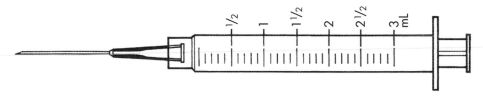

8. Dilute a vial containing 100,000 U of Polycillin (ampicillin) so that each milliliter contains 50,000 U. Approximately how much distilled water will you need to add to the vial to get 50,000 U/mL?

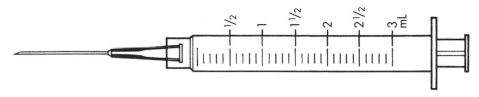

9. Ordered: Carbenicillin 200,000 U IM q6h. Available: a vial containing 500,000 U of carbenicillin. The directions read: *Add 4.8 mL of distilled water to make 5 mL of carbenicillin.* Each milliliter will contain 100,000 U. How many milliliters will you administer?

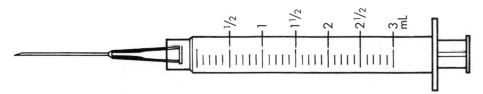

10. Ordered: Keflin 400,000 U. Available: a vial with 600,000 U/mL. How many milliliters will you administer?

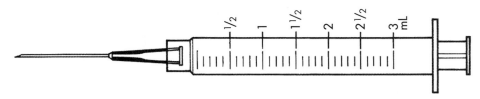

Basic IV Calculations

6

OBJECTIVES

- Calculate intravenous (IV) flow rates for gtt/min, mL/hr, and infusion time.
- Interpret IV labels.
- Identify various electronic IV infusion devices.
- Identify IV sets: primary, primary with a port, IVPB extension tubing, transfusion sets, and venous access devices for intermittent use.
- Calculate the amount of saline or heparin for use in keeping venous access patent.
- Calculate the grams of NaCl or dextrose in IV bags.
- Analyze IV orders for safe administration using critical thinking skills.
- Check IV order for type of solution, amount, additives, and rate.

INTRODUCTION

It is the nurse's responsibility to calculate the milliliters per hour or drops per minute to regulate the intravenous infusion. Knowledge of electronic infusion devices is required, as well as knowledge of the basic hand-regulated primary sets. The nurse is responsible for calculating the intravenous piggyback (IVPB) infusions that are timed for shorter periods.

● IV INFUSIONS

Intravenous (IV) infusions are used more frequently today than intramuscular (IM) injections. Continuous medication therapy can be delivered via an IV route, minimizing multiple injections via the IM route. Intermittent medication therapy can be delivered through a saline/heparin lock (Figure 6-1), which allows the patient free movement until the next scheduled dose. The heparin lock is used for short durations in acute care, long-term care, and home care.

Medications (additives) can be added to the IV by the manufacturer, pharmacist, or nurse. The physician orders the medication, strength, and amount, as well as the type and amount of diluent. It is important that the person responsible for the IV understand the actions of the medication, flow rate, adverse reactions, and antidotes. IV fluids flow directly into the vein, resulting in immediate action, and cannot be retrieved. Therefore it is imperative that the correct calculations, medications, and flow rate be administered.

FIGURE 6-1
Saline/heparin lock. *(From Elkin M, Perry P, Potter A: Nursing interventions and clinical skills, ed 2, St Louis, 2000, Mosby.)*

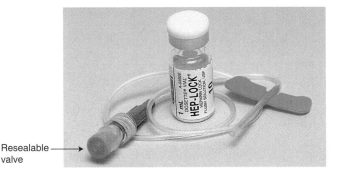

Resealable valve

Intermittent IV locks, also known as *saline lock, buff cap,* or *PRN cap* have needleless resealable valves.

● TYPES OF IV LINES

Peripheral	IV line inserted in the hand, arm, or possibly the leg if the hand or arm cannot be accessed.
Peripheral inserted central catheter	PICC line (Figure 6-2) is inserted in the ante-cubital region vein in the arm and is advanced into the superior vena cava. The catheter is approximately 22 inches in length and is inserted by a PICC-certified RN.

Central line

Inserted by an MD directly into the jugular or subclavian veins into the superior vena cava.

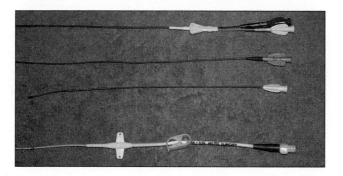

FIGURE 6-2 Peripheral inserted central catheter (PICC lines). The double-lumen catheter is used to draw blood samples.

Table 6-1 is a guide that can be used to maintain patency by flushing intermittent access locks. Always refer to hospital protocol for type of solution, volume, and frequency.

Table 6-1 Intermittent Flushing Ranges

Catheter	Flush Solution	Volume (mL)
Peripheral	Normal saline	1-3 mL
Central venous	Heparinized saline	2-5 mL
Peripherally inserted central catheter (PICC)	Normal saline	3-5 mL

● IV CALCULATIONS

Check IV orders before beginning calculations. There are two steps in IV calculations. The first step is to find out how many *milliliters per hour* (volume) the IV is ordered to infuse. The second step is to calculate the *drops per minute* needed to infuse the ordered volume.

Analyze your problem. If the order reads to infuse the IV for 24 hours, calculate the mL/hr by beginning with Step 1. If the order reads to infuse the IV at 75 mL/hr, begin with Step 2.

STEP 1 mL/hr

◉◀◀◀◀◀◀◀◀RULE When the total volume is given, calculate the mL/hr.

$$\frac{\text{Total volume (TV)}}{\text{Total time (TT) in hours}} = \text{mL/hr}$$

EXAMPLE Ordered: 2000 mL D5W (dextrose 5% in water) to be infused for 24 hours. The problem is to find out how many mL/hr the patient must receive for the 2000 mL to be infused in 24 hours.

FORMULA

$$\frac{\text{Total volume (TV)}}{\text{Total time (TT) in hours}} = \text{mL/hr}$$

CALCULATION

$$\frac{\text{TV}}{\text{TT}} = \frac{2000}{24} \div 24 = 83 \text{ mL/hr}$$

We now know that to infuse 2000 mL of fluid in 24 hours, the patient must receive 83 mL/hr. IV pumps are calibrated for mL/hr.

Drop Factor Calculations

The drop factor is needed to calculate gtt/min. The drop factor is the number of drops in 1 mL (or 1 cc). The diameter of the needle where the drop enters the drip chamber varies from one manufacturer to another. The bigger the needle, the fatter the drop (Figure 6-3, *A*); it takes only 10 drops to make a milliliter. The smallest unit is the microdrop (60 gtt/mL) (Figure 6-3, *B*). This is used for people who can tolerate only small amounts of fluid, such as pediatric and geriatric patients or patients who require fluid restrictions. Drop factors of 10, 15, and 60 (microdrip) are the most common. The drop factor is determined by the manufacturer and is found on the IV tubing package.

◀◀◀◀◀◀◀◀**RULE** When the mL/hr is given, calculate the gtt/min.

$$\frac{\text{Drop factor or gtt/mL (from IV package)}}{\text{Time in minutes}} \times \text{Total hourly volume (V/hr)} = \text{gtt/min}$$

EXAMPLE Ordered: D5W to infuse at 83 mL/hr. The drop factor (Df) is 10.

$$\frac{\text{Df}}{\text{Time (min)}} \times \text{V/hr} = \frac{10 \text{ (Df)}}{60 \text{ (min)}} \times 83 \text{ (V/hr)}$$

$$\frac{10}{60} \times \frac{83}{1} = \frac{1}{6} \times \frac{83}{1} = \frac{83}{6} = 13.8 \text{ or } 14 \text{ gtt/min}$$

Drops cannot be timed in tenths, only in whole numbers. If the decimal is greater than 0.5, round to the next higher number.

EXAMPLE Ordered: Antibiotic to infuse at 100 mL in 30 min. The drop factor is 15.

$$\frac{\text{Df}}{\text{Time (min)}} \times \text{V/hr} = \frac{15 \text{ (Df)}}{30 \text{ (min)}} \times 100 \text{ (V/hr)}$$

$$\frac{15}{30} \times \frac{100}{1} = \frac{1}{2} \times \frac{100}{1} = \frac{100}{2} = 50 \text{ gtt/min}$$

SUMMARY Two-step IV flow rate calculations

Step 1 $\frac{\text{TV}}{\text{TT in hr}} = \text{mL/hr}$

Step 2 $\frac{\text{Df}}{\text{Time in min}} \times \text{V/hr} = \text{gtt/min}$

✷ **REMEMBER** ● Reduce the fraction Df/min *before* multiplying by the volume.

EXAMPLE Which would you rather calculate?

$$\frac{12}{60} \times 60 \quad \text{or} \quad \frac{1}{5} \times 60$$

The reduced fraction is easier to calculate.

✷ **REMEMBER** ● When the IV tubing is microdrip, 60 gtt/mL, the gtt/min will be the same as the mL/hr.

EXAMPLE 1000 mL to infuse in 8 hours with a microdrip set.

Step 1 $\dfrac{\text{TV}}{\text{TT in hr}} = \dfrac{1000}{8} = 125 \text{ mL/hr}$

Step 2 $\dfrac{\text{Df}}{\text{Time in min}} \times \text{V/hr} = \dfrac{60}{60} \times 125 = 125 \text{ gtt/min}$

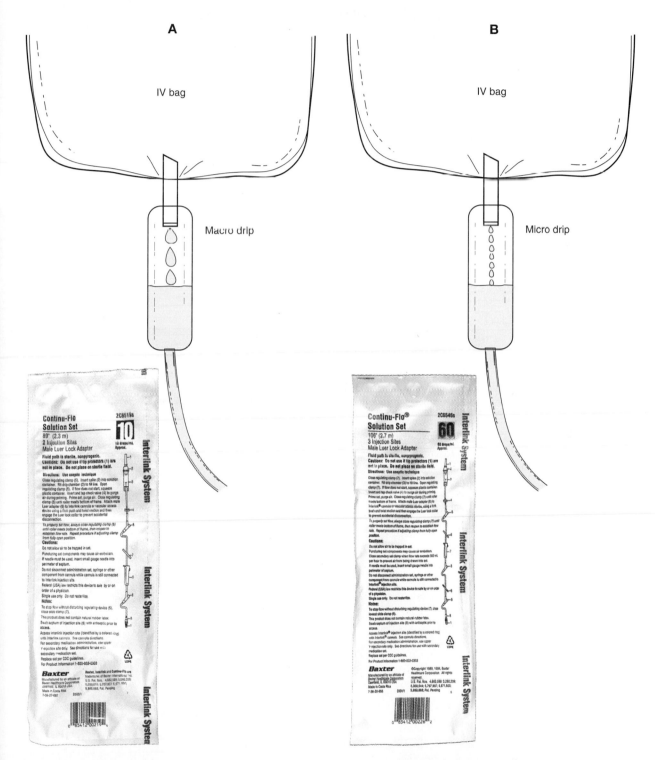

FIGURE 6-3 Drops per minute must be calibrated for gravity flow. **A,** Interlink® System Continu-Flo® Solution Set with drop factor of 10 (10 gtt = 1 mL). **B,** Interlink® System Continu-Flo® Solution Set with drop factor of 60 (60 gtt = 1 mL). *(From Baxter Healthcare Corporation, Deerfield, IL. All rights reserved.)*

■ Drops Per Minute by Manufacturer

A simple approach to calculate gtt/min after you have determined the mL/hr is to memorize the reduced fraction numbers. Manufacturers have established rates for their products. Below is an example.

PRODUCT DRIP RATES	MINUTES	Df	=	REDUCED NUMBER
60 gtt/mL	60	60	=	1
20 gtt/mL	60	20	=	3
15 gtt/mL	60	15	=	4
10 gtt/mL	60	10	=	6

You may only have to memorize one number because most facilities purchase equipment from one company.

EXAMPLE　If you know you are using a set that delivers 20 gtt/mL, divide 3 into the mL/hr.

$$\frac{125}{3} = 41.6 = 42 \text{ gtt/min}$$

As you already know, the formula for calculating gtt/min is:

$$\frac{\text{Df}}{\text{Time in min}} \times \text{V/hr} \quad \text{or} \quad \frac{20}{60} \times 125 = \frac{1}{3} \times 125 = 41.6 = 42 \text{ gtt/min}$$

Now you know two different methods for calculating gtt/min.

CLINICAL ALERT!

Check the IV every hour, even if an infusion device is used. Recheck drops per minute rate frequently because the IV rate can be positional.

ANSWERS ON PAGE 361

WORKSHEET
6A   IV Calculations

Use either the Step 1 or Step 2 formula to calculate mL/hr or gtt/min to answer the following questions.

Step 1 $\dfrac{TV}{TT \text{ in hr}}$ = mL/hr

Step 2 $\dfrac{Df}{Time \text{ in min}} \times$ V/hr = gtt/min   or $\dfrac{mL/hr}{reduced \ gtt \ rate}$

1. Ordered: 1000 mL to be infused for 8 hr. How many gtt/min will be administered if the drop factor is 10?

2. Ordered: 200 mL to be infused for 1 hr. If the drop factor is 15, how many gtt/min will be administered?

3. Ordered: 100 mL to be infused for 30 min. How many gtt/min is this if the drop factor is 10?

4. Ordered: 1500 mL to be infused for 12 hr. If the drop factor is 15, how many gtt/min is this?

5. Ordered: 50 mL to be infused for 1 hr. How many gtt/min will be administered with microdrip?

6. Ordered: 1500 mL to be infused for 8 hr. How many mL/hr will be administered?
   a. How many gtt/min is this with a drop factor of 10?
   b. How many gtt/min is this with a drop factor of 15?

7. Ordered: 75 mL to be infused for 45 min. The drop factor is 10. How many gtt/min will be administered?

8. Ordered: 250 mL to be infused for 90 min. The drop factor is microdrip. How many gtt/min will be administered?

9. Ordered: 150 mL to be infused for 40 min. The drop factor is 15 gtt/mL. How many gtt/min is this?

10. Ordered: 1000 mL to be infused at 150 mL/hr. The drop factor is 20. How many gtt/min is this?

ANSWERS ON PAGE 361

WORKSHEET 6B Additional Practice in IV Calculations

Use either the Step 1 or Step 2 formula to calculate mL/hr or gtt/min to answer the following questions.

1. You have 2000 mL D5W being infused for 24 hr. How many mL/hr is this?

2. You have 1500 mL normal saline (NS). The drop factor is 15. The solution is to be given for an 8-hr period.
   a. How many mL/hr is this?
   b. How many gtt/min is this?

3. A solution of 3000 mL D5W is being infused for 24 hr with 1.5 g carbenicillin. The drop factor is 60 (microdrip). How many gtt/min will be administered?

4. You have 500 mL 0.45% NS infusing for 4 hr. The drop factor is 15. How many gtt/min is this?

5. Ordered: 1000 mL to be infused for 12 hr on microdrip. At how many gtt/min will you regulate the flow?

6. Ordered: 100 mL gentamicin to be infused for 30 min. The drop factor is 20.
   a. With which step will you begin?
   b. How many gtt/min will be administered?

7. Ordered: 2000 mL for 24 hr. The drop factor is 15. How many gtt/min will be administered?

8. Ordered: 250 mL D5W is to be infused for 10 hr on a microdrip. How many gtt/min will be administered?

9. Ordered: 1500 mL of Ringer's lactate solution to be infused for 12 hr.
   a. How many mL/hr is this?
   b. The drop factor is 15. How many gtt/min is this?

10. Write your two-step formula again.
    Step 1   **Step 2**

ANSWERS ON PAGE 362

WORKSHEET
6C Additional Practice in IV Calculations

Use either the Step 1 or Step 2 formula to calculate mL/hr or gtt/min to answer the following questions.

1. Ordered: 100 mL/hr. How many gtt/min is this if the drop factor is 10?

2. Ordered: 1000 mL to be infused for 6 hr. How many gtt/min will be administered if the drop factor is 15?

3. Ordered: 50 mL to be infused for 30 min. How many gtt/min is this if the drop factor is 10?

4. Ordered: 100 mL to be infused for 60 min. How many gtt/min will be administered if a microdrip is used?

5. Ordered: 2000 mL to be infused for 12 hr. The drop factor is 60.
   a. How many mL/hr is this?
   b. How many gtt/min is this?

6. Ordered: 100 mL to be infused for 30 min. The drop factor is 15. How many gtt/min will be administered?

7. Ordered: 1500 mL 0.45% NS for 24 hr. The drop factor is 10. How many gtt/min is this?

8. Ordered: 500 mL for 8 hr by microdrip. How many gtt/min is this?

9. Ordered: 1000 mL Ringer's lactate solution at 75 mL/hr. The drop factor is 15. How many gtt/min will be administered?

10. Ordered: D5W continuous infusion at 85 mL/hr. The drop factor is 20. How many gtt/min is this?

● ABBREVIATIONS FOR COMMON INTRAVENOUS SOLUTIONS

NS	Normal saline; 0.9% sodium chloride (Figure 6-4)
$\frac{1}{2}$ NS	Normal saline; 0.45% saline or $\frac{1}{2}$ strength sodium chloride (Figure 6-5)
D5W or 5% D/W	Dextrose 5% in water (Figure 6-6)
D5RL	Dextrose 5% in Ringer's lactate (Figure 6-7)
RL or RLS	Ringer's lactate solution (Figure 6-8)
D5NS	Dextrose 5% in 0.9% normal saline (Figure 6-9)
D5 and $\frac{1}{2}$ NS (0.45% NS)	Dextrose 5% in $\frac{1}{2}$ normal saline or 0.45% sodium chloride (Figure 6-10)

● PERCENTAGE OF SOLUTE IN IV BAGS

The percentage numbers of the IV bags indicate the amount of dextrose, normal saline, or other constituents in the infusion. To determine the number of milliliters of dextrose or normal saline the percentage (%) represents, use the following formula. The dissolved substance or solute (dextrose, sodium chloride) is represented by a weight measurement (g). However, one mL of water weighs 1g. Therefore g and mL can be used interchangeably.

REMEMBER ● percentage is based on 100.

EXAMPLE How many mL of dextrose are in 1000 mL of D5W?
Know   *Want to Know*

5 g (solute) : 100 mL :: x g (solute) : 1000 mL

$$\text{or } \frac{5}{100} \times \frac{x}{1000} = \frac{1\cancel{00}x}{5 \times 1\cancel{000}} = \frac{1}{50} = 50 \text{ g or mL}$$

$100x = 5 \times 1000 = 5000$
$1\cancel{00}x = 5\cancel{000}$
$\quad x = 50$ g (solute) or mL of dextrose in 1000 mL

PROOF
$100 \times 50 = 5000$
$5 \times 1000 = 5000$

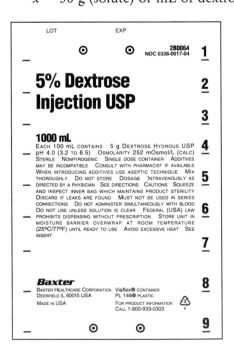

ANSWERS ON PAGE 363

WORKSHEET
6D
IV Solute Calculations

Calculate the g of NaCl in the following intravenous fluids:

1.

LOT   EXP

2B1064
NDC 0338-0089-04   **1**

5% Dextrose and
0.9% Sodium Chloride
Injection USP

— **2**

— **3**

— **4**

1000 mL
EACH 100 mL CONTAINS   5 g DEXTROSE HYDROUS USP
900 mg SODIUM CHLORIDE USP   pH 4.0 (3.2 TO 6.5)
mEq/L   SODIUM 154   CHLORIDE 154   HYPERTONIC
OSMOLARITY 560 mOsmol/L (CALC)   STERILE   NONPYROGENIC
SINGLE DOSE CONTAINER   ADDITIVES MAY BE INCOMPATIBLE
CONSULT WITH PHARMACIST IF AVAILABLE   WHEN INTRODUCING
ADDITIVES USE ASEPTIC TECHNIQUE   MIX THOROUGHLY   DO NOT
STORE   DOSAGE   INTRAVENOUSLY AS DIRECTED BY A PHYSICIAN
SEE DIRECTIONS   CAUTIONS   SQUEEZE AND INSPECT INNER BAG
WHICH MAINTAINS PRODUCT STERILITY   DISCARD IF LEAKS ARE
FOUND   MUST NOT BE USED IN SERIES CONNECTIONS   DO NOT
USE UNLESS SOLUTION IS CLEAR   FEDERAL (USA) LAW PROHIBITS
DISPENSING WITHOUT PRESCRIPTION   STORE UNIT IN MOISTURE
BARRIER OVERWRAP AT ROOM TEMPERATURE (25°C/77°F) UNTIL
READY TO USE   AVOID EXCESSIVE HEAT   SEE INSERT

— **5**

— **6**

— **7**

Baxter
BAXTER HEALTHCARE CORPORATION   Viaflex® CONTAINER
DEERFIELD IL 60015 USA   PL 146® PLASTIC
MADE IN USA   FOR PRODUCT INFORMATION
CALL 1-800-933-0303

— **8**

— **9**

g _____ NaCl
g _____ dextrose

2.

LOT   EXP

2B1073
NDC 0338-0085-03   **1**

5% Dextrose and
0.45% Sodium
Chloride Injection USP

— **2**

500 mL
EACH 100 mL CONTAINS   5 g DEXTROSE HYDROUS USP   450 mg SODIUM
CHLORIDE USP   pH 4.0 (3.2 TO 6.5)   mEq/L   SODIUM 77   CHLORIDE 77
HYPERTONIC   OSMOLARITY   406 mOsmol/L (CALC)   STERILE
NONPYROGENIC   SINGLE DOSE CONTAINER   ADDITIVES MAY BE INCOMPATIBLE
CONSULT WITH PHARMACIST IF AVAILABLE   WHEN INTRODUCING ADDITIVES USE
ASEPTIC TECHNIQUE   MIX THOROUGHLY   DO NOT STORE   DOSAGE
INTRAVENOUSLY AS DIRECTED BY A PHYSICIAN   SEE DIRECTIONS   CAUTIONS
SQUEEZE AND INSPECT INNER BAG WHICH MAINTAINS PRODUCT STERILITY
DISCARD IF LEAKS ARE FOUND   MUST NOT BE USED IN SERIES CONNECTIONS
DO NOT USE UNLESS SOLUTION IS CLEAR   FEDERAL (USA) LAW PROHIBITS
DISPENSING WITHOUT PRESCRIPTION   STORE UNIT IN MOISTURE BARRIER
OVERWRAP AT ROOM TEMPERATURE (25°C/77°F) UNTIL READY TO USE
AVOID EXCESSIVE HEAT   SEE INSERT

— **3**

— **4**

Baxter
BAXTER HEALTHCARE CORPORATION   Viaflex® CONTAINER
DEERFIELD IL 60015 USA   PL 146® PLASTIC
MADE IN USA   FOR PRODUCT INFORMATION
CALL 1-800-933-0303

g _____ dextrose
g _____ NaCl

3.

LOT   EXP

2B1163
NDC 0338-0095-03   **1**

10% Dextrose and
0.9% Sodium Chloride
Injection USP

— **2**

500 mL
EACH 100 mL CONTAINS   10 g DEXTROSE HYDROUS USP   900 mg SODIUM
CHLORIDE USP   pH 4.0 (3.2 TO 6.5)   mEq/L   SODIUM 154
CHLORIDE 154   OSMOLARITY   813 mOsmol/L (CALC)   HYPERTONIC   MAY
CAUSE VEIN DAMAGE   STERILE   NONPYROGENIC   SINGLE DOSE CONTAINER
ADDITIVES MAY BE INCOMPATIBLE   CONSULT WITH PHARMACIST IF AVAILABLE
WHEN INTRODUCING ADDITIVES USE ASEPTIC TECHNIQUE   MIX THOROUGHLY
DO NOT STORE   DOSAGE   INTRAVENOUSLY AS DIRECTED BY A PHYSICIAN   SEE
DIRECTIONS   CAUTIONS   SQUEEZE AND INSPECT INNER BAG WHICH MAINTAINS
PRODUCT STERILITY   DISCARD IF LEAKS ARE FOUND   MUST NOT BE USED IN
SERIES CONNECTIONS   DO NOT USE UNLESS SOLUTION IS CLEAR   FEDERAL
(USA) LAW PROHIBITS DISPENSING WITHOUT PRESCRIPTION   STORE UNIT IN
MOISTURE BARRIER OVERWRAP AT ROOM TEMPERATURE (25°C/77°F) UNTIL
READY TO USE   AVOID EXCESSIVE HEAT   SEE INSERT

— **3**

— **4**

Baxter
BAXTER HEALTHCARE CORPORATION   Viaflex® CONTAINER
DEERFIELD IL 60015 USA   PL 146® PLASTIC
MADE IN USA   FOR PRODUCT INFORMATION
CALL 1-800-933-0303

g _____ dextrose
g _____ NaCl

Continued

ANSWERS ON PAGE 363

WORKSHEET
6D IV Solute Calculations—cont'd

Calculate the g of NaCl in the following intravenous fluids:

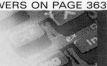

4. FIGURE 6-4
Normal saline 0.9%.

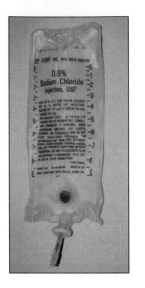

LOT   EXP

2B1324
NDC 0338-0049-04
DIN 00060208

1

0.9% Sodium Chloride Injection USP

2

3

4

1000 mL
EACH 100 mL CONTAINS   900 mg SODIUM CHLORIDE USP
pH 5.0 (4.5 TO 7.0)   mEq/L SODIUM 154 CHLORIDE 154
OSMOLARITY   308 mOsmol/L (CALC)   STERILE
NONPYROGENIC SINGLE DOSE CONTAINER ADDITIVES MAY BE
INCOMPATIBLE CONSULT WITH PHARMACIST IF AVAILABLE WHEN
INTRODUCING ADDITIVES USE ASEPTIC TECHNIQUE   MIX
THOROUGHLY   DO NOT STORE DOSAGE INTRAVENOUSLY AS
DIRECTED BY A PHYSICIAN   SEE DIRECTIONS CAUTIONS
SQUEEZE AND INSPECT INNER BAG WHICH MAINTAINS PRODUCT
STERILITY   DISCARD IF LEAKS ARE FOUND   MUST NOT BE USED
IN SERIES CONNECTIONS   DO NOT USE UNLESS SOLUTION IS
CLEAR   FEDERAL (USA) LAW PROHIBITS DISPENSING WITHOUT
PRESCRIPTION   STORE UNIT IN MOISTURE BARRIER OVERWRAP AT
ROOM TEMPERATURE (25°C/77°F) UNTIL READY TO USE   AVOID
EXCESSIVE HEAT   SEE INSERT

5

6

7

Baxter
BAXTER HEALTHCARE CORPORATION
DEERFIELD IL 60015 USA

8

MADE IN USA
DISTRIBUTED IN CANADA BY
BAXTER CORPORATION
TORONTO ONTARIO CANADA

Viaflex® CONTAINER
PL 146® PLASTIC
FOR PRODUCT INFORMATION
CALL 1-800-933-0303

9

g _____ NaCl

5. FIGURE 6-5
Normal saline 0.45%.

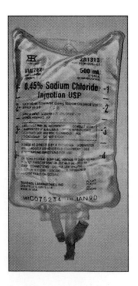

LOT   EXP

2B1313
NDC 0338-0043-03

1

0.45% Sodium Chloride Injection USP

2

500 mL
EACH 100 mL CONTAINS   450 mg SODIUM CHLORIDE USP
pH 5.0 (4.5 TO 7.0)   mEq/L SODIUM 77 CHLORIDE 77 HYPOTONIC
OSMOLARITY   154 mOsmol/L (CALC) STERILE NONPYROGENIC SINGLE
DOSE CONTAINER   ADDITIVES MAY BE INCOMPATIBLE   CONSULT WITH
PHARMACIST IF AVAILABLE   WHEN INTRODUCING ADDITIVES USE ASEPTIC
TECHNIQUE   MIX THOROUGHLY   DO NOT STORE   DOSAGE INTRAVENOUSLY
AS DIRECTED BY A PHYSICIAN   SEE DIRECTIONS   CAUTIONS   SQUEEZE AND
INSPECT INNER BAG WHICH MAINTAINS PRODUCT STERILITY   DISCARD IF LEAKS
ARE FOUND   MUST NOT BE USED IN SERIES CONNECTIONS   DO NOT USE
UNLESS SOLUTION IS CLEAR   FEDERAL (USA) LAW PROHIBITS DISPENSING
WITHOUT PRESCRIPTION   STORE UNIT IN MOISTURE BARRIER OVERWRAP AT
ROOM TEMPERATURE (25°C/77°F) UNTIL READY TO USE   AVOID EXCESSIVE
HEAT   SEE INSERT

3

4

Baxter
BAXTER HEALTHCARE CORPORATION
DEERFIELD IL 60015 USA
MADE IN USA

Viaflex® CONTAINER
PL 146® PLASTIC
FOR PRODUCT INFORMATION
CALL 1-800-933-0303

g _____ NaCl

ANSWERS ON PAGE 363

WORKSHEET

6D   IV Solute Calculations—cont'd

Calculate the g of NaCl in the following intravenous fluids:

6. **FIGURE 6-6**
5% Dextrose.

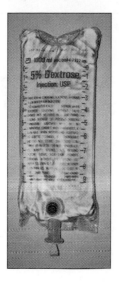

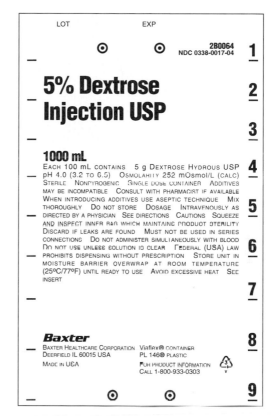

LOT   EXP

2B0064
NDC 0338-0017-04   **1**

2

3

5% Dextrose
Injection USP

1000 mL
EACH 100 mL CONTAINS   5 g DEXTROSE HYDROUS USP
pH 4.0 (3.2 TO 6.5)   OSMOLALITY 252 mOsmol/L (CALC)
STERILE NONPYROGENIC SINGLE DOSE CONTAINER ADDITIVES
MAY BE INCOMPATIBLE   CONSULT WITH PHARMACIST IF AVAILABLE
WHEN INTRODUCING ADDITIVES USE ASEPTIC TECHNIQUE   MIX
THOROUGHLY   DO NOT STORE   DOSAGE   INTRAVENOUSLY AS
DIRECTED BY A PHYSICIAN   SEE DIRECTIONS   CAUTIONS   SQUEEZE
AND INSPECT INNER BAG WHICH MAINTAINS PRODUCT STERILITY
DISCARD IF LEAKS ARE FOUND   MUST NOT BE USED IN SERIES
CONNECTIONS   DO NOT ADMINISTER SIMULTANEOUSLY WITH BLOOD
DO NOT USE UNLESS SOLUTION IS CLEAR   FEDERAL (USA) LAW
PROHIBITS DISPENSING WITHOUT PRESCRIPTION   STORE UNIT IN
MOISTURE BARRIER OVERWRAP AT ROOM TEMPERATURE
(25°C/77°F) UNTIL READY TO USE   AVOID EXCESSIVE HEAT   SEE
INSERT

4

5

6

7

Baxter
BAXTER HEALTHCARE CORPORATION   Viaflex® CONTAINER
DEERFIELD IL 60015 USA   PL 146® PLASTIC
MADE IN USA   FOR PRODUCT INFORMATION
CALL 1-800-933-0303

8

9

g _____ dextrose

7. **FIGURE 6-7**
Lactated Ringer's and
5% Dextrose.

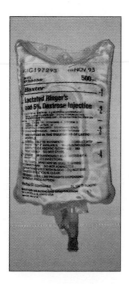

LOT   EXP

2B2073
NDC 0338-0125-03   **1**

Lactated Ringer's
and 5% Dextrose
Injection USP

2

3

500 mL
EACH 100 mL CONTAINS   5 g DEXTROSE HYDROUS USP
600 mg SODIUM CHLORIDE USP   310 mg SODIUM LACTATE
30 mg POTASSIUM CHLORIDE USP   20 mg CALCIUM CHLORIDE USP
pH 5.0 (4.0 TO 6.5)   mEq/L SODIUM 130   POTASSIUM 4   CALCIUM 2.7
CHLORIDE 109   LACTATE 28   HYPERTONIC   OSMOLARITY 525 mOsmol/L
(CALC)   STERILE NONPYROGENIC SINGLE DOSE CONTAINER   NOT FOR USE
IN THE TREATMENT OF LACTIC ACIDOSIS   ADDITIVES MAY BE INCOMPATIBLE
CONSULT WITH PHARMACIST IF AVAILABLE   WHEN INTRODUCING ADDITIVES USE
ASEPTIC TECHNIQUE   MIX THOROUGHLY   DO NOT STORE   DOSAGE
INTRAVENOUSLY AS DIRECTED BY A PHYSICIAN   SEE DIRECTIONS   CAUTIONS
SQUEEZE AND INSPECT INNER BAG WHICH MAINTAINS PRODUCT STERILITY
DISCARD IF LEAKS ARE FOUND   MUST NOT BE USED IN SERIES CONNECTIONS
DO NOT ADMINISTER SIMULTANEOUSLY WITH BLOOD   DO NOT USE UNLESS
SOLUTION IS CLEAR   FEDERAL (USA) LAW PROHIBITS DISPENSING WITHOUT
PRESCRIPTION   STORE UNIT IN MOISTURE BARRIER OVERWRAP AT ROOM
TEMPERATURE (25°C/77°F) UNTIL READY TO USE   AVOID EXCESSIVE HEAT
SEE INSERT

4

Baxter
BAXTER HEALTHCARE CORPORATION   Viaflex® CONTAINER
DEERFIELD IL 60015 USA   PL 146® PLASTIC
MADE IN USA   FOR PRODUCT INFORMATION
CALL 1-800-933-0303

g _____ dextrose

Continued

6D IV Solute Calculations—cont'd

Calculate the g of NaCl in the following intravenous fluids:

8. FIGURE 6-8
Lactated Ringer's
solution.

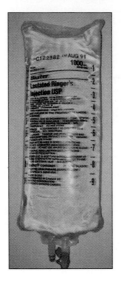

LOT   EXP

2B2324
NDC 0338-0117-04
DIN 00061085

1

Lactated Ringer's Injection USP

2

3

1000 mL

EACH 100 mL CONTAINS   600 mg SODIUM CHLORIDE USP
310 mg SODIUM LACTATE   30 mg POTASSIUM CHLORIDE USP
20 mg CALCIUM CHLORIDE USP   pH 6.5 (6.0 TO 7.5)   mEq/L
SODIUM 130 POTASSIUM 4 CALCIUM 2.7 CHLORIDE 109
LACTATE 28   OSMOLARITY 273 mOsmol/L (CALC)   STERILE
NONPYROGENIC SINGLE DOSE CONTAINER   **NOT FOR USE IN THE TREATMENT OF LACTIC ACIDOSIS**   ADDITIVES MAY BE
INCOMPATIBLE   CONSULT WITH PHARMACIST IF AVAILABLE   WHEN
INTRODUCING ADDITIVES USE ASEPTIC TECHNIQUE   MIX
THOROUGHLY   DO NOT STORE   DOSAGE   INTRAVENOUSLY AS
DIRECTED BY A PHYSICIAN   SEE DIRECTIONS   CAUTIONS
SQUEEZE AND INSPECT INNER BAG WHICH MAINTAINS PRODUCT
STERILITY   DISCARD IF LEAKS ARE FOUND   MUST NOT BE USED IN
SERIES CONNECTIONS   DO NOT ADMINISTER SIMULTANEOUSLY
WITH BLOOD   DO NOT USE UNLESS SOLUTION IS CLEAR   FEDERAL
(USA) LAW PROHIBITS DISPENSING WITHOUT PRESCRIPTION
STORE UNIT IN MOISTURE BARRIER OVERWRAP AT ROOM
TEMPERATURE (25ºC/77ºF) UNTIL READY TO USE   AVOID
EXCESSIVE HEAT   SEE INSERT

4

5

6

7

Baxter
BAXTER HEALTHCARE CORPORATION
DEERFIELD IL 60015 USA

MADE IN USA
DISTRIBUTED IN CANADA BY
BAXTER CORPORATION
TORONTO ONTARIO CANADA

Viaflex® CONTAINER
PL 146® PLASTIC
FOR PRODUCT INFORMATION
CALL 1-800-933-0303

8

9

g _____ sodium chloride

Calculate the g of NaCl in the following intravenous fluids:

9. FIGURE 6-9
5% Dextrose in
normal saline.

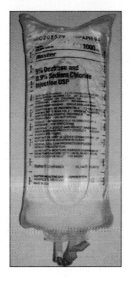

LOT   EXP

2B1064
NDC 0338-0089-04   **1**

**5% Dextrose and
0.9% Sodium Chloride
Injection USP**   **2**

3

1000 mL   **4**
EACH 100 mL CONTAINS   5 g DEXTROSE HYDROUS USP
900 mg SODIUM CHLORIDE USP   pH 4.0 (3.2 TO 6.5)
mEq/L   SODIUM 154   CHLORIDE   154   HYPERTONIC
OSMOLARITY   560 mOsmol/L (CALC)   STERILE   NONPYROGENIC   **5**
SINGLE DOSE CONTAINER   ADDITIVES MAY BE INCOMPATIBLE
CONSULT WITH PHARMACIST IF AVAILABLE   WHEN INTRODUCING
ADDITIVES USE ASEPTIC TECHNIQUE   MIX THOROUGHLY   DO NOT
STORE   DOSAGE   INTRAVENOUSLY AS DIRECTED BY A PHYSICIAN
SEE DIRECTIONS   CAUTIONS   SQUEEZE AND INSPECT INNER BAG   **6**
WHICH MAINTAINS PRODUCT STERILITY   DISCARD IF LEAKS ARE
FOUND   MUST NOT BE USED IN SERIES CONNECTIONS   DO NOT
USE UNLESS SOLUTION IS CLEAR   FEDERAL (USA) LAW PROHIBITS
DISPENSING WITHOUT PRESCRIPTION   STORE UNIT IN MOISTURE
BARRIER OVERWRAP AT ROOM TEMPERATURE (25°C/77°F) UNTIL   **7**
READY TO USE   AVOID EXCESSIVE HEAT   SEE INSERT

8
Baxter
BAXTER HEALTHCARE CORPORATION   Viaflex® CONTAINER
DEERFIELD IL 60015 USA   PL 146® PLASTIC
MADE IN USA   FOR PRODUCT INFORMATION
                               CALL 1-800-933-0303
9

g _____ dextrose
g _____ NaCl

10. FIGURE 6-10
5% Dextrose in ½
normal saline.

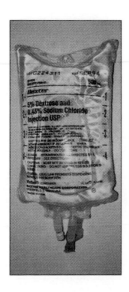

LOT   EXP

2B1073
NDC 0338-0085-03   **1**

**5% Dextrose and
0.45% Sodium
Chloride Injection USP**   **2**

500 mL   **3**
EACH 100 mL CONTAINS   5 g DEXTROSE HYDROUS USP   450 mg SODIUM
CHLORIDE USP   pH 4.0 (3.2 TO 6.5)   mEq/L SODIUM 77   CHLORIDE 77
HYPERTONIC   OSMOLARITY   406 mOsmol/L (CALC)   STERILE
NONPYROGENIC   SINGLE DOSE CONTAINER   ADDITIVES MAY BE INCOMPATIBLE
CONSULT WITH PHARMACIST IF AVAILABLE   WHEN INTRODUCING ADDITIVES USE
ASEPTIC TECHNIQUE   MIX THOROUGHLY   DO NOT STORE   DOSAGE   **4**
INTRAVENOUSLY AS DIRECTED BY A PHYSICIAN   SEE DIRECTIONS   CAUTIONS
SQUEEZE AND INSPECT INNER BAG WHICH MAINTAINS PRODUCT STERILITY
DISCARD IF LEAKS ARE FOUND   MUST NOT BE USED IN SERIES CONNECTIONS
DO NOT USE UNLESS SOLUTION IS CLEAR   FEDERAL (USA) LAW PROHIBITS
DISPENSING WITHOUT PRESCRIPTION   STORE UNIT IN MOISTURE BARRIER
OVERWRAP AT ROOM TEMPERATURE (25°C/77°F) UNTIL READY TO USE
AVOID EXCESSIVE HEAT   SEE INSERT

Baxter
BAXTER HEALTHCARE CORPORATION   Viaflex® CONTAINER
DEERFIELD IL 60015 USA   PL 146® PLASTIC
MADE IN USA   FOR PRODUCT INFORMATION
                               CALL 1-800-933-0303

g _____ dextrose
g _____ NaCl

		NURSING CARE RECORD
	HOSPITAL	Medical/Surgical
	DATA FLOW RECORD	Date _1-12-02_

TIME	0600	1600													
PULSE	84	80													
RESPIRATION	20	22													
BLOOD PRESSURE	150/92	152/90													
COUGH/ DEEP BREATH	✓	✓													
INITIALS	JG	CB													

The IV flow sheet may record the vital signs prior to initiating IV therapy and again on every shift. The IV site and location is recorded along with the time and date it was started. The catheter type and needle size are recorded next to the type and rate of the IV solution. Additional IV solutions are recorded in the date/time inserted column. When the IV is discontinued, the reason is recorded under the comments column.

IV THERAPY

SITE	DATE/TIME INSERTED	SITE LOCATION	CATH TYPE/ SIZE	IV SOLUTION	RATE	DEVICE	TUBING CHANGE	APPEARANCE 7-3	3-11	11-7	SITE D/C'd	COMMENTS
R	1-12-02 0600	LPF	22 angio	1000 D5W	75°			1				
R	1-12-02 1900	LPF	22 angio	1000 D5W	75°		△		1			
R	1-12-02 2200	LPF	22 angio						2		✓	Slight redness noted at site pt denies pain or tenderness.

HEALTH DEVIATION NEEDS

DCP ASSESSED: In Progress ☐   Revise Plan ☐
DCP Conference ☐ _____
_____
_____

REFERRAL MADE: SS ☐   HHC ☐   Dietary ☐   Pharmacy ☐
Other _____

PATIENT/FAMILY TEACHING:
Pt/Other _____
_____
_____
_____
_____

	PT/FAMILY TEACHING RESPONSE CODES
	1 = Received Literature
	2 = Communicates Understanding
	3 = Requires Reinforcement
	4 = Previous Experience
	5 = Return Demonstration
	6 = Objective Achieved
	7 = Referral Initiated
	8 = Refused
	9 = Preprinted Teaching Protocol

IV CODES
Site Location
L = Left
R = Right
S = Scalp
Ft = Foot
F = Femoral
H = Hand
W = Wrist

AC = Antecubital
UA = Upper Arm
UPF = Upper Posterior Forearm
LPF = Lower Posterior Forearm

UAF = Upper Anterior Forearm
LAF = Lower Anterior Forearm
IJ = Internal Jugular
SC = Subclavian

Catheter
S.G. = Swan Ganz
H.D. = Hemodialysis
Hick = Hickman
G = Groshong
Port = Port-A-Cath or other implanted port
I = Introducer
PP = Pace Port

Appearance
1 = Asymptomatic
2 = Red
3 = Swollen
4 = Ecchymotic
5 = Warm
6 = Cool
7 = Draining
8 = Leaking
Lumen
d = distal
m = middle
p = proximal

EMOTIONAL SUPPORT CODES
1 = Active Listening
2 = Reassurance/Comfort
3 = Relaxation
   A = Breathing
   B = Visualization/Imagery
4 = Coping Skills Review

△ = Change

PROCEDURES

TIME	DEPT.	MODE	TRANSPORTER	RETURN

INITIAL	SIGNATURE/TITLE	INITIAL	SIGNATURE/TITLE
J	J Jahle, RN		

FIGURE 6-11 Example of an IV therapy medication administration record (MAR).

IV DELIVERY SETS

Figure 6-12, *A* shows a primary set. This is the basic set that delivers IV fluids for a short duration. It does not have a port for additions. This is a needleless connector.

Figure 6-12, *B* shows a primary set with a port for adding piggyback medications. This set has a manual dial for the mL/hr rate.

A
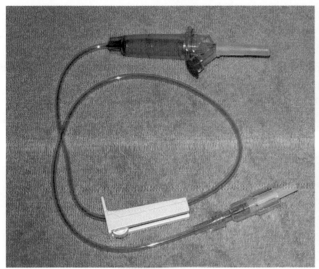
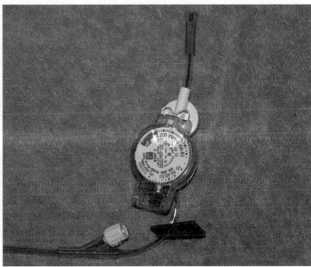
R

FIGURE 6-12 **A,** Primary set with a roller clamp to regulate the IV set. **B,** Primary set with a port for adding piggyback.

Needleless IV Systems

Needleless IV systems (Figure 6-13) are designed to protect caregivers from accidental punctures by contaminated needles.

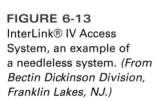

FIGURE 6-13
InterLink® IV Access System, an example of a needleless system. *(From Bectin Dickinson Division, Franklin Lakes, NJ.)*

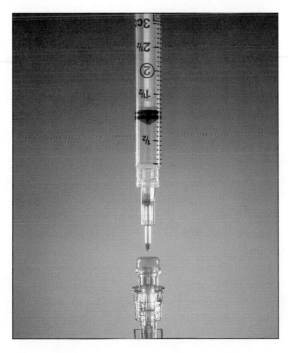

Gravity Piggyback Infusions

The acronym for intravenous piggyback is IVPB (Figure 6-14). When special medications are ordered intermittently, the primary IV can be bypassed by introducing the medication through a special entry or portal. Piggyback (PB) medications are infused intermittently via the existing IV line. A secondary IV tube with a needle attachment is inserted into the portal or entry site. The PB infusion amount is usually 50 to 250 mL of medicated solution.

Elevating the IVPB 12 inches above the existing IV allows the PB to infuse by gravity (Figure 6-15). When all of the medication has been infused, the existing IV will resume to the rate set for the PB infusion. The nurse must remember to regulate the primary IV to the previous rate. If an infusion device is used, the IV can be programmed to resume to the primary infusion rate at the completion of the PB.

Piggyback medications are premixed by the pharmacy, drug manufacturer, or nurse. The manufacturer's insert provides recommended times for IVPBs to infuse if the physician does not state the rate in the order.

 REMEMBER ● **Gravity flow sets are delivered in drops per minute.**

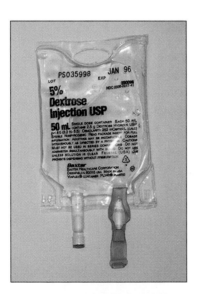

FIGURE 6-14 Fifty milliliters of solution for IV piggyback infusion.

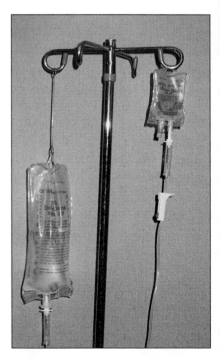

FIGURE 6-15 Gravity flow IV piggyback. The IV piggyback is elevated above the existing IV, allowing it to infuse by gravity.

Piggyback Premixed IVs

Piggyback IV additions are premixed by the pharmacy or the manufacturer. The medication is diluted in 50 to 250 mL of an iso-osmotic sterile solution. The amount of solution used depends on the type of medication, any fluid restrictions, and the weight of the patient.

IVPB admixtures (Figure 6-16) are usually prepared in bulk by the pharmacist for greater efficiency of time. If more than one day's supply is prepared, the IVPB can be frozen without altering the stability.

Premixed frozen IVPBs should be thawed in the refrigerator or at room temperature. Never thaw in a microwave oven or in hot or warm water.

All IVPB admixtures must be visually inspected before starting. Check the order, label, medication, strength, and quantity. Make sure the admixture is clear and free from particles and within the expiration date.

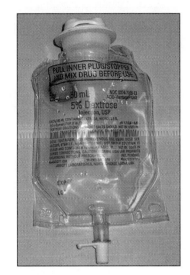

FIGURE 6-16
Fifty milliliters of dextrose. Medication can be added for infusion as an IV piggyback.

Nurse-Activated Piggyback Systems

Abbott ADD-VANTAGE and the Baxter Mini-Bag Plus (Figure 6-17) are used in home care, as well as in hospitals and long-term care centers. The IVPB minibag has a vial of medication attached to a special port. The pharmacy dispenses

A

B

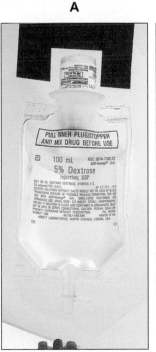

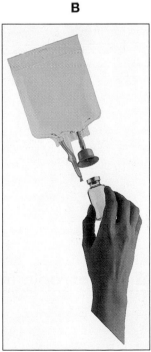

FIGURE 6-17 A, Abbott ADD-VANTAGE® System, 100 mL of 5% dextrose. *(From Abbott Laboratories, Inc., Abbott Park, IL.)* **B,** The Mini-Bag™ Plus Container is a "Ready-to-Mix" drug delivery system for reconstituting and administering IV drug dosages. The system consists of a Mini-Bag™ container with a built-in vial adaptor that fits powered drug vials with standard 20-mm closures. The system can be assembled without immediately mixing the drug and diluent. The drug admixture may be prepared just before administration by breaking the seal between the vial and the IV solution container. The medication vial remains attached to the Mini-Bag™ Plus Container, which reduces the potential for medication errors. The Mini-Bag™ Plus Container may be used in home care, as well as in hospitals and long-term care centers. *(From Baxter Healthcare Corporation, Deerfield, IL.)*

the IVPB with the unreconstituted drug vial attached to the mini-bag. At the time of delivery, the nurse breaks the seal between the vial and the mini-bag. This allows the medication to flow into the mini-bag. The medication vial remains attached to the mini-bag, which is a safety feature created to decrease potential medication errors. Figure 6-18 shows the steps for assembling and using the ADD-VANTAGE system.

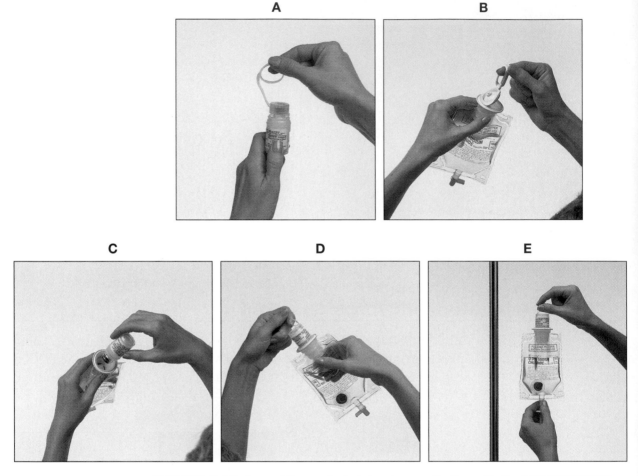

FIGURE 6-18 Assembling and administering medication with the ADD-VANTAGE® system. **A,** Swing the pull ring over the top of the vial, and pull down far enough to start the opening. Then pull straight up to remove the cap. Avoid touching the rubber stopper and vial threads. **B,** Hold diluent container, and gently grasp the tab on the pull ring. Pull up to break the tie membrane. Pull back to remove the cover. Avoid touching the inside of the vial port. **C,** Screw the vial into the vial port until it will go no further. Recheck the vial to ensure that it is tight. Label appropriately. **D,** Mix container contents thoroughly to ensure complete dissolution. Look through bottom of vial to verify complete mixing. Check for leaks by squeezing container firmly. If leaks are found, discard unit. **E,** When ready to administer, remove the white administration port cover and pierce the container with the piercing pin. *(From Abbott Laboratories, Inc., Abbott Park, IL.)*

Electronic Infusion Devices

Electronic infusion devices are used in hospitals, extended care facilities, home care, and ambulatory care settings. They deliver a set amount of intravenous fluids per hour. Some examples of electronic infusion devices are shown in Figure 6-19. They are individually programmed to deliver a set amount of intravenous solution per hour.

CADD-Prizm (Figure 6-19, *A*) is a battery-operated pump that provides IV medications to confined or ambulatory patients. There are four delivery modes:

- Patient-controlled analgesia (PCA)
- Continuous infusion
- Intermittent infusion
- Total parenteral nutrition

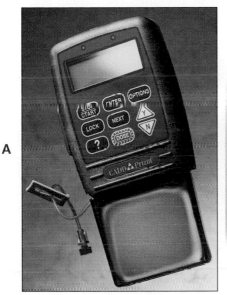

A

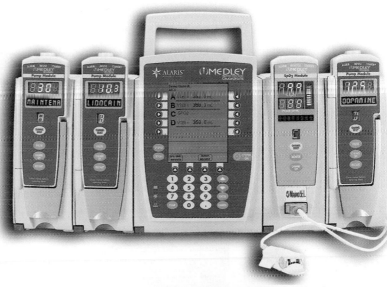

B

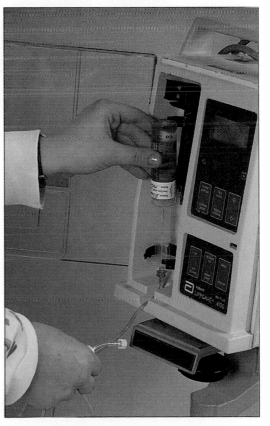

C

FIGURE 6-19 Electronic infusion devices. **A,** CADD-Prizm VIP ambulatory battery-operated infusion device used for IV parenteral nutrition. *(From SIMS Deltec, Inc., St Paul, MN.)* **B,** Medley™ Medication Safety System. *(From ALARIS Medical Systems, Inc., San Diego, CA.)* **C,** Nurse using a PCA electronic infusion device. *(From Potter P, Perry A:* Basic nursing: essentials for practice, *ed 5, St Louis, 2003, Mosby.)*

Total Parenteral Nutrition Tubing

The total parenteral (TPN) delivery mode allows the infusion of nutritional elements slowly at the beginning of the administration. This keeps the glucose level from rising too rapidly. The system slowly tapers up and then tapers down toward the end of the infusion.

Pressure-Flow Infusion Device

The ambulatory infusion device system was developed for ambulatory use. It can be put in a pocket, inside a shirt, or in any other convenient place where it can be concealed. The flow rate is pre-set. Figure 6-20 shows an example of an ambulatory infusion device.

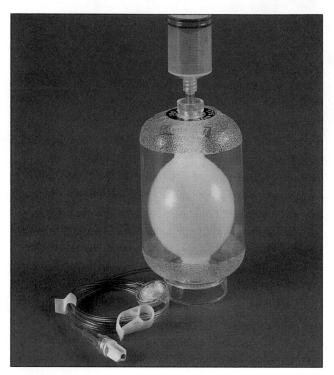

FIGURE 6-20 MedFlo® postoperative pain management system ambulatory infusion device. *(From Smith & Nephew Endoscopy, Andover, MA.)*

Piggyback Infusions

■ Ordered: Cefazolin 1 g IV in 50 mL for 30 min. At how many mL/hr should the infusion pump be set?

Know   *Want to Know*

50 mL : 30 min :: x mL : 60 min   **OR** $\frac{50}{30} \times \frac{x}{60} = \frac{300}{3} = 100$ mL/hr

$30\,x = 3000$

$x = 100$ mL/hr

> **PROOF**
> $30 \times 100 = 30$
> $50 \times 60 = 30$

Set the infusion pump for 100 mL/hr.

■ Ordered: Ampicillin 500 mg IV in 100 mL NS for 45 min. At how many mL/hr should the infusion pump be set?

Know   *Want to Know*

100 mL : 45 min :: x mL : 60 min   Convert minutes into a decimal

$45\,x = 100 \times 60 = 6000$ **OR**   45 min $\div$ 60 = 0.75

$45\,x = 6000$

$x = 133.3 = 133$ mL/hr   100 mL $\div$ 0.75 = 133 mL/hr

> **PROOF**
> $45 \times 133.3 = 5998.5$
> $60 \times 100 = 6000$

Set the infusion pump at 133 mL/hr.

CLINICAL ALERT!

Electronic infusion devices are set to infuse mL/hr. When administering a small amount of medication for less than 1 hour, the device must be set at mL/hr even though the medication will infuse in less than 1 hour.

ANSWERS ON PAGE 366

WORKSHEET 6E   Infusion Device and Solute g/mL Calculations

Use the two-step formula to answer the following questions.

1. Ordered: Gentamicin 80 mg in 50 mL IVPB to be infused for 30 min.
    a. At how many mL/hr will you set an infusion device?
    b. How many gtt/min will infuse for a gravity flow if the drop factor is 60?

2. Ordered: Aqueous penicillin 600,000 U in 100 mL IVPB to be infused for 1 hr. The drop factor is 15. How many gtt/min will you infuse?

3. Ordered: 250 mL NS to be infused at 150 mL/hr. The drop factor is 15 gtt/mL. How long will it take to infuse?

4. Ordered: Ampicillin 1 g in 50 mL IVPB ADD-VANTAGE system to be infused for 20 min.
    a. At how many mL/hr would you set an infusion device?
    b. How many gtt/min will be administered on a gravity flow if the drop factor is 15?

5. Ordered: Keflin 2 g in 100 mL IVPB to be infused for 1 hr. The drop factor is 15. How many gtt/min is this?

6. Ordered: 100 mL with 1 g cephalothin to be infused for 30 min by microdrip.
    a. How many gtt/min will infuse?
    b. How many mL/hr will you set the infusion pump?

7. Ordered: 200 mL Foscavir to infuse for 90 min. The drop factor is microdrip.
    a. How many gtt/min will infuse?
    b. At how many mL/hr will you set the infusion pump?

8. Ordered: 1000 mL 0.9% saline to infuse for 12 hr. The drop factor is 15 gtt/mL.
    a. How many gtt/min will infuse?
    b. At how many mL/hr will you set the infusion pump?
    c. How many milliliters of sodium chloride will the patient receive?

9. Ordered: 2000 mL D5W to be infused for 8 hr. The drop factor is 15 gtt/mL.
    a. How many mL/hr will infuse?
    b. How many gtt/min will infuse?
    c. How many milliliters of dextrose will the patient receive in 8 hours?

10. Ordered: Kantrex 300 mg in 150 mL IVPB. Label reads to infuse for 40 to 60 min. The drop factor is microdrip.
    a. What is the fastest rate for the IVPB to infuse? At what rate will you set the infusion device?
    b. What is the slowest rate for the IVPB to infuse? At what rate will you set the device?

ANSWERS ON PAGE 367

WORKSHEET

6F   **Multiple-Choice Practice**

Circle the letter of the correct answer in the following problems.
Remember to convert tenths of an hour to minutes, multiply by 60.
Example: 0.65 hr × 60 = 39 min

1. Ordered: 50 mL piggyback to be infused for 30 min. The drop factor is 20. At how many gtt/min will you set the rate?
   a. 17 gtt/min   **b.** 100 gtt/min   **c.** 20 gtt/min   **d.** 33 gtt/min

2. Ordered: Dobutrex 150 mg in 150 mL Ringer's lactate (RL). The infusion device is set at 12 mL/hr. How long will it take to infuse?
   a. 6 hr, 15 min   **b.** 12 hr, 50 min   **c.** 8 hr, 15 min   **d.** 12 hr, 30 min

3. Ordered: 2500 mL to be infused for 24 hr. Available: An IV tubing with 15 gtt/mL. At what rate will you set the IV device?
   a. 52 gtt/min   **b.** 35 gtt/min   **c.** 26 gtt/min   **d.** 104 gtt/min

4. Ordered: 300 mL of 0.9% NS for 6 hr. The IV set is microdrip. At how many gtt/min will you set the rate?
   a. 60 gtt/min   **b.** 50 gtt/min   **c.** 30 gtt/min   **d.** 45 gtt/min

5. Administer 50 mL of an IV antibiotic for 15 min. The IV set is calibrated at 15 gtt/mL. At how many gtt/min will you set the rate?
   a. 100 gtt/min   **b.** 60 gtt/min   **c.** 25 gtt/min   **d.** 50 gtt/min

6. Calculate the infusion time for an IV of 1000 mL of D5W infusing at 25 gtt/min with a drop factor of 10 gtt/mL.
   a. 6 hr, 40 min   **b.** 6 hr, 10 min   **c.** 5 hr, 57 min   **d.** 4 hr, 17 min

7. The IV is infusing at 30 gtt/min. The drop factor is 20 gtt/mL. The IV bag label reads 500 mL of $\frac{1}{4}$% NS. How many hours will it take to infuse the IV?
   a. 5 hr, 50 min   **b.** 3 hr, 36 min   **c.** 4 hr, 40 min   **d.** 5 hr, 30 min

8. A pint of blood (500 mL) is hung at 1100 hours. The flow rate is 42 gtt/min. The drop factor on the administration set is 10 gtt/mL. When will the infusion be completed?
   a. 1733 hours   **b.** 1920 hours   **c.** 1300 hours   **d.** 1654 hours

9. Tridil is infusing at 30 mL/hr. The IV label reads: *500 mL D5W with Tridil 5 μg/3 mL.* How many hours will it take to infuse?
   a. 15 hr, 10 min   **b.** 18 hr, 45 min   **c.** 16 hr, 40 min   **d.** 12 hr, 48 min

10. Ordered: Amicar 5 g in 250 mL for 2 hr. Calculate how many mL/hr to set the infusion device.
    a. 150 mL/hr   **b.** 100 mL/hr   **c.** 175 mL/hr   **d.** 125 mL/hr

Refer to the Calculating Dosages, Intravenous (IV) Dosages section of the enclosed CD-ROM for additional practice problems.

CRITICAL THINKING EXERCISES

It is the change of shift. The patient with congestive heart failure (CHF) has an IV of 1000 mL D5W infusing. The patient complains of being very short of breath. After checking the IV rate, you find that it is infusing at 175 mL/hr. Taking into consideration the patient's diagnosis, you check the IV order and it reads 500 mL D5W in 24 hr.

- Order:
- Given:
- Error:
- Preventive measures:
- Potential injury:

Discussion
- What would your first action be?
- What other factors relate to this incident?
- At what rate shoud the IV be infusing?

ANSWERS ON PAGE 369

CHAPTER 6 FINAL

1. Ordered: 3000 mL for 24 hr. The drop factor is 15. How many gtt/min will infuse via gravity pump?

2. Ordered: 75 mL to be infused for 45 min. The drop factor is 10. At how many mL/hr will you set the infusion device? How many gtt/min will infuse via gravity pump?

3. Ordered: 1000 mL to be infused for 12 hr IV. At how many mL/hr will you set the infusion device? How many gtt/min will be administered via gravity pump if the drop factor is 20?

4. Ordered: 1200 mL to be infused for 8 hr. The drop factor is microdrip. How many gtt/min will infuse?

5. Infuse 2000 mL D5W for 24 hr. The drop factor is 10. At how many mL/hr will you set the infusion device? How many gtt/min will be administered?

6. Ordered: 1500 mL NS to infuse for 12 hr. The drop factor is 15. How many mL/hr will be administered? How many gtt/min will infuse?

7. Ordered: 3000 mL D5W to infuse for 24 hr with 0.5 g of penicillin in each 1000 mL. The drop factor is 60, by microdrip. How many mL/hr will infuse? How many gtt/min will be administered?

8. Ordered: 200 mL cefazolin to infuse for 45 min on the infusion device. At how many mL/hr will you set the infusion device?

9. Ordered: 1000 mL to run for 12 hr on microdrip. At how many gtt/min will you regulate the flow?

10. Ordered: 250 mL to infuse for 90 min. How many mL/hr will infuse if the electronic infusion device is used? How many gtt/min will infuse with microdrip?

Advanced IV Calculations

7

INTRODUCTION

This chapter builds on the mastery of basic IV calculations in Chapter 6. Taking the time to work through each set of problems will facilitate the acquisition of the logic needed to solve complex IV solution calculations. When each step has been mastered, you will be able to identify and use basic safe calculation shortcuts.

● ADVANCED IV CALCULATIONS

Advanced IV calculations are used to determine the amount of IV drug and flow rate per minute and/or per hour for potent medications based on the patient's weight, condition, and response to treatment. If an infusion device is not available, microdrip tubing should be used with a volume-control device. (See Figure 11-4 on page 264 for an illustration of equipment.) Some medications are delivered directly into a vein with a syringe.

The choice of administration and equipment depends not only on the orders and the patient's condition but also on hospital policy, state board policy, the literature and pharmacy recommendations, and the equipment available.

The nurse must be able to evaluate orders and existing solutions for safe and correct dose/flow rate, preferred routes, and compatibilities with existing solutions.

● TITRATED INFUSIONS

Dose/flow rate adjustments may be made, particularly with powerful solutions of medications, based on the patient's condition, weight, and physiologic response to the medication. For example, an order may call for an IV to be **titrated** (adjusted) to maintain a certain blood pressure range. The most potent IV medications are administered and adjusted in micrograms per kilogram per minute or milligrams per kilogram per minute. For purposes of reducing errors and simplifying mathematics in flow rate calculations, many of these infusions now have a standardized **total drug/total volume ratio** of 1:1, 1:2, and 1:4 (e.g., 250 mg/250 mL [1:1]; 250 mg/500 mL [1:2], 250 mg/1000 mL [1:4]). If the patient needs fluid restriction, the physician may order a stronger concentration of drug to solution (4:1, or 2:1 drug in solution, such as 1 g/250 mL [4:1] or 500 mg:250 mL [2:1].

Figure 7-1 shows an infusion with 500 mg of aminophylline to 1000 mL or 1:2 ratio of total drug to total volume ratio.

CLINICAL ALERT!

If you consult flow rate and compatibility charts, examine the source and the date published. If the publisher is a reputable source, such as the laboratory that furnishes the IV solutions in use, and if the chart is current, then take further care to examine the layout and content of the tables to ensure that the information needed is selected.

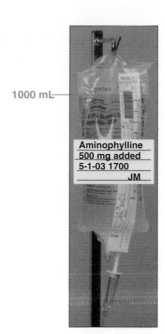

1000 mL

FIGURE 7-1
An infusion with aminophylline. *(From Potter P, Perry A:* Basic nursing: essentials for practice, *ed 5, St Louis, 2003, Mosby.)*

Aminophylline
500 mg added
5-1-03 1700
JM

Note Label
500 mg aminophylline
in 1000 mL D5W

$$\frac{\text{Total drug} \ : \ \text{Total volume}}{500 \text{ mg} \quad : \quad 1000 \text{ mL}}$$

$$\frac{\text{Reduced ratio}}{1 \text{ mg} : 2 \text{ mL}}$$

Solving Titrated Infusion Problems

STEPS Calculate the recommended drug dose per kilogram per minute (μg/kg/min or mg/kg/min) from the literature.

Compare the recommended drug dose in the literature with the physician's order using the same terms (micrograms or milligrams) and evaluate for the safe dose range (SDR) as shown on p. 166.

If the order is safe, calculate the hourly drug and flow rate using the formula below.

Hourly Drug and Flow Rate Formula for Titrated Infusions

$$\text{TD} \quad : \quad \text{TV} \quad :: \quad \text{HD} \quad : \quad \text{HV}$$

Total drug : Total volume :: Hourly drug : Hourly volume

in
Lowest reduced ratio

One of these will be *x*.
One of these will be known.

CLINICAL ALERT!

Titrated infusions seldom require a high flow rate. It is essential that the flow rates be correct. Speeding up or slowing down an IV without a physician's order to compensate for incorrect flow rate is hazardous. Be aware that abrupt changes in IV fluid and therefore medication levels can cause serious side effects.

🌟 REMEMBER ● **This may necessitate converting mg or μg/min to mg or μg/hr.**

EXAMPLE Ordered: 0.3 mg/min of Intropin (dopamine). Available: 500 mg dissolved in 500 mL D5W. The literature recommends an initial dose of 2 to 5 μg/kg/min, not to exceed a total of 50 μg/kg/min. Titrate to patient response. The patient weighs 242 lb. What flow rate should be set on the infusion device?

Step 1   **a. Convert** pounds to kilograms using a calculator.
242 lb ÷ 2.2 = 110 kg
b. Calculate the SDR from the literature.

Know *Want to Know*	**PROOF**
2 μg : 1 kg :: x μg : 110 kg	$2 \times 110 = 220$
$x = 220$ μg/min (low therapeutic dose)	$1 \times 220 = 220$

Know *Want to Know*	**PROOF**
50 μg : 1 kg :: x μg : 110 kg	$5 \times 110 = 550$
$x = 550$ μg/min (high therapeutic dose)	$1 \times 550 = 550$

The SDR is 220 to 550 μg/min for this patient.

Step 2   **Compare** the SDR recommended in the literature with the order:
SDR: 220 to 550 μg/min
Ordered: 0.3 mg
Need to convert milligrams to micrograms to compare.
1000 × 0.3 or 0.300.
300 μg/min ordered.
Decision: Safe to give.

Step 3   **a. Calculate** the ordered hourly drug dose in milligrams (same as drug on hand) using a calculator.
0.3 mg × 60 min = 18 mg/hr

b. Calculate hourly rate after reducing the total drug/total volume ratio to lowest terms.

TD : TV :: HD : HV
500 mg : 500 mL :: 18 mg : x mL   **PROOF** $1 \times 18 = 18$
      1 : 1 :: 18 : x $1 \times 18 = 18$
$x = 18$ mL/hr
Set the flow rate on the IV infusion device to 18 mL/hr.

Alternative Step 3   If the hourly volume is known but the hourly drug dose is not, just place the unknown (*x*) under the hourly drug dose and fill in the hourly volume ordered in this equation. Then check the answer with the literature for the SDR (e.g., the order was for 18 mL/hr or is infusing at 18 mL/hr when you arrive; how much drug is the patient receiving per hour and per minute so that you can compare with SDR in literature?).

Use the same formula. You read the total drug and total volume and hourly volume on the IV set in the room:

$$TD : TV :: HD : HV$$
$$500 \text{ mg} : 500 \text{ mL} :: x \text{ mg} : 18 \text{ mL}$$
$$1 : 1 :: x : 18$$

Reduce ratio:

$x = 18$ mg/hr (1 : 1 ratio)

18 mg : 60 min : x mg : 1 min

$60x = 18$

$x = 0.3$ mg/min

PROOF $18 \times 1 = 18$
$60 \times 0.3 = 18$

Now you know that the order was followed properly. (You have already checked the literature for the SDR for this patient.)

ANSWERS ON PAGE 370

WORKSHEET
7A   Advanced IV Calculation Practice

1. Change the drug per minute to drug per hour in micrograms, then in milligrams, for each given weight. The use of a calculator is permissible, or a ratio of given drug × kg : 1 min :: *x* drug : 60 min (1000 µg = 1 mg).

		DRUG/kg/min	RECOMMENDED	µg/hr	mg/hr
EXAMPLE	a.	5 µg/kg/min	Wt: 5 kg	$5 \times 5 \times 60 = 1500$	1.500. = 1.5
	b.	8 µg/kg/min	Wt: 20 kg	_____	_____
	c.	3 µg/kg/min	Wt: 121 lb	_____	_____
	d.	4 µg/kg/min	Wt: 50 kg	_____	_____
	e.	20 µg/kg/min	Wt: 60 kg	_____	_____

2. Reduce the total drug/total volume ratio to lowest terms (e.g., 1000 : 250 = 4 : 1)

		TD : TV	LOWEST RATIO
EXAMPLE	a.	250 mg : 1000 mL	1 : 4
	b.	500 mg : 500 mL	_____
	c.	100 mg : 1000 mL	_____
	d.	250 mg : 500 mL	_____
	e.	500 mg : 1000 mL	_____

Continued

ANSWERS ON PAGE 370

WORKSHEET
7A **Advanced IV Calculation Practice—cont'd**

3. Estimate the value of x (hourly volume) after reducing the ratio of total drug to total volume. The ratio of hourly drug to hourly volume will be the same as total drug to total volume.

	TD : TV :: HD : HV	ANSWER
EXAMPLE a.	250 mg : 1000 mL :: 10 mg : x mL	<u>1 : 4 :: 10 : 40</u> mL/hr
b.	500 mg : 500 mL :: 30 mg : x mL	_____ mL/hr
c.	100 mg : 1000 mL :: 5 mg : x mL	_____ mL/hr
d.	250 mg : 500 mL :: 3 mg : x mL	_____ mL/hr
e.	500 mg : 250 mL :: 10 mg : x mL	_____ mL/hr

4. If you came on duty and evaluated these IV solutions and rates in a patient-care setting, you would estimate the hourly drug after first reducing the total drug/total volume ratio and then examining the rate set on the infusion device.

Estimate the hourly drug (x).

	TD : TV :: HD : HV	ANSWER
EXAMPLE a.	250 mg : 250 mL :: x mg : 20 mL	<u>1 : 1 :: 20 : 20</u> (20 mg/hr)
b.	1000 mg : 500 mL :: x mg : 6 mL	_____ ___ mg/hr
c.	250 mg : 500 mL :: x mg : 18 mL	_____ ___ mg/hr
d.	400 mg : 1000 mL :: x mg : 10 mL	_____ ___ mg/hr
e.	500 mg : 250 mL :: x mg : 18 mL	_____ ___ mg/hr

5. Change micrograms to milligrams by moving the decimal three places to the left. Reduce the total drug/total volume ratio to the lowest terms. Finally, estimate the hourly volume. (The hourly drug must always be calculated in the same terms as the total drug.)

	TD : TV :: HD : HV	ANSWER
EXAMPLE a.	250 mg : 1000 mL :: (4000 µg) 4 mg : x mL	<u>1 : 4 :: 4 : 16</u> mL/hr
b.	500 mg : 500 mL :: (9000 µg) ___ mg : x mL	_____ mL/hr
c.	1000 mg : 500 mL :: (20,000 µg) ___ mg : x mL	_____ mL/hr
d.	250 mg : 500 mL :: (15,000 µg) ___ mg : x mL	_____ mL/hr
e.	400 mg : 250 mL :: (8000 µg) ___ mg : x mL	_____ mL/hr

ANSWERS ON PAGE 370

WORKSHEET
7B   **IV Drug/Flow Rates**

Tip: **Being able to convert drug, weight, time, and volume parameters within the metric system with ease facilitates advanced IV calculations.**

1. Fill in the table by using a calculator and/or by moving decimals.

	mg/hr	μg/hr	mg/min	μg/min
a.	0.050.	50	0.050 ÷ 60 = 0.0008	0.8
b.			4	
c.	30			
d.				20
e.	7.5			

2. Fill in the table using a calculator.

	kg	mg/hr	mg/kg/min	μg/kg/min
a.	85	25	25 ÷ 85 ÷ 60 = 0.005	5
b.	70		10	
c.	62			0.1
d.	55	75		
e.	48			5

3. Fill in the table for these IV drug/flow rate calculations using the TD : TV :: IID : IIV formula.

IV contents	TD : TV reduced ratio	HD (mg/hr)	HV (mL/hr)	mg/mL
a. 500 mg/1000 mL	1 : 2	5	1 : 2 :: 5 : 10	500 ÷ 1000 = 0.5
b. 250 mg/500 mL			30	
c. 400 mg/250 mL		24		
d. 500 mg/500 mL			75	
e. 500 mg/250 mL		16		

CLINICAL ALERT!

Remember that the difference between a microgram (μg or mcg) and a milligram (mg) is "× 1000." The difference between drug per minute and hourly drug is "× 60."

The difference between μg/kg/min and μg/min is equal to "× the weight in kilograms." Manipulating these differences is critical for safe medication administration.

ANSWERS ON PAGE 371

WORKSHEET
7C

Medication Dosages Infusing in Existing Solutions

It is often necessary to verify the amount of drug being delivered in an existing solution. The amount of drug in the IV solution is frequently a milligram dose, whereas the amount of drug the patient is receiving is a microgram dose or microgram/kilogram dose.

Note the example in Problem 1 and do the following in the remaining problems.

- Set up your TD : TV :: HD : HV ratio and determine mg/hr. Prove your answer.

- Move decimals to change milligrams to micrograms (×1000).

- Use a calculator to change hourly drug (HD) to drug/minute (divide by 60).

- Use a calculator to determine kilograms, and divide micrograms by kilogram weight to obtain μg/kg/min.

EXAMPLE 1. An IV of Drug X 100 mg in 1000 mL is infusing at 20 mL/hr. The physician asks, How many *mg/hr* is the patient receiving? How many *μg/min*? How many *μg/kg/min*? The patient weighs 143 lb today.

  a. TD : TV reduced ratio: 100 : 1000 = 1 : 10
  b. TD : TV :: HD : HV   1 mg : 10 mL :: 2 mg : 20 mL
  c. mg/hr: 2
  d. μg/hr: 2 × 1000 = 2000
  e. μg/min: 2000 ÷ 60 = 33.3
  f. μg/kg/min: 33.3 ÷ 65 kg = 0.5

PROOF 1 × 20 = 20
           10 × 2 = 20

2. An IV of Drug X 250 mg in 500 mL is infusing at 15 mL/hr. The patient weighs 110 lb today.
  a. TD : TV :: HD : HV reduced ratio: **PROOF**
  b. μg/hr:
  c. μg/min:
  d. μg/kg/min:

3. An IV of Drug X 400 mg in 1000 mL is infusing at 5 mL/hr. The patient weighs 121 lb today.
  a. TD : TV :: HD : HV reduced ratio: **PROOF**
  b. μg/hr:
  c. μg/min:
  d. μg/kg/min:

4. An IV of Drug X 1000 mg in 250 mL is infusing at 10 mL/hr. The patient weighs 132 lb today.
  a. TD : TV :: HD : HV reduced ratio: **PROOF**
  b. μg/hr:
  c. μg/min:
  d. μg/kg/min:

ANSWERS ON PAGE 371

WORKSHEET
7C
Medication Dosages Infusing in Existing Solutions—cont'd

5. An IV of Drug X 500 mg in 250 mL is infusing at 8 mL/hr. The patient weighs 175 lb today. (Calculate kilograms to nearest tenth.)
  a. TD : TV :: HD : HV reduced ratio:
  b. μg/hr:
  c. μg/min:
  d. μg/kg/min:

PROOF

ANSWERS ON PAGE 371

WORKSHEET
7D
Evaluating Critical Care IV Orders

Evaluate the following orders and infusions for safety. Use a calculator to determine kilogram weights to the nearest tenth. Change micrograms to milligrams when applicable by moving decimals. Use a calculator to determine the SDR when applicable. Double check and label all calculations. Provo the hourly flow rate calculation. Decide whether the order/infusion is:

1. Safe/Correct.

2. Unsafe/Incorrect. Consult with physician.

EXAMPLE **1.** Ordered: Dopamine 200 μg/min for a 110 lb patient. The literature states that the usual dose is 2 to 5 μg/kg/min. Available: Dopamine 250 mg in 250 mL D5W.

  a. Patient's weight in kg: 110 ÷ 2.2 = 50
  b. SDR/min: 100 − 250 μg/min
  c. Is order safe?   Safe to continue.
  d. TD : TV reduced ratio: 1 : 1 (250 : 250)
  e. Hourly drug order in μg: 12,000 (200 × 60)
  f. Hourly drug order in mg: 12
  g. Hourly flow rate to be set on infusion device: 12 (1 : 1 or 12 : 12)

2. Ordered: Dobutamine 100 μg/min. Available: Dobutamine 250 mg in 250 mL D5W. The flow rate is currently infusing at 5 mL/hr.
  a. TD : TV reduced ratio:
  b. Hourly drug order in μg:
  c. Hourly drug order in mg:
  d. Is current infusion correct?
  e. Evaluation and decision:

Continued

ANSWERS ON PAGE 371

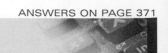

WORKSHEET 7D	Evaluating Critical Care IV Orders—cont'd

 REMEMBER ● **If catching up is allowed by the physician for an IV that is behind or ahead in flow rate and if a new flow rate is *not* ordered, confirm that the flow rate can be recalculated based on the *original order* and the *remaining volume*.**

EXAMPLE   If an IV of 1000 mL is ordered for 100 mL/hr (to last 10 hr) and 4 hr later has 700 mL remaining for infusion instead of 600 mL, then the remaining volume divided by the desired remaining hours would provide the new adjusted flow rate to complete the IV in 10 hr as originally ordered—700 divided by 6 = 116 4/6 or 117 mL/hr would infuse the volume in 10 hr total time.

It is never wise to increase an IV by more than 10% of original flow rate at a time. The patient's condition may not permit an increase in flow rate so this decision must be made by an experienced nurse in collaboration with the physician, taking into consideration the patient's hydration and cardiopulmonary and renal status among other factors.

3. Ordered: Lidocaine 4 mg/min. Available: 1 g of lidocaine in 500 mL of D5W.
   a. TD : TV reduced ratio (mg : mL):
   b. Hourly drug ordered:
   c. Hourly flow rate to be set on infusion device:

4. Ordered: Isuprel (isoproterenol hydrochloride) 5 µg/min. Available: Isoproterenol hydrochloride 1 mg in 250 mL D5W.
   a. TD : TV reduced ratio:
   b. Hourly drug ordered in µg and in mg: **PROOF**
   c. TD : TV :: HD : HV ratio:
   d. Hourly flow rate to be set on infusion device:

5. Ordered: Initial infusion of norepinephrine at 50 mL/hr. Available: Norepinephrine 1 mg in 250 mL normal saline (NS). The SDR is 8 to 12 µg/min initially.
   a. TD : TV : HD : HV ratio:
   b. Hourly drug being infused in mg: **PROOF**
   c. Hourly drug order in µg/hour:
   d. Hourly drug order in µg/min:
   e. SDR for this patient:
   f. Evaluation and decision:

ANSWERS ON PAGE 371

WORKSHEET
7E IV Calculations with Aminophylline

Calculate and evaluate the following infusion problems.

EXAMPLE 1. Ordered: Aminophylline 50 mL/hr. Available: Aminophylline 250 mg in 1000 mL D5W on an infusion device. The literature states that the SDR is 0.1 to 0.5 mg/kg/hr for aminophylline. The patient weighs 60 kg.
   a. SDR for this patient: 6–30 mg/hr
   b. TD : TV reduced ratio: 250 : 1000 = 1 mg : 4 mL (1 : 4)
   c. mg/hr aminophylline ordered: 1 : 4 :: x mg : 50 mL, x = 12.5 mg/hr **PROOF** 1 × 50 = 50
   d. Evaluation and decision: Safe to give 4 × 12.5 = 50

2. Ordered: Aminophylline 45 mg/hr. Available: Aminophylline 500 mg in 1000 mL D5W. The literature states that the SDR is 0.5 to 0.7 mg/kg/hr for the first 12 hr. The patient weighs 80 kg.
   a. SDR for this patient (mg/hr):
   b. Ordered dose:
   c. Evaluation and decision:
   d. TD : TV reduced ratio:
   e. TD : TV :: HD : HV ratio: **PROOF**
   f. If safe, mL/hr to be infused:

3. Ordered: Aminophylline 50 mL/hr. Available: Aminophylline 250 mg in 500 mL of D5W. The recommended maintenance dose is 0.1 to 0.5 mg/kg/hr. The patient weighs 70 kg.
   a. SDR for this patient (mg/hr):
   b. TD : TV reduced ratio:
   c. TD : TV :: HD : HV ordered: **PROOF**
   d. Ordered mg/hr:
   e. Evaluation and decision:

4. Ordered: Aminophylline 20 mg/hr. Available: Aminophylline 250 mg in 500 mL D5W. The maximum dose for maintenance is 0.5 mg/kg/hr. The patient weighs 50 kg.
   a. Safe maximum dose for this patient (mg/hr):
   b. Evaluation and decision:
   c. TD : TV reduced ratio:
   d. TD : TV :: HD : HV ordered: **PROOF**
   e. If safe, mL/hr to be infused:

5. Ordered: Aminophylline 15 mg/hr. The patient's IV is set at 50 mL/hr on an infusion device. The IV is labeled "Aminophylline 500 mg/1000 mL D5W." The SDR is 0.1 to 0.5 mg/kg/hr. The patient weighs 154 lb.
   a. SDR for this patient (mg/hr):
   b. Evaluation and decision:
   c. TD : TV :: HD : HV ordered:
   d. TD : TV :: HD : HV infusing: **PROOF**
   e. Evaluation and decision regarding existing IV:

ANSWERS ON PAGE 372

WORKSHEET
7F IV Calculations for Obstetrics

Calculate and evaluate the following orders. Remember that the terms must be the same in your TD : TV :: HD : HV ratio and proportion.

EXAMPLE **1.** Ordered: Magnesium sulfate 2 g/hr IV. Available: Magnesium sulfate 40 g/250 mL Lactated Ringer's solution on an infusion device infusing at 13 mL/hr.

    a. TD : TV :: HD : HV   40 g : 250 mL :: 2 g : x mL
    b. mL/hr ordered (HV): $4x = 50$, $x = 12.5$ mL/hr
    c. mL/hr infusing: 13 mL/hr
    d. Evaluation and decision: Rate is correct.

PROOF $4 \times 12.5 = 50$
               $25 \times 2 = 50$

2. Ordered: Pitocin (oxytocin) 20 mU/min. Available: 1000 mL D5 N/S with 10 U of Pitocin (1000 mU = 1 U). The IV is infusing at 100 mL/hr.
    a. TD : TV reduced ratio:
    b. TD (mU) : TV :: HD (mU) : HV ordered: **PROOF**
    c. Evaluation and decision:

3. Ordered: Terbutaline 10 µg/min for 30 min. Available. Terbutaline 5 mg in 500 mL/D5W.
    a. TD : TV reduced ratio:
    b. Hourly drug ordered in µg:
    c. Hourly drug ordered in mg:
    d. TD : TV :: HD : HV ratio: **PROOF**
    e. Hourly flow rate to be set on infusion device:

4. Ordered: Magnesium sulfate 25 mL/hr. Call the doctor when 2 g have been infused. Available: 500 mL D5W with 20 g of magnesium sulfate on infusion device.
    a. TD (g) : TV reduced ratio in infusion:
    b. TD : TV :: HD : HV (existing infusion):   **PROOF**
    c. g/hr ordered at 25 mL/hr:
    d. Length of time 2 g to be infused:

5. Ordered: Pitocin (oxytocin) 2 mU/min. Available: 10 U Pitocin in 1000 mL of D5 N/S.
    a. mU/mL of Pitocin in IV container:
    b. TD : TV reduced ratio:
    c. Hourly drug ordered:
    d. TD : TV :: HD : HV ratio: **PROOF**
    e. Flow rate on infusion device to be set:

ANSWERS ON PAGE 373

WORKSHEET
7G   More IV Practice Problems

Calculate and evaluate the following infusion problems.

1. Ordered: Esmolol hydrochloride at 39 mL/hr. Available: 5 g in 500 mL
   5% D Lactated Ringer's solution. The patient weighs 143 lb. The SDR is
   50 to 200 µg/kg/min.
   a. Patient's weight in kg:
   b. SDR for this patient in µg/min:
   c. SDR in mg/hr:
   d. TD : TV : HD : HV ratio ordered:
   e. Hourly drug delivered in mg:
   f. mg/min ordered:
   g. µg/min ordered:
   h. µg/kg/min ordered:
   i. Evaluation and decision:

2. Ordered: Nitroglycerin IV at 10 µg/min. Available: Nitroglycerin IV
   50 mg in 500 mL D5W. The infusion is flowing at 6 mL/hr.
   a. TD : TV :: HD : HV ratio ordered:
   b. Hourly drug ordered in mg:
   c. TD : TV :: HD : HV infusing
   d. µg/min being delivered:
   e. Is flow rate correct?
   f. Evaluation and decision:

3. Ordered: Pronestyl (procainamide hydrochloride) at 50 mL/hr. Available:
   1 g in 500 mL D5W. The SDR for maintenance is 1 to 6 mg/min.
   a. TD : TV :: HD : HV ratio:
   b. Hourly drug delivered in mg:
   c. mg/min ordered:
   d. Evaluation and decision:

4. Ordered: Nipride (sodium nitroprusside) at 0.3 µg/kg/min. Available:
   50 mg sodium nitroprusside in 250 mL NS. The infusion is flowing at
   15 mL/hr. The patient weighs 220 lb.
   a. Weight in kg:
   b. Hourly drug ordered in mg:
   c. TD : TV :: HD : HV ratio ordered:
   d. TD : TV :: HD : HV ratio infusing:
   e. Hourly drug infusing in mg:
   f. Evaluation and decision:

5. Ordered: Cardizem (diltiazem hydrochloride) at 15 mg/hr. Available:
   Diltiazem hydrochloride 125 mg in 25 mL diluent to be added to
   100 mL D5W. Infusion is flowing at 15 mL/hr.
   a. TD : TV :: HD : HV ratio:
   b. Evaluation and decision:

● DIRECT IV (BOLUS) ADMINISTRATION WITH A SYRINGE

Direct IV administration (IV push) is used to administer small amounts of diluted or undiluted medication over a brief period (seconds or minutes).

Medications such as meperidine, Dilantin, or furosemide may be prepared in a syringe and then delivered directly via a vein, intermittent heparin lock, or proximal port of an existing continuous IV.

It is crucial that the literature be consulted for safe-dose limits, rates of flow, dilutions, compatible solutions, and routes and that the patient's response be closely monitored during the administration and afterward (Figure 7-2).

A
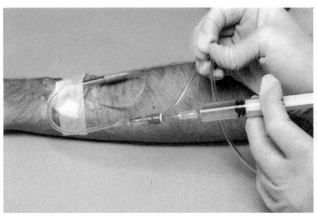
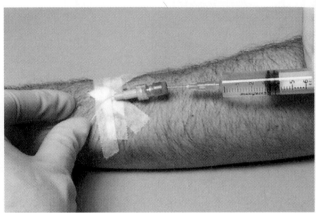

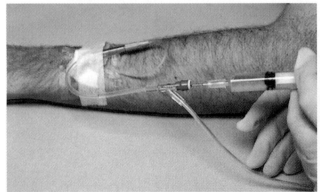

FIGURE 7-2 A, Occlude IV line by pinching tubing just above injection port. Pull back gently on syringe's plunger to aspirate for blood return. **B, C,** Insert needle of syringe containing prepared drug through center of diaphragm. Inject medication bolus slowly over several minutes. Each medication has a recommended rate for bolus administration. Check package directions or a reliable pharmacology reference. *(From Skidmore L: Mosby's drug guide for nurses, ed 3, St Louis, 1999, Mosby.)*

There are two ways to time IV push medications for direct administration with a syringe. Regardless of the method you select, the first step is always to calculate and prepare the correct volume.

● Timing IV Push Medications—Method 1

RULE   Divide the number of seconds of total time to be administered by the number of calibrated increments in prepared syringe with medication (lines on the syringe within each milliliter). This will yield the seconds per increment to be pushed.

FORMULA $\dfrac{\text{Total seconds}}{\text{Total increments}}$ = Seconds to deliver each increment

EXAMPLE   Give 0.5 mg digoxin IV over 5 min. Directions say to dilute to 4 mL of sterile water for injection. There are 20 calibrations in 4 mL on this syringe.

$$\frac{300 \text{ seconds}}{20 \text{ calibrations (0.2 mL ea)}} = 15 \text{ seconds per calibration}$$

Use the second hand on your watch and/or count each cycle (1-15) as you administer the medication, 1 calibration (0.2/mL) every 15 seconds.

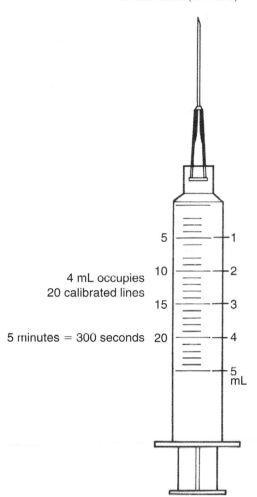

4 mL occupies
20 calibrated lines

5 minutes = 300 seconds

Timing IV Push Medications—Method 2

This method calculates the amount in milliliters to be slowly and gradually pushed over each minute.

FORMULA
$$\text{TV} \quad : \quad \text{TM} \quad :: \quad x \text{ mL} \quad : 1 \text{ min}$$
$$\text{Total volume : Total minutes :: } x \text{ volume (mL) : 1 min}$$

EXAMPLE   Ordered: Digoxin 0.5 mg IV over 5 min. Dilute to 4 mL sterile water for injection.

$$\text{TV : TM :: } x \text{ mL : 1 min}$$
$$4 \text{ mL : 5 min :: mL : 1 min}$$

$$\frac{\cancel{5}}{\cancel{5}} x = \frac{4}{5}$$

$x = 0.8$ mL to be pushed slowly each minute

PROOF $4 \times 1 = 4$
$5 \times 0.8 = 4.0$

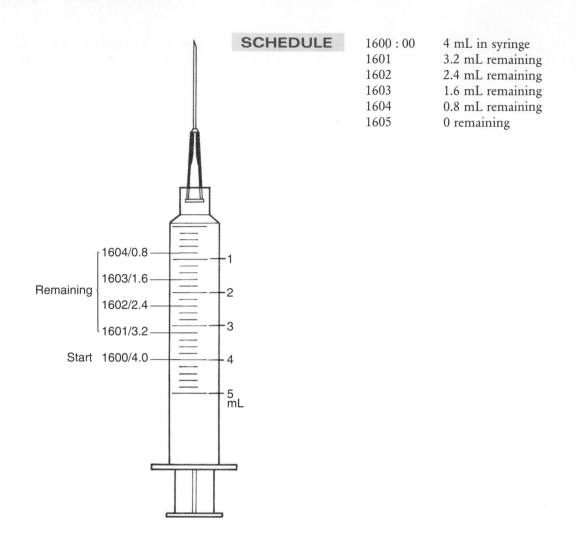

SCHEDULE

1600 : 00	4 mL in syringe
1601	3.2 mL remaining
1602	2.4 mL remaining
1603	1.6 mL remaining
1604	0.8 mL remaining
1605	0 remaining

The schedule above reflects a start time of 1600 hours. It is helpful to write your start time and a schedule of "markers" (increments of time and volume) when you need to push over several minutes. Write this before beginning to inject and have it in front of you to avoid errors caused by distraction.

ANSWERS ON PAGE 373

WORKSHEET

7H   IV Push Calculations

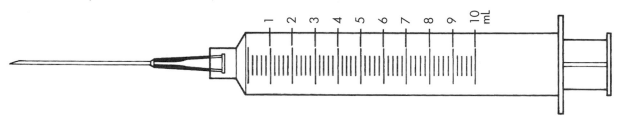

Solve the following problems, using the syringes provided to calculate the seconds per calibration, if applicable, and mL/min to be administered.

1. Ordered: 10% calcium chloride (10 mL) over 5 min.
   a. How many seconds will you administer each calibration?
   b. How many mL/min will be injected?

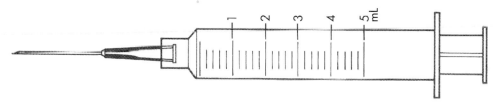

2. Ordered: Digoxin 0.5 mg IV over 10 min. (The literature specifies a minimum of 5 min for administration.) Available: Digoxin 250 µg/mL.
   a. Total mL you will inject:
   b. Total seconds for injection:
   c. Seconds per calibration:
   d. mL/min to be injected:

3. Ordered: Phenytoin sodium IV loading dose of 900 mg at 50 mg/min on an infusion device (Figure 7-3). Available: Phenytoin 100 mg/mL.
   a. Total mL to be injected:
   b. Total time for injection:
   c. mL/min to be administered:

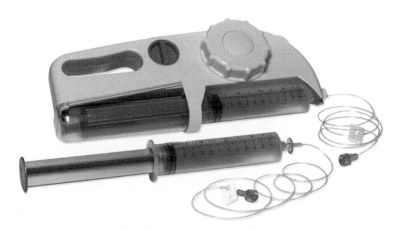

FIGURE 7-3 Freedom 60 syringe infusion device system for direct IV medications. *(From Repro-med Systems, Inc., Chester, NY.)*   *Continued*

ANSWERS ON PAGE 373

4. Ordered: Furosemide 20 mg IV over 2 min. Available:
   Furosemide 10 mg/mL.
   a. Total mL to be injected:
   b. Total time in seconds:
   c. Seconds per calibration:
   d. mL/min to be administered:

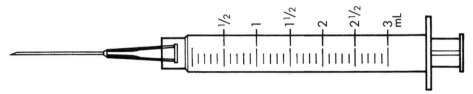

5. Ordered: Meperidine HCl 10 mg IV. The literature states that a single
   dose should be administered over 5 min and that it must be diluted
   to at least 5 mL of sterile water or normal saline for injection. Available:
   Meperidine 50 mg/mL.
   a. Total mL to be injected:
   b. Total time in seconds.
   c. Seconds per calibration:
   d. mL/min to be administered:

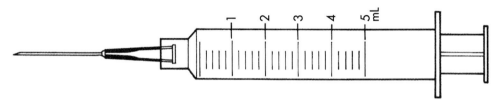

ANSWERS ON PAGE 374

WORKSHEET

71 Multiple-Choice Practice

Use a calculator. Estimate your answers for each applicable step in the mathematics. Establish the reduced total drug/total volume ratio for the infusions, move decimals to convert between micrograms and milligrams, and use logical shortcuts such as multiplying by 60 to change minutes to hours where applicable.

1. Ordered: Isoproterenol HCl IV at 5 μg/min. How many mg/hr would be infused?
   a. 0.5 mg
   b. 50 mg
   c. 0.3 mg
   d. 300 mg

2. Available: Aminophyllinc 250 mg in 1000 mL of D5W. How many milligrams are in each milliliter of the IV solution (mg/mL)?
   a. 0.25 mg
   b. 0.5 mg
   c. 1 mg
   d. 4 mg

3. Available: 1 g of lidocainc in 500 mL of D5W. What is the total drug ratio to the total volume of IV solution?
   a. 2:1
   b. 4:1
   c. 1:2
   d. 1:4

4. Available: Norepinephrine 1 mg in 250 mL of N/S. The SDR is 8 to 12 μg/min initially. What is the minimum flow rate recommendation in mL/hr? *Hint: Change the SDR to milligrams after you obtain the SDR in μg/hr so that you can compare milligrams to milligrams.*
   a. 48 mL/hr
   b. 60 mL/hr
   c. 120 mL/hr
   d. 480 mL/hr

5. Ordered: Furosemide 30 mg IV push over 2 min. Available: Furosemide 10 mg/mL. How many mL/min are to be administered?
   a. 0.5 mL/min
   b. 0.7 mL/min
   c. 1 mL/min
   d. 1.5 mL/min

6. Ordered: Lanoxin IV push 0.5 mg over 5 min. Available: Lanoxin 250 μg/mL. How many mL/min will be injected?
   a. 0.25 mL/min
   b. 0.4 mL/min
   c. 1 mL/min
   d. 1.5 mL/min

Continued

ANSWERS ON PAGE 374

WORKSHEET
71
Multiple-Choice Practice—cont'd

7. Procainamide hydrochloride is infusing at 40 mL/hr for maintenance of an arrhythmia in an adult. Available: 1 g in 500 mL D5W. The SDR for maintenance is 1 to 6 mg/min. What decision will the nurse make?
   a. The order is within SDR. Proceed with the IV.
   b. The order is above the SDR. Hold the infusion and clarify with the physician.
   c. The order is below SDR. Start the infusion and consult with the physician.
   d. The order is unclear. Consult with a knowledgable colleague.

8. Ordered: Procainamide hydrochloride at 60 mg/hr on an infusion device. Available: 1 g in 1000 mL D5W. What flow rate in mL/hr will the nurse set?
   a. 30 mL/hr
   b. 60 mL/hr
   c. 100 mL/hr
   d. 120 mL/hr

9. Ordered: Magnesium sulfate 30 mL/hr. Call the physician when 3 g has been infused. Available: 500 mL D5W with 20 g of magnesium sulfate on an infusion device. In how much time will you expect to call the physician at this flow rate? *Hint: Determine how much drug per hour is infusing.*
   a. 30 min
   b. 1 hr 50 min
   c. 2 hr 30 min
   d. 3 hr

10. Ordered: Dobutamine HCl 2.5 μg/kg/min for a 70-kg patient. Available: Dobutamine HCl IV concentration 500 mcg/mL. What flow rate will you set in mL/hr?
    a. 10 mL/hr
    b. 11 mL/hr
    c. 20 mL/hr
    d. 21 mL/hr

 Refer to the Calculating Dosages, Critical Medications and Titrating Medications sections of the enclosed CD-ROM for additional practice problems.

CRITICAL THINKING EXERCISES

During a bedside emergency for ventricular fibrillation, a physician called for several medications to be given IV direct push. Also ordered were two IV sites to be maintained (both arms), one with D5W. As the orders were called out, one nurse prepared the medications and handed them to the nurse who was assisting, who then gave the medications. At one point, the nurse was handed two syringes of medication. She was told one was bretylium tosylate, and the other syringe contained KCl 30 mEq. The KCl was administered undiluted to the patient direct push, and the bretylium was placed in D5W.

- ■ Error:
- ■ Causes of error:
- ■ Potential injury:
- ■ Nursing actions:
- ■ Preventive measures:

ANSWERS ON PAGE 376

CHAPTER 7 FINAL

Calculate and solve the following problems using a calculator, moving decimals, reducing ratios, and labeling your answers. Prove your work.

Make a decision:

A. Safe to give.   OR

B. Unsafe, consult with physician.

1. Ordered: Potassium chloride 10 mEq to be administered to a 44 lb child with hypokalemia. Administer over 4 hr. Dilute in 100 mL of D5W. The literature states that the rate should not exceed 3 mEq/kg/24 hr for a child.

    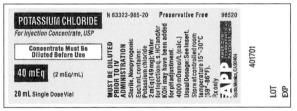

    a. Patient's weight in kg:

    b. SDR for this child per 24 hr:

    c. Total drug ordered:

    d. Decision (Safe/Unsafe):

    e. Amount of drug in mL to be added to IV (refer to label):

    f. Hourly flow rate on infusion device in mL:

2. Ordered: Dobutamine HCl 5 mcg/kg/min. Available: Dobutamine HCl 2000 mcg/mL in an infusion device. Patient's weight is 50 kg.

    a. μg/hr needed:

    b. Flow rate to be set on IV infusion device: _____ hr

3. Ordered: Dopamine HCl at 2 µg/kg/min. Infusing when you enter room: Dopamine HCl at 15 mL/hr. Available: Dopamine HCl 400 mg/500 mL. Patient's weight is 80 kg.

   a. mg/hr needed:

   b. Actual mg/hr infusing:

   c. Flow rate ordered:

   d. Actual flow rate in mL/hr:

   e. Decision (Correct or needs order for change):

4. Ordered: Dopamine IV at 4 µg/kg/min for a patient in septic shock who weighs 110 lb today. The SDR is 2 to 10 µg/kg/min. The IV solution contains 200 mg in 250 mL of solution. The IV is flowing at 15 mL/hr when you enter the room.

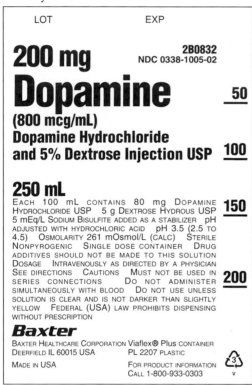

   a. Patient's weight in kg:

   b. SDR for this patient:

   c. Ordered drug rate/minute:

   d. Decision (Safe/Unsafe):

   e. TD : TV ratio:

   f. mg/hr of drug ordered:

   g. Hourly flow rate needed:

   h. Decision (Correct or needs order for change):

5. Ordered: Meperidine HCl 30 mg IV to be administered for pain at the rate of 10 mg/min. Must be diluted to at least 5 mL with sterile water for injection.

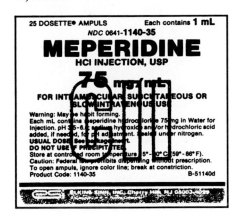

a. Total amount of meperidine to be prepared (in mL, round to nearest tenth):

b. Total amount of diluted volume to be administered in mL:

c. Total number of minutes for injection:

d. Use the syringe provided to calculate the number of seconds per calibration to be administered to nearest whole number of seconds:

e. Amount in mL/min to be administered gradually:

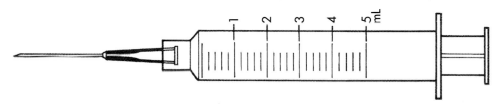

Parenteral Nutrition

8

OBJECTIVES

- Calculate grams of protein, dextrose, and lipids per order.
- Calculate the percentage of protein, dextrose, and lipids per infusion.
- Calculate the percentage of additives per infusion.
- Calculate the kilocalories for protein, dextrose, and lipids per infusion.
- Calculate the total kilocalories per infusion.
- Compare the ordered amount of parenteral nutrition with the infusion label.

INTRODUCTION

The IV requirements for patients who are unable to ingest food are calculated on a daily basis. Concentrations of nutrients are calculated to show the differing strengths and percentages of additives for peripheral and central lines. Percentage of additives is calculated to ensure that the mineral requirements are being met. Standard orders for peripheral and central lines are compared. Medication administration records are discussed. The importance of parenteral orders and verification of the labels on the bag are stressed.

• TOTAL PARENTERAL NUTRITION

Total parenteral nutrition (TPN) permits the venous administration of dextrose, amino acid, electrolytes, lipids, and vitamins to sustain life when the gastrointestinal system must be bypassed. A TPN bag is shown in Figure 8-1.

A routine maintenance IV solution of 1000 mL with 5% dextrose delivered over an 8-hour period only provides approximately 200 calories derived from dextrose. If an NPO patient received 3 L of D5W a day, the 600 total calories received would not be enough to promote or maintain health for a sustained period. In contrast, TPN may deliver as much as 1 cal/mL depending on the concentration of nutrients.

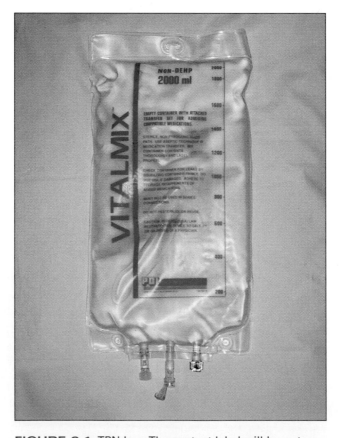

FIGURE 8-1 TPN bag. The content label will be put on the bag by the pharmacist.

TPN is administered via a central vein such as the subclavian or internal jugular. This is known as *central parenteral nutrition (CPN)*. The peripheral administration known as *peripheral parenteral nutrition (PPN)* is given via peripheral veins. The choice depends on the patient, the vein condition, and how long the patient will need the therapy. The larger central veins are selected for longer-term therapy and higher concentrations of nutrients. The contents of TPN are customized according to the patient's condition and need, the venous route, relevant laboratory values, and weight. Orders for the contents may be changed daily.

PPN is used for nutritional therapy of 2 weeks or less. PPN solution must be kept at the following concentration levels to prevent vein irritation: amino acids, 5.5%; dextrose, 10%; lipids, 10%. CPN permits high levels of concentration because it is infused into large veins. CPN is used for nutrition therapy needed for longer than 2 weeks. CPN maximum concentrations are as follows: amino acids, 8.5% to 10%; dextrose, 20% to 70%; lipids, 20%.

A three-in-one solution, or total nutrition admixture, combines lipids, amino acids, and dextrose. The solution is white because of the lipids, which make precipitation difficult to observe. The three-in-one solution is used for both hospital and home therapy. The lipids can also be administered separately (Figure 8-3).

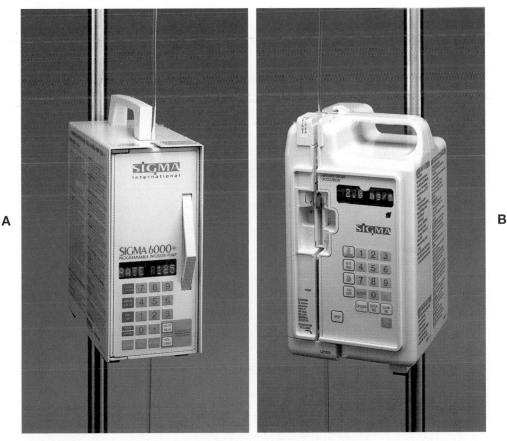

FIGURE 8-2 A, Sigma international 6000 programmable infusion device. **B,** Sigma 8000 automatic dose-related calculation device. *(From Sigma International, Inc., Medina, NY.)*

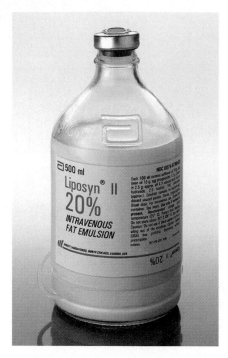

FIGURE 8-3 Liposyn II (fat emulsion) 20% for parenteral nutrition. Notice the opaque contents contrasted with the parenteral infusion without lipids. *(From Abbott Laboratories, Abbott Park, IL.)*

The nurse's responsibility is to check the physician's order to determine whether the pharmacy has filled the order according to the directions. Figure 8-4 shows a physician order for TPN. Calculate grams, percentage of concentration, and kilocalories per bag of TPN.

EXAMPLE (Refer to Figure 8-4, a sample physician's order form)

◼ Total Grams Per Bag

Formula: % × mL = g/L

Step 1
Amino acids (AA) 10% in 425 mL

0.10 × 425 = 42.5 g/L

Formula: g/L × TV/L = g/bag

Step 2
42.5 g/L × 1.307 TV/L = 55.5 g/bag

There are 55.5 g of AA in 1307 mL of TPN.

Shortcut method: % × mL = g/L × TV/L = g/bag

Dextrose 70% in 357 mL

0.70 × 357 = 249.9 g/L × 1.307 TV/L = 326.6 g/bag

To calculate the answer for g/L, multiply by the TV to determine the total g/bag.

There are 326.6 g of dextrose in 1307 mL of TPN.

TPN ORDER SHEET

HOME HEALTH	DATE
PATIENT	ADDRESS

TPN FORMULA:

AMINO ACIDS: ☐ 5.5% ☐ 8.5% ☑ 10%	ml	*425*
☐ WITH STANDARD ELECTROLYTES		
DEXTROSE: ☐ 10% ☐ 20% ☐ 40% ☐ 50% ☑ 70%	ml	*357*
(check one)		
LIPIDS: ☐ 10% ☑ 20%	ml	*125*
FOR ALL-IN-ONE FORMULA		

FINAL VOLUME		
qsad STERILE WATER FOR INJECTION *400 mL*	*1307* ml	

Calcium Gluconate	0.465 mEq/ml	*5*	mEq
Magnesium Sulfate	4 mEq/ml	*5*	mEq
Potassium Acetate	2 mEq/ml		mEq
Potassium Chloride	2 mEq/ml		mEq
Potassium Phosphate	3 mM/ml	*22*	mM
Sodium Acetate	2 mEq/ml		mEq
Sodium Chloride	4 mEq/ml	*35*	mEq
Sodium Phosphate	3 mM/ml		mM
TRACE ELEMENTS CONCENTRATE	☐ 4 ☐ 5 ☐ 6		ml

Patient Additives:

☐ MVC 9 + 3 10 ml Daily

☐ HUMULIN-R _*10*_ u DAILY

☐ FOLIC ACID _____ mg
_____ times weekly

☐ VITAMIN K _____ mg
_____ times weekly

☐ OTHER: *MVI 12 10 mL/daily*

☐ OTHER: _____

Directions:

INFUSE: ☑ DAILY

☐ _____ TIMES WEEKLY

OTHER DIRECTIONS:

_____

_____

_____

_____

Rate: ☐ CYCLIC INFUSION:	"	☐ CONTINUOUS INFUSION:	"	☑ STANDARD RATE:	
OVER _____ HOURS	"	AT _____ ml PER HOUR	"	AT _*110*_ ml PER HOUR	
(TAPER UP AND DOWN)	"		"	FOR _*12*_ HOURS	

LAB ORDERS:

☐ STANDARD LAB ORDERS
SMAC-20, CO2, Mg+2 TWICE WEEKLY
CBC WITH AUTO DIFF WEEKLY
UNTIL STABLE, THEN:
SMAC-20, CO2, Mg+2 WEEKLY
CBC WITH AUTO DIFF MONTHLY

☐ OTHER: _____

_____

_____

VALIDATION:

_____

DOCTOR'S SIGNATURE

Print Name: _____

Office Address: _____

_____

Phone: _____

WHITE: Home Health   CANARY: Physician

FIGURE 8-4 Sample physician's order form for TPN example calculation on p. 190.

Lipids 20% in 125 mL

$0.20 \times 125 = 25$ g/L $\times$ TV/L $1.307 = 32.68$ g/bag

There are 32.68 g of lipids in 1307 mL of TPN.

Percentage of Concentration Per Bag

Formula: $\frac{\text{g/bag}}{\text{TV}} = \%/\text{bag}$

AA $\frac{55.5}{1307} = 0.04246 = 4.25\%$ of bag is AA (PRO)

Dextrose $\frac{326.6}{1307} = 0.2498 = 25\%$ dextrose (CHO)

Lipids $\frac{32.8}{1307} = 0.02509 = 2.5\%$ lipids (FAT)

Percentage of Additives

| **Formula:** | **Step 1** | **mEq/L × TV/L = mEq/bag** |
| | **Step 2** | **mEq/bag ÷ TV = % in bag** |

| **Shortcut method:** | mEq/L × TV/L ÷ TV = % in bag |

Calcium gluconate   5 mEq × 1.307 TV = 6.53 mEq/bag
                     6.53 ÷ 1307 = 0.00499 = 0.5% in bag

Magnesium sulfate   5 mEq × 1.307 = 6.53 ÷ 1307 = 0.5% in bag

Potassium phosphate 22 mEq × 1.307 = 28.75 ÷ 1307 = 2.2% in bag

Sodium chloride   35 mEq × 1.307 = 45.75 ÷ 1307 = 3.5% in bag

A milliequivalent (mEq) is a measurement of weight that represents 1000th of a gram.

mL/Hour to Set the Pump

$$\frac{\text{TV}}{\text{Total Time (hr)}} = \text{mL/hr} \quad \frac{1307}{12} = 109 \text{ mL/hr}$$

Kilocalories (Kcal) Per Bag

Formula: kcal/g × g/bag = kcal/bag

1 g CHO = 4 kcal   326.6 g × 4 kcal = 1306 kcal of CHO
1 g PRO = 4 kcal   55.5 g × 4 kcal = 222 kcal of PRO
1 g FAT = 9 kcal   32.68 g × 9 kcal = 294 kcal of FAT

Total kcal = 1822/bag of TPN

CLINICAL ALERT!

Begin TPN at a slow rate of 40 to 50 mL/hr and gradually increase by 25 mL/hr q6h to the ordered rate. Maintain a steady rate of infusion (within 10% of the ordered dose) to reduce the sudden onset of hyperglycemia.

■ Validation of TPN Label With Physician's Order

Validate the contents listed on the TPN bag label (Figure 8-5), with the physician's order (Figure 8-6).

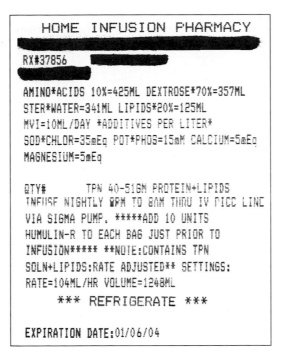

FIGURE 8-5
TPN bag label.

The 341 mL of qsad (quantity sufficient additive) sterile water includes the volume for the additives of calcium gluconate, magnesium sulfate, potassium phosphate, sodium chloride, and multivitamins. In this order, the pharmacist included all of the additives (except for the 10 units of insulin, which the nurse will add immediately before administration).

EXAMPLE   Refer to Figure 8-6, a sample physician's order form.

1. $\dfrac{\% \text{ of AA} \times \text{mL} = \text{g/L}}{0.10 \times 425 = 42.50 \text{ g/L}} \rightarrow \dfrac{\text{g/L} \times \text{TV/L} = \text{g/bag}}{42.50 \times 1.248 = 53 \text{ g/bag}}$

   $\dfrac{\text{g/bag} \div \text{TV} = \% \text{ of concentration/bag}}{53 \div 1248 = 4.25\% \text{ of concentration of AA/bag}}$

2. $\dfrac{\% \text{ of dextrose} \times \text{mL} = \text{g/L}}{0.70 \times 357 = 250 \text{ g/L}} \rightarrow \dfrac{\text{g/L} \times \text{TV/L} = \text{g/bag}}{250 \times 1.248 = 312 \text{ g/bag}}$

   $\dfrac{\text{g/bag} \div \text{TV} = \% \text{ of concentration/bag}}{312 \div 1248 = 25\% \text{ of concentration of dextrose (CHO)/bag}}$

3. $\dfrac{\% \text{ of lipids} \times \text{mL} = \text{g/L}}{0.20 \times 125 = 25 \text{ g/L}} \rightarrow \dfrac{\text{g/L} \times \text{TV/L} = \text{g/bag}}{25 \times 1.248 = 31.2 \text{ g/bag}}$

   $\dfrac{\text{g/bag} \div \text{TV} = \% \text{ of concentration/bag}}{31.2 \div 1248 = 2.5\% \text{ of concentration of lipids/bag}}$

TPN ORDER SHEET

HOME HEALTH		DATE
PATIENT	ADDRESS	

TPN FORMULA:

AMINO ACIDS: ☐ 5.5% ☐ 8.5% ☑ 10% ☐ WITH STANDARD ELECTROLYTES	*425*	ml
DEXTROSE: ☐ 10% ☐ 20% ☐ 40% ☐ 50% ☑ 70% (check one)	*357*	ml
LIPIDS: ☐ 10% ☑ 20% FOR ALL-IN-ONE FORMULA	*125*	ml

FINAL VOLUME qsad STERILE WATER FOR INJECTION	*400 mL*	*1248*	ml

Calcium Gluconate	0.465 mEq/ml	*5*	mEq
Magnesium Sulfate	4 mEq/ml	*5*	mEq
Potassium Acetate	2 mEq/ml		mEq
Potassium Chloride	2 mEq/ml		mEq
Potassium Phosphate	3 mM/ml	*15*	mM
Sodium Acetate	2 mEq/ml		mEq
Sodium Chloride	4 mEq/ml	*35*	mEq
Sodium Phosphate	3 mM/ml		mM
TRACE ELEMENTS CONCENTRATE	☐ 4 ☐ 5 ☐ 6		ml

Patient Additives:

☐ MVC 9 + 3 10 ml Daily

☐ HUMULIN-R *10* u DAILY

☐ FOLIC ACID _____ mg
_____ times weekly

☐ VITAMIN K _____ mg
_____ times weekly

☐ OTHER: *MVI 10 mL/daily*

☐ OTHER: _____

Directions:

INFUSE: ☐ DAILY

☐ _____ TIMES WEEKLY

OTHER DIRECTIONS:

_____

_____

_____

_____

Rate: ☐ CYCLIC INFUSION:
OVER _____ HOURS
(TAPER UP AND DOWN)

☐ CONTINUOUS INFUSION:
AT _____ ml PER HOUR

☑ STANDARD RATE:
AT *104* ml PER HOUR
FOR *12* HOURS

LAB ORDERS:

☐ STANDARD LAB ORDERS
SMAC-20, CO2, Mg+2 TWICE WEEKLY
CBC WITH AUTO DIFF WEEKLY
UNTIL STABLE, THEN:
SMAC-20, CO2, Mg+2 WEEKLY
CBC WITH AUTO DIFF MONTHLY

☐ OTHER: _____

_____

_____

VALIDATION:

_____
DOCTOR'S SIGNATURE

Print Name: _____

Office Address: _____

_____

Phone: _____

WHITE: Home Health   CANARY: Physician

FIGURE 8-6 Sample physician's order form and TPN example calculation on page 193.

Additives

$$mEq/L \times TV/L = mEq/bag$$
Calcium gluconate 5 mEq $\times$ 1.248 = 6.24 mEq/bag
Magnesium sulfate 5 mEq $\times$ 1.248 = 6.24 mEq/bag
Potassium phosphate 15 mEq $\times$ 1.248 = 18.72 mEq/bag
Sodium chloride 35 mEq $\times$ 1.248 = 43.68 mEq/bag

$$mEq/bag \div TV = \%/bag$$
6.24 $\div$ 1248 = 0.5%/bag
6.24 $\div$ 1248 = 0.5%/bag
18.72 $\div$ 1248 = 1.5%/bag
43.68 $\div$ 1248 = 3.5%/bag

Remember to add the 10 units of regular insulin.

Kilocalories

Formula: kcal/g $\times$ g/bag = kcal/bag
1 kcal of PRO = 4 g   53 g of PRO $\times$ 4 = 212 kcal
1 kcal of CHO = 4 g   312 g of CHO $\times$ 4 = 1248 kcal
1 kcal of FAT = 9 g   31.2 g of FAT $\times$ 9 = 281 kcal
Total kcal = 1739/bag of TPN

Nursing Considerations for TPN

- Patients receiving TPN must be monitored for hyperglycemia and serum potassium levels.
- TPN and lipid administration set should be changed every 24 hours.
- TPN and lipid solutions should be refrigerated at 39° F or 4° C until time of administration.
- TPN solutions should be filtered with a 0.22-micron filter.
- Fat emulsions filter should be a 1.2-micron size.

◀◀◀◀◀◀◀◀◀RULE   Always compare the order with the label to ensure correct percentage of nutritional elements.

CLINICAL ALERT!

The admixture of fat emulsions with the dextrose and amino acids may produce bacterial growth. Discard after 24 hours.

ANSWERS ON PAGE 377

WORKSHEET 8A Central Parenteral Nutrition Calculations

Use Figure 8-7 to answer the following:

1. What are the total grams per bag for:
   a. Amino acids (AA)
   b. Dextrose
   c. Lipids

2. What are the percentages of concentration per bag for:
   a. AA
   b. Dextrose
   c. Lipids

3. What are the percentages of concentration per bag for:
   a. Calcium gluconate
   b. Magnesium sulfate
   c. Potassium acetate
   d. Potassium phosphate
   e. Sodium chloride

4. How many kilocalories per bag for:
   a. CHO
   b. PRO
   c. FAT
   d. What is the total number of kilocalories per bag?

5. For how many mL/hr will you set the infusion device?

A sample MAR for parenteral nutrition is shown in Figure 8-11 on page 203.

TPN ORDER SHEET

HOME HEALTH	DATE

PATIENT	ADDRESS

TPN FORMULA:

AMIN0 ACIDS: ☑ 5.5% ☐ 8.5% ☐ 10% ☐ WITH STANDARD ELECTROLYTES	ml *400*	
DEXTROSE: ☑ 10% ☐ 20% ☐ 40% ☐ 50% ☐ 70% (check one)	ml *350*	
LIPIDS: ☑ 10% ☐ 20% FOR ALL-IN-ONE FORMULA	ml *200*	

FINAL VOLUME qsad STERILE WATER FOR INJECTION *400 mL*	*1350* ml

Calcium Gluconate	0.465 mEq/ml	*5*	mEq
Magnesium Sulfate	4 mEq/ml	*10*	mEq
Potassium Acetate	2 mEq/ml		mEq
Potassium Chloride	2 mEq/ml	*20*	mEq
Potassium Phosphate	3 mM/ml		mM
Sodium Acetate	2 mEq/ml		mEq
Sodium Chloride	4 mEq/ml	*30*	mEq
Sodium Phosphate	3 mM/ml		mM
TRACE ELEMENTS CONCENTRATE	☐ 4 ☐ 5 ☐ 6		ml

Patient Additives:

☐ MVC 9 + 3 10 ml Daily

☐ HUMULIN-R _____ u DAILY

☐ FOLIC ACID _____ mg
_____ times weekly

☐ VITAMIN K _____ mg
_____ times weekly

☐ OTHER: _____

☐ OTHER: _____

Directions:

INFUSE: ☐ DAILY

☐ _____ TIMES WEEKLY

OTHER DIRECTIONS:

_____

_____

_____

_____

Rate:	☐ CYCLIC INFUSION: OVER _____ HOURS (TAPER UP AND DOWN)	" " "	☐ CONTINUOUS INFUSION: AT _____ ml PER HOUR	" " "	☑ STANDARD RATE: AT _____ ml PER HOUR FOR _*12*_ HOURS

LAB ORDERS:

☐ STANDARD LAB ORDERS
SMAC-20, CO2, Mg+2 TWICE WEEKLY
CBC WITH AUTO DIFF WEEKLY
UNTIL STABLE, THEN:
SMAC-20, CO2, Mg+2 WEEKLY
CBC WITH AUTO DIFF MONTHLY

☐ OTHER: _____

_____

_____

VALIDATION:

_____

DOCTOR'S SIGNATURE

Print Name: _____

Office Address: _____

_____

Phone: _____

WHITE: Home Health   CANARY: Physician

FIGURE 8-7 Sample physician's order for Worksheet 8A.

ANSWERS ON PAGE 377

WORKSHEET
8B
Peripheral Parenteral Nutrition Calculations

Use Figure 8-8 to answer the following:

1. What are the total grams per bag for:
   a. Amino acids (AA)
   b. Dextrose
   c. Lipids

2. What are the percentages of concentration per bag for:
   a. AA
   b. Dextrose
   c. Lipids

3. What are the percentages of concentration per bag for:
   a. Calcium gluconate
   b. Magnesium sulfate
   c. Potassium chloride
   d. Sodium chloride

4. How many kilocalories per bag for:
   a. PRO
   b. CHO
   c. FAT
   d. What is the total number of kilocalories per bag?

5. For how many mL/hr will you set the infusion device?

TPN ORDER SHEET

HOME HEALTH	DATE
PATIENT	ADDRESS

TPN FORMULA:

AMINO ACIDS: ☐ 5.5% ☑ 8.5% ☐ 10% ☐ WITH STANDARD ELECTROLYTES	*500*	ml
DEXTROSE: ☐ 10% ☐ 20% ☐ 40% ☑ 50% ☐ 70% (check one)	*500*	ml
LIPIDS: ☑ 10% ☐ 20% FOR ALL-IN-ONE FORMULA	*250*	ml

FINAL VOLUME qsad STERILE WATER FOR INJECTION	*1500*	ml

Calcium Gluconate	0.465 mEq/ml	*5*	mEq
Magnesium Sulfate	4 mEq/ml	*15*	mEq
Potassium Acetate	2 mEq/ml	*8.3*	mEq
Potassium Chloride	2 mEq/ml		mEq
Potassium Phosphate	3 mM/ml	*35*	mM
Sodium Acetate	2 mEq/ml		mEq
Sodium Chloride	4 mEq/ml	*35*	mEq
Sodium Phosphate	3 mM/ml		mM
TRACE ELEMENTS CONCENTRATE	☐ 4 ☐ 5 ☐ 6		ml

Patient Additives:

☐ MVC 9 + 3 10 ml Daily

☐ HUMULIN-R *10* u DAILY

☐ FOLIC ACID _____ mg
    _____ times weekly

☐ VITAMIN K _____ mg
    _____ times weekly

☑ OTHER: *MVI 12 1.5mL/daily*

☐ OTHER: _____

Directions:

INFUSE: ☑ DAILY

          ☐ _____ TIMES WEEKLY

OTHER DIRECTIONS:

_____

_____

_____

_____

Rate:	☐ CYCLIC INFUSION: OVER *12* HOURS (TAPER UP AND DOWN)	"	☐ CONTINUOUS INFUSION: AT _____ ml PER HOUR	"	☑ STANDARD RATE: AT _____ ml PER HOUR FOR *12* HOURS	

LAB ORDERS:

☑ STANDARD LAB ORDERS
SMAC-20, CO2, Mg+2 TWICE WEEKLY
CBC WITH AUTO DIFF WEEKLY
UNTIL STABLE, THEN:
SMAC-20, CO2, Mg+2 WEEKLY
CBC WITH AUTO DIFF MONTHLY

☐ OTHER: _____
_____
_____

VALIDATION:

_____

DOCTOR'S SIGNATURE

Print Name: _____

Office Address: _____

_____

Phone: _____

WHITE: Home Health   CANARY: Physician

FIGURE 8-8 Sample physician's order form for Worksheet 8B.

ANSWERS ON PAGE 378

WORKSHEET 8C
Central Parenteral Nutrition Calculations

Refer to Figure 8-9 to answer the following questions. Use the formulas on pages 190-192.

1. Total grams per bag
   a. How many total grams of amino acids (AA) per bag?
   b. How many total grams of dextrose per bag?

2. Percentage of concentrations per bag
   a. What is the percentage of amino acids per bag?
   b. What is the percentage of dextrose per bag?

3. Percentage of additives per bag
   a. Sodium chloride
   b. Potassium phosphate
   c. Potassium chloride
   d. Magnesium sulfate
   e. Calcium gluconate

4. Kilocalories per bag
   a. AA
   b. CHO
   c. Total kcal

5. How many hours will it take for the parenteral nutrition bag to be infused?

Amino Acid 10%	**(900 ML)**
Dextrose 70%	**(430 ML)**
Sterile Water For Injection	**(70 ML)**
Sodium Chloride Conc 140 MEQ	**(35 ML)**
Potassium Phosphate 41 MEQ	**(9.318 ML)**
Potassium Chloride 43 MEQ	**(21.5 ML)**
Magnesium Sulfate 7 MEQ	**(1.75 ML)**
Calcium Gluconate 7 MEQ	**(14.98 ML)**
Insulin Humulin Regular 20 U	**(0.2 ML)**
Infuvite Multivitamin A 10 ML	**(10 ML)**

Total: 1492.748

** Continued **

DO NOT START AFTER 24 HOURS

Rate: 55 ml/hr   Freq: Q24H
Modified Central TPN
Hang Date/Time: 1800 11/19/02
Expir:
Init: DF
Refrigerate
Prep. By: /_____

DO NOT START AFTER 24 HOURS

FIGURE 8-9 Sample CPN label for Worksheet 8C. Notice that the three-in-one formula with lipids is not used. The time to hang the CPN is 1800 hours.

ANSWERS ON PAGE 379

WORKSHEET
8D

Peripheral Parenteral Nutrition Calculations

Refer to Figure 8-10 to answer the following questions. Use the formulas on pages 190-192.

1. Total grams per bag
  a. Amino acids
  b. Dextrose

2. Percentage of concentrations per bag
  a. Amino acids
  b. Dextrose

3. Percentage of additives per bag
  a. Sodium chloride
  b. Potassium phosphate
  c. Potassium acetate
  d. Calcium gluconate
  e. Magnesium sulfate

4. Kilocalories per bag
  a. AA
  b. CHO
  c. Total kcal

5. How many hours will it take to be infused?

Amino Acid 8% (Hepatic)	(600 ML)
Dextrose 20%	(600 ML)
Sodium Chloride Conc 42 MEQ	(10.5 ML)
Potassium Phosphate 26 MEQ	(6.909 ML)
Potassium Acetate 10 MEQ	(5 ML)
Calcium Gluconate 6 MEQ	(12.84 ML)
Magnesium Sulfate 6 MEQ	(1.5 ML)
Infuvite Multivitamin A 10 ML	(10 ML)
Insulin Humulin Regular 24 U	(0.24 ML)

Total: 1245.989

** Continued **

DO NOT START AFTER 24 HOURS

Rate: 50 ml/hr   Freq: Q24H
Peripheral

Hang Date/Time: 1800 11/19/02
Expir:
Init: MM

Prep. By: /_____

DO NOT START AFTER 24 HOURS

FIGURE 8-10 Sample PCN label for Worksheet 8D.
Peripheral central line is to be infused at 1800 hours.

ANSWERS ON PAGE 380

WORKSHEET

8E **Multiple-Choice Practice**

1. Have: CPN solution with 8.5% AA in 375 mL. The total volume (TV) is 1500 mL. How many grams of protein are in the solution?
   a. 50 g/bag   **b.** 77.7 g/bag   **c.** 62 g/bag   **d.** 47.8 g/bag

2. What is the percentage of concentration of grams per bag of the AA in question 1?
   a. 4.6%   **b.** 3%   **c.** 8.2%   **d.** 4.7%

3. Have: CPN solution with 40% dextrose in 400 mL. The TV is 1450. How many grams of dextrose are in the solution?
   a. 232 g/bag   **b.** 130 g/bag   **c.** 160 g/bag   **d.** 260 g/bag

4. What is the percentage of concentration per bag for dextrose in question 3?
   a. 18%   **b.** 16%   **c.** 160%   **d.** 180%

5. Have: A three-in-one TPN solution with 20% lipids in 175 mL. The TV is 1200 mL. How many grams of lipids are in the solution?
   a. 42 g/bag   **b.** 48 g/bag   **c.** 52 g/bag   **d.** 36 g/bag

6. What is the percentage of concentration of grams per bag for lipids in question 5?
   a. 2.7%   **b.** 3.5%   **c.** 5.6%   **d.** 7%

7. Have: Calcium gluconate additive of 6 mEq/L. The TV of the TPN is 1350 mL. What is the percentage of calcium gluconate in the bag?
   a. 0.3%   **b.** 1%   **c.** 0.4%   **d.** 0.6%

8. Have: Magnesium sulfate additive 10 mEq/L. The TV is 1258 mL. What is the percentage of magnesium sulfate in the bag?
   a. 1%   **b.** 10.2%   **c.** 1.8%   **d.** 11%

9. Have: Potassium acetate 12 mEq/L. The TV is 1385 mL. What is the percentage of potassium acetate in the bag?
   a. 2.2%   **b.** 3.6%   **c.** 1.2%   **d.** 2.6%

10. The TV of the parenteral nutrition (PN) solution is 1275 mL. The infusion rate is 110 mL/hr. The infusion is started at 1800 hr. What time will it be completed?
    a. 0659 hr   **b.** 0459 hr   **c.** 0535 hr   **d.** 0345 hr

Acct: Admitted: Att Phys: Diagnosis: Allergies:			MR#: Age: HT: WT:			M A R	MEDICATION AMINISTRATION RECORD

Page:3
From:10/10/02 0730
Thru:10/11/02 0730

Start Date/Time	Stop Date/Time	RN/ LPN	Medication		0731-1530	1531-2330	2331-0730
10/05 1800	11/04 1759		.PICC Line Flush FLush Q12H IV Flush PICC Q 12 HRS with NS 10 ML when PICC line used for TPN	(1 Inject) #022		1800	0600
10/09 1800	11/08 1759		Amino Acid 8.5% 600 ML Dextrose 50% 600 ML Sodium Chloride CO 58 MEQ Potassium Acetate 12 MEQ Magnesium Sulfate 6 MEQ	(600 ML) (600 ML) (14.5 ML) (6 ML) (1.5 ML)		1800	
			Calcium Gluconate 8 MEQ Infuvlte Multivitamin 10 ML Trace Elements 1 ML Sodium Phosphate 26 MEQ Insulin Humulin Regu 21 U	(12.84 ML) (10 ML) (1 ML) (6.5 ML) (0.21 ML)			
			50 ML/HR Q24H IV Central	#047			
			Store in Refrigerator				

The preprinted MAR from the pharmacy shows the contents of the TPN, the time it is to
be started and the times and amount of NS to be used to flush the Central and PICC Lines.
The nurse will initial next to the pre-printed time as well as initial and sign the bottom of
the MAR. The MAR is for 24 hours only.

Order Date	RN INIT.	Date/Time To Be Given	One Time Orders and Pre-Operatives Medication-Dose-Route	Actual Time Given	Site Codes			Dose Omission Code
					Arm	LA	RA	A = pt absent
					Deltoid	LD	RD	H = hold
					Ventrogluteal	LVG	RVG	M = med absent
					Gluteal	LG	RG	N = NPO
					Abdomen	LUQ	RUQ	O = other
					Abdomen	LLQ	RLQ	R = refused
								U = unable to tolerate

INIT	Signature	INIT	Signature

60321 (8/98)A   CHART

FIGURE 8-11 Sample medication administration record (MAR).

▨ CRITICAL THINKING EXERCISES

Your patient, Mary Braun, is receiving peripheral parenteral nutrition (PPN). On assessment, she complains that the IV site burns. When the site is checked, the solution is infusing well and infusing at the correct rate. The label on the solution is 8.5% amino acids and 70% dextrose. When you check the original order, it specifies 5.5% amino acids and 10% dextrose.

- ■ Error:
- ■ Causes of error:
- ■ Nursing interventions:
- ■ Preventive measures:

Discussion
What will your first action be?
Why are the percentages of amino acids and dextrose important?
What is the percentage difference?

ANSWERS ON PAGE 380

CHAPTER 8 FINAL

Calculate and solve the following problems using a calculator, moving decimals, reducing ratios, and labeling your answers. Prove your work.*

1. A TPN order reads amino acids 8.5% in 550 mL. The total volume of the TPN infusion is 1430 mL.
   a. How many grams of AA will the patient receive through the central line?
   b. How many kilocalories of protein will the patient receive?

2. A TPN order reads dextrose 10% in 475 mL.
   a. How many grams of dextrose will be infused?
   The total volume is 1550 mL in the peripheral line.
   b. How many kilocalories of dextrose will the patient receive?

3. A PPN order reads: Amino acids 5% in 350 mL. The TV is 1280 mL.
   a. How many grams of AA will the patient receive?
   b. How many kilocalories of protein will the patient receive?

4. The TPN order reads: Dextrose 40% in 400 mL. The TV is 1325 mL.
   a. How many grams of dextrose will the patient receive?
   b. How many kilocalories of carbohydrate will the patient receive?

5. The TPN formula has potassium chloride 4 mEq. The TV is 1250 mL.
   What is the percentage of potassium chloride in the bag?

6. The parenteral nutrition formula has 25 mEq of sodium chloride (NaCl). The TV of the bag is 1425 mL.
   What is the percentage of NaCl in the bag?

7. A TPN solution has 48 g of protein, 255 g of carbohydrate, and 38.6 g of fat.
   How many total kilocalories will the patient receive?

8. A three-in-one TPN solution has lipids 20% in 110 mL. The TV is 1145 mL.
   a. How many grams of lipids will the patient receive?
   b. How many kilocalories of fat will the patient receive?

9. The TPN of 1420 mL is to start at 1800 hr. The rate is 108 mL/hr.
   What time will the infusion be completed?

10. A TPN of 1320 mL is infusing at 120 mL/hr.
    How many hours will it take to infuse?

*It may be acceptable to withdraw small amounts of large-volume IV solutions equal to the amount of milliliters of drug to be added to simplify calculations and flow rates. Follow your institution's policy.

Insulin 9

- Identify sites for insulin injections.
- Identify the different types of insulin.
- Compare the actions of fast-, intermediate-, and long-acting insulins.
- Read calibrations on 30-, 50-, and 100-unit insulin syringes.
- Prepare single- and mixed-dose insulin injections.
- Interpret the sliding scale using the BMBG method.
- Calculate IV insulin for U/hr and mL/hr and duration.
- Understand insulin pumps.
- Analyze medication errors using critical thinking.

INTRODUCTION

The importance of measuring the correct amount of insulin is stressed. Different types of insulin syringes are shown for the practice of selecting the most appropriate syringe for the ordered dose. Mixing two types of insulin is shown in drawings. The Bedside Monitor Blood Glucose (BMBG) flow sheet shows how to use the sliding scale to chart hourly insulin needs. IV infusions are calculated for units per hour based on the BMBG level.

● INSULIN

Insulin is an aqueous solution of the principal hormone of the pancreas. Insulin affects metabolism by allowing glucose to leave the blood and enter the body cells, preventing hyperglycemia.

● DIABETES MELLITUS

Diabetes mellitus is a deficiency of insulin and is classified according to etiology. Type 1, which has an onset usually before the age of 30 years, occurs when the pancreatic beta cells do not produce insulin. Insulin injections must be taken every day to control blood glucose levels.

The onset of type 2 diabetes usually occurs after 30 years of age. The pancreas produces *some* insulin but not enough to metabolize the glucose. In some cases, the insulin that is produced is not effective, which is known as *insulin resistance*. Ninety-five percent of people with diabetes are type 2, and 40% of type 2 people with diabetes take insulin injections in conjunction with oral diabetes medications.

The most common complication of insulin therapy is hypoglycemia. This may be caused by injecting too much insulin (a risk in home care), missed or delayed meals, or more physical activity than usual. To treat hypoglycemia, the patient should always carry sugar in some form. The treatment of choice, if the patient can swallow, is glucose tablets (5 g CHO per tablet). If the blood glucose level gets very low, unconsciousness may occur. At that point, the patient will need a glucagon injection. Emergency kits are available for home use (Figure 9-1).

FIGURE 9-1
Glucagon emergency kit for home use. *(From Eli Lilly and Company, Indianapolis, IN.)*

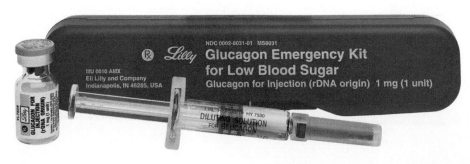

● INJECTION SITES

The abdomen is the preferred site for insulin injections. When insulin injections are required on a daily basis, it is important to rotate within that site (Figure 9-2). The abdomen absorbs insulin more rapidly and is safer as an injection site than the upper arm, back, or thigh. If use of the abdomen is medically contraindicated, alternate sites may be used.

● TYPES OF INSULIN

The source of insulin is either human or animal. This is known as the *species* of the insulin. Human insulin is manufactured to be the same as insulin produced by the body. Human insulin is made in one of two ways:

- Recombinant DNA technology, a chemical process used to produce unlimited amounts of human insulin
- A process that chemically changes pork insulin to make human insulin

Humalog insulin (lispro) is another recombinant DNA insulin with a rapid action of 15 minutes, allowing patients to dose and eat.

Insulin made from pork is seldom used. Recombinant DNA insulins, Lantus (glargine) cause fewer allergies than those from animal sources. Beef insulin is no longer available.

All insulin is supplied in units denoting strength. Insulin is given with special insulin syringes (Figure 9-3) and pens (Figure 9-4). Figure 9-5 shows examples of the different types of cartridges used with insulin pens.

Insulin is supplied in 10 mL vials labeled U-100, which means there are 100 units/mL (Figure 9-5). Insulin is also supplied in 10 mL vials of U 500, which means there are 500 units/mL. This strength is used for those whose blood glucose fluctuates to very high levels. This type of insulin is rarely used. Table 9-1 lists the duration of activity of different types of insulins. See examples of various U-100 insulins on pages 210 and 211.

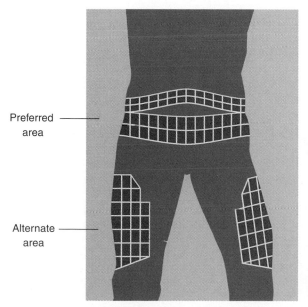
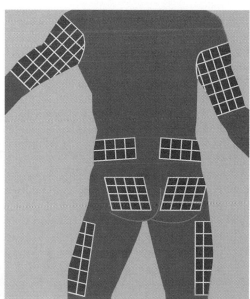

Preferred area

Alternate area

Alternate areas

FIGURE 9-2 Insulin injection areas. *(From Eli Lilly and Company, Indianapolis, IN.)*

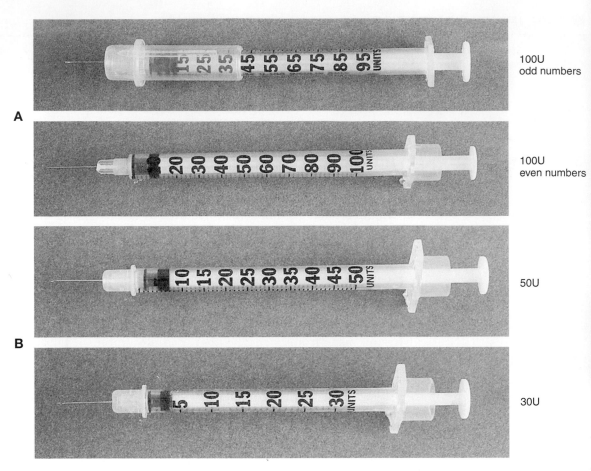

FIGURE 9-3 Insulin syringes. **A,** 100-unit syringes with odd and even numbers. **B,** 50-unit and 30-unit syringes. *(From Becton, Dickinson and Company, Franklin Lakes, NJ.)*

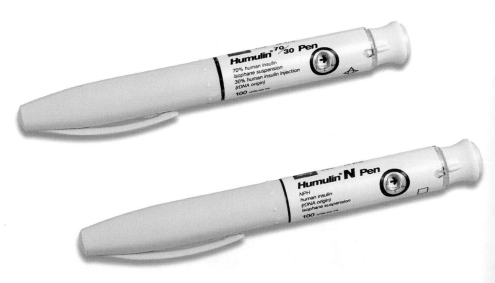

FIGURE 9-4 Insulin pens. *(From Eli Lilly and Company, Indianapolis, IN.)*

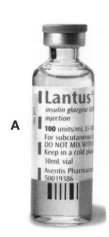
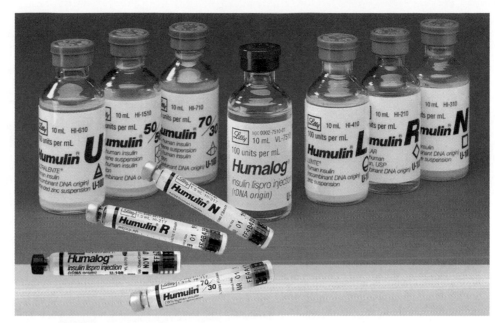

FIGURE 9-5 A, Lantus (insulin glargine). The Lantus vial is taller and narrower than the NPH, Lente, Regular, and Humalog vials. Lantus is written in purple letters. *(From Aventis Pharmaceuticals Inc., Bridgewater, NJ.)* **B,** Insulin vials and cartridges used in insulin pens. *(From Eli Lilly and Company, Indianapolis, IN.)*

Table 9-1 Insulin Chart

Type	Onset	Peak	Effective Duration	Maximum Duration
RAPID ACTING:				
• Humalog (lispro)	Within 15 minutes	0.5-1.5 hours	3-4 hours	4-6 hours
• Novolog (aspart)*	Within 15 minutes	1-3 hours		
SHORT ACTING:				
• Regular (R)	$1/2$-1 hour	2-3 hours	3-6 hours	6-8 hours
INTERMEDIATE-ACTING:				
• NPH (N)	2-4 hours	6-10 hours	10-16 hours	14-18 hours
• Lente (L)	3-4 hours	6-12 hours	12-18 hours	16-20 hours
LONG ACTING:				
• Ultralente (U)	6-10 hours	10-16 hours	18-20 hours	20-24 hours
• Glargine (lantus)	2 hours	Peakless	24 hours	24 hours
FIXED COMBINATIONS OF N AND R				
• 70/30 = 70% N and 30% R	$1/2$-1 hour	Dual	10-16 hours	14-18 hours
• 50/50 = 50% N and 50% R	$1/2$-1 hour	Dual	10-16 hours	14-18 hours
FIXED COMBINATION OF NEUTRAL PROTAMINE LISPRO AND LISPRO				
• 75/25 = 75% NPL and 25% lispro	Within 15 minutes	1-6.5 hours (average 2.6 hours)	Refer to N and lispro	Refer to N and lispro

Note: Unopened vials are good through the expiration date and should be stored in the refrigerator. Opened insulin vials are good for 30 days after opening. Lantus is good for 28 days.

References: PDR; Package inserts; Campbell RK, White JR: *Medications for the treatment of diabetes,* ed 3, Alexandria, VA, 2000, American Diabetes Association; Lebovitz HE. *Therapy for diabetes and related disorders,* ed 3, Alexandria, VA, 1998, American Diabetes Association.
This sheet is designed as a medication overview. Please refer to the packaging insert for complete drug information.
*FDA approved, anticipate prescribing availability 2001.
(From American Healthways, Nashville, TN.)

TYPES OF U-100 INSULINS

Fast-Acting

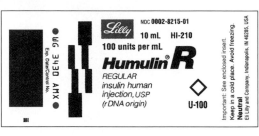

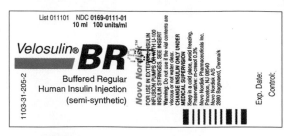

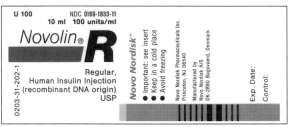

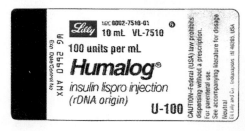

CLINICAL ALERT!

Regular insulin should always be clear. Discard if unclear.

Only mix insulins with the same name because there may be differing amounts of preservatives. For example, Humulin R should only be combined with Humulin L or N.

Intermediate-Acting

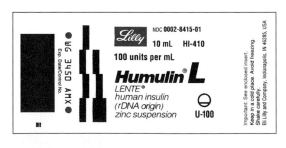

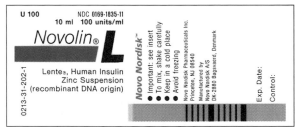

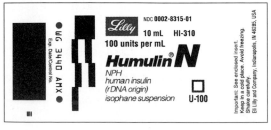

● Intermediate- and Fast-Acting Mixtures

The insulin combination of NPH and Regular is used to give a 24-hour effect.

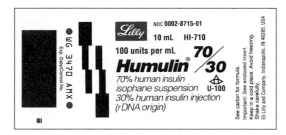

In 1 mL of Humulin 70/30, there are 70 units of intermediate-acting insulin and 30 units of fast-acting insulin. In 1 mL of Humulin 50/50, there are 50 units of intermediate-acting insulin and 50 units of fast-acting insulin.

Note: Mix before administration by rolling gently between the palms.

CLINICAL ALERT!

Insulin comes in various strengths (e.g., U-100 and U-500). Read labels carefully to avoid giving the wrong strength.

● Long-Acting

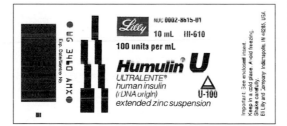

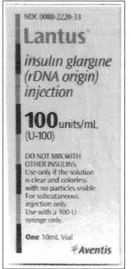

CLINICAL ALERT!

Lantus must NOT be mixed in the same syringe with any other insulin or be diluted. It is NOT intended for IV administration. Caution: Lantus is clear like Regular Humalog. Lantus is given at bedtime for 24-hour coverage without a peak.

● INSULIN SYRINGES

Insulin is usually given in a 1 mL or 0.5 mL insulin syringe calibrated to U-100 insulin. The 0.5 mL insulin syringe is used for smaller doses because the calibrations are larger and easier to read. The most commonly used insulin syringes are 50 and 100 unit syringes, as shown in Figure 9-3.

● Types of U-100 Insulin Syringes

Each calibration in the syringe shown in Figure 9-6 represents 1 unit. This syringe is used for small doses of 50 units or less and is used with U-100 insulin only.

FIGURE 9-6
50-unit syringe.

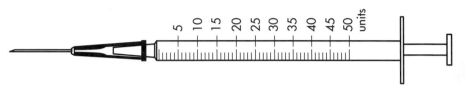

Each calibration in the syringe shown in Figure 9-7 equals 2 units. This syringe is for use with U-100 insulin only.

FIGURE 9-7
100-unit syringe.

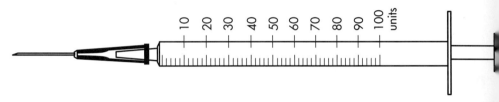

Each calibration in the syringe shown in Figure 9-8 represents 1 unit. This syringe is used for small doses of 30 units or less as a safety feature for people with diabetes who have vision problems or for children who require small doses of insulin. This syringe is for use with U-100 insulin only.

FIGURE 9-8
30-unit syringe.

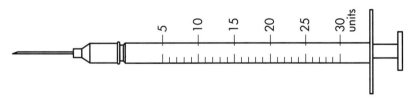

● INSULIN ORDERS

A typical order for insulin must include the following:
    A. The *name* of insulin: Humulin, Novolin, Lantus.
    B. The *type* of the insulin: regular, lispro, Lente, NPH, Ultra Lente, or Glargine.
    C. The *number* of units or amount the patient will receive. 10 units.
    D. The *time* to be given: AM, $\frac{1}{2}$ hr ac.
    E. The *route* is subcutaneous unless IV is specified.

EXAMPLE Give 30 units of U-100 Humulin R insulin sc $\frac{1}{2}$ hr ac. Using a U-100 syringe, fill the syringe to the 30 units calibration (Figure 9-9).

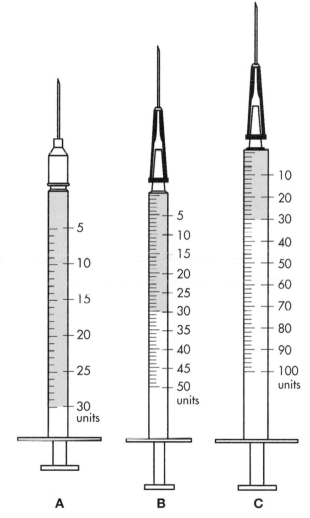

FIGURE 9-9
Comparison of 30 units in different size insulin syringes. **A,** 30-unit syringe filled to 30 units. **B,** 50-unit syringe filled to 30 units. **C,** 100-unit syringe filled to 30 units.

CLINICAL ALERT!

Units must be spelled out (not abbreviated "U") because this can be a source of medication errors (i.e., mistaking the "U" for a zero).

ANSWERS ON PAGE 381

WORKSHEET

9A   **Single-Dose Measures**

Read the syringes and write your answer in the space provided.

1. Units measured: _____

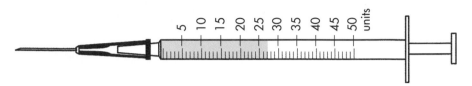

2. Units measured: _____

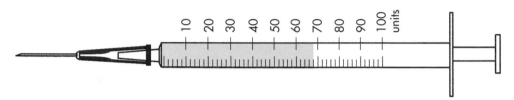

3. Units measured: _____

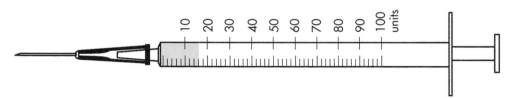

4. Units measured: _____

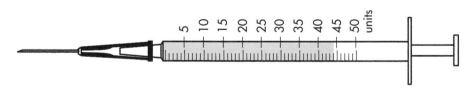

5. Units measured: _____

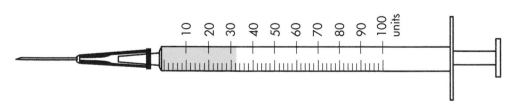

ANSWERS ON PAGE 381

WORKSHEET
9A Single-Dose Measures—cont'd

6. Units measured: _____

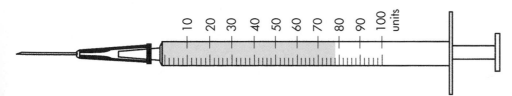

7. Units measured: _____

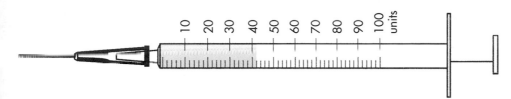

8. Units measured: _____

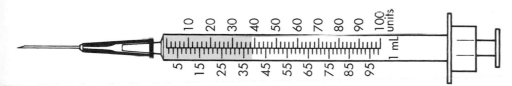

9. Units measured: _____

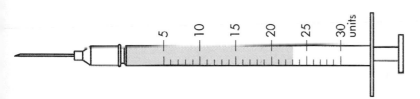

10. Units measured: _____

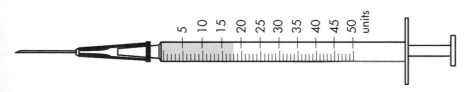

ANSWERS ON PAGE 381

WORKSHEET 9B

Additional Practice in Single-Dose Measures

Circle the letter of the syringe with the *correct* ordered amount.

1. Ordered: 28 units of Novolin Regular SC 30 min ac.

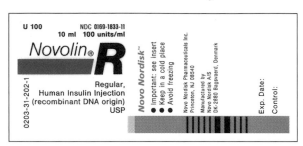

a.

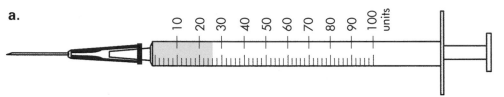

b.

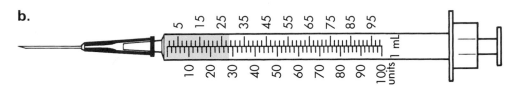

2. Ordered: 57 units of Humulin Regular SC $\frac{1}{2}$ hr ac.

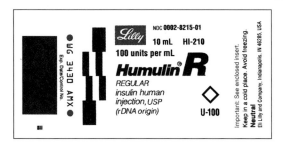

a.

b.

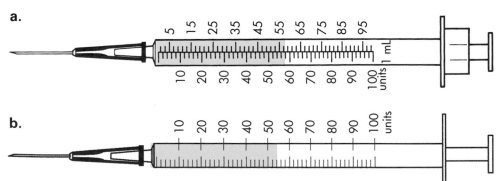

ANSWERS ON PAGE 381

WORKSHEET 9B — Additional Practice in Single-Dose Measures—cont'd

3. Ordered: 13 units of Humulin NPH SC at 11:00 AM.

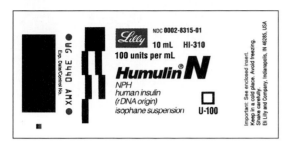

a.

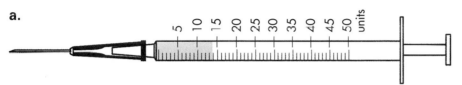

b.

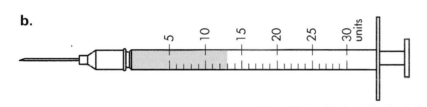

4. Ordered: 12 units of Humulin Ultra Lente SC at 0900.

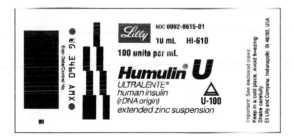

a.

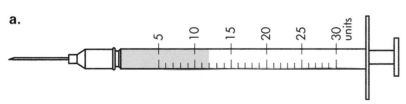

b.

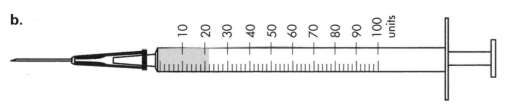

Continued

ANSWERS ON PAGE 381

WORKSHEET 9B

Additional Practice in Single-Dose Measures—cont'd

5. Ordered: 62 units of Humulin Lente SC at 0930.

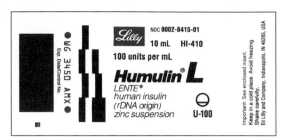

a.

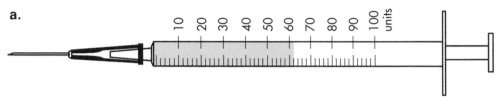

b.

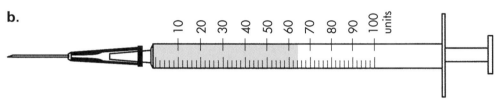

● MIXING INSULIN

Insulin dosages are drawn up *exactly* as ordered. An incorrect dosage could be devastating to the patient. Frequently, regular or fast-acting insulin is combined with an intermediate-acting insulin. This gives insulin coverage (glucose control) within 15 to 20 minutes and lasts 14 to 20 hours. This technique of combining the two types of insulin is important for the nurse, patient, and family to master. The regular insulin vial should *not* be contaminated with the longer-acting insulin; therefore the regular insulin should be drawn up first. The mixing procedure is illustrated in Figures 9-10 and 9-11.

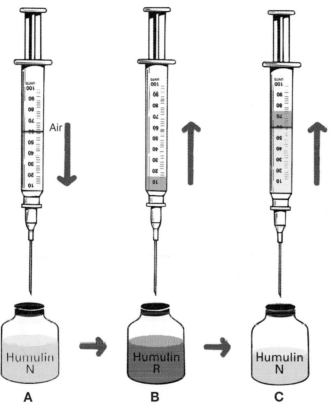

FIGURE 9-10
A, Inject 60 units of air into Humulin N first. Do not allow needle to touch insulin. Withdraw needle.
B, Inject 15 units of air into Humlin R and withdraw 15 units. Withdraw needle.
C, Insert needle into vial of Humulin N and withdraw 60 units. Total equals 75 units.

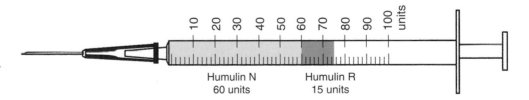

FIGURE 9-11
100-unit syringe showing the mixing of two insulins. Remember: clear to cloudy when drawing up insulins.

Humulin N
60 units

Humulin R
15 units

EXAMPLE   Ordered: 15 units of Humulin Regular and 60 units of Humulin NPH.

EXAMPLE Ordered: 10 units of Novolin Regular and 20 units of Novolin Lente. (Use U-100 strength.)
Total units: 30 units
Source: DNA and DNA
Which insulin will you draw up first? *Regular* (see Figure 9-10)

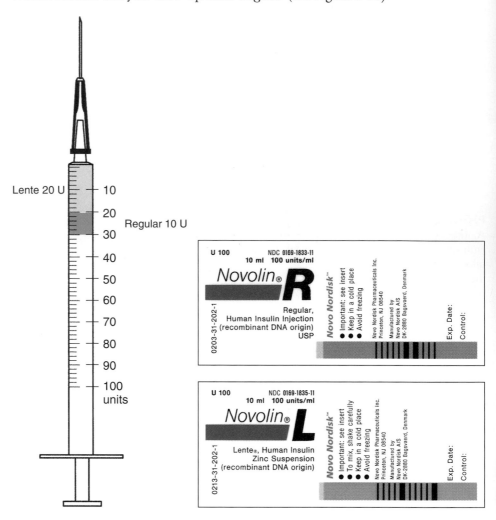

Lente 20 U

Regular 10 U

| 10 |
| 20 |
| 30 |
| 40 |
| 50 |
| 60 |
| 70 |
| 80 |
| 90 |
| 100 units |

U 100   NDC 0169-1833-11
10 ml   100 units/ml

Novolin® **R**

Regular,
Human Insulin Injection
(recombinant DNA origin)
USP

0203-31-202-1

Novo Nordisk™
● Important: see insert
● ● Keep in a cold place
● ● Avoid freezing

Novo Nordisk Pharmaceuticals Inc.
Princeton, NJ 08540
Manufactured by
Novo Nordisk A/S
DK-2880 Bagsvaerd, Denmark

Exp. Date:
Control:

U 100   NDC 0169-1835-11
10 ml   100 units/ml

Novolin® **L**

Lente®, Human Insulin
Zinc Suspension
(recombinant DNA origin)

0213-31-202-1

Novo Nordisk™
● Important: see insert
● ● To mix, shake carefully
● ● Keep in a cold place
● ● Avoid freezing

Novo Nordisk Pharmaceuticals Inc.
Princeton, NJ 08540
Manufactured by
Novo Nordisk A/S
DK-2880 Bagsvaerd, Denmark

Exp. Date:
Control:

Insulin will not stay separated as pictured in the syringe.

CLINICAL ALERT!

Draw up regular insulin first before NPH is added (see Figure 9-10).

Regular insulin should not be contaminated with Humulin NPH or any NPH insulin. A multiple-dose vial of regular insulin can be used for IV infusion, and contamination with intermediate-acting insulin could be fatal.

ANSWERS ON PAGE 381

WORKSHEET
9C   Mixing Insulin

Calculate the total number of units in the following problems. (All problems use U-100 strength.) Circle the letter of the syringe with the correct amount.

1. Ordered: 20 units of Humulin R and 38 units Humulin L $\frac{1}{2}$ hr ac breakfast. Total units: _____

a.

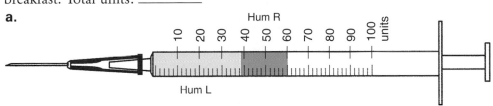

b.

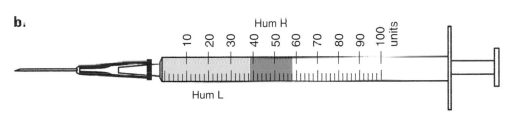

2. Ordered: Humulin R 18 units and Humulin N 25 units. Total units:

a.

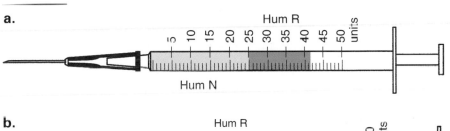

b.

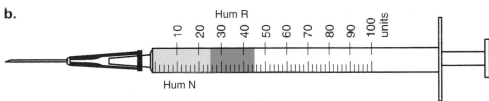

3. Ordered: Novolin R 8 units and Novolin L 15 units. Total units:

a.

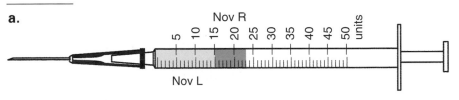

b.

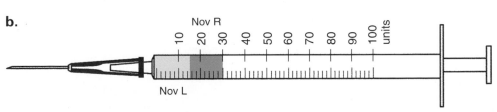

Continued

ANSWERS ON PAGE 381

WORKSHEET
9C Mixing Insulin–cont'd

4. Ordered: Novolin Regular 22 units and Novolin Lente 30 units. Total units: _____

a.

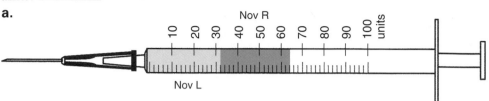

b.

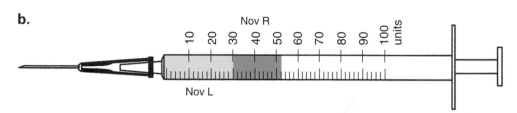

5. Ordered: Humulin Regular insulin 8 units and Humulin NPH 60 units $\frac{1}{2}$ hr ac breakfast. Total units: _____

a.

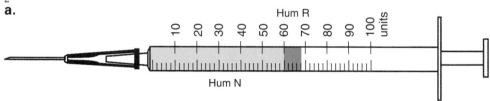

b.

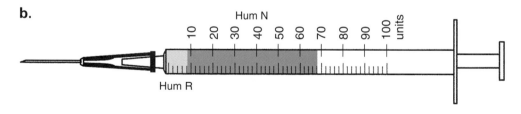

ANSWERS ON PAGE 381

WORKSHEET
9C   Mixing Insulin–cont'd

Shade in insulin dose on syringe. All orders are for U-100 insulin.

6. Ordered: 35 units of Humalog insulin at 0830 ac. Available: Humalog insulin U-100. How many units will you administer? When will it peak?

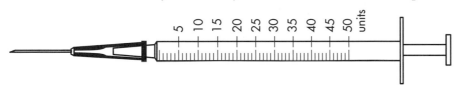

7. Ordered: 20 units of Humalog insulin ac tid. Available: Humalog insulin U-100. How many units will you give? When will the action begin (onset)?

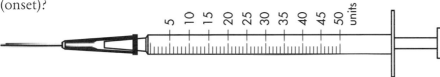

8. Ordered: Humulin 70/30 44 units qd. Available: Humulin 70/30. How many units will you give? When will it peak? What is the duration?

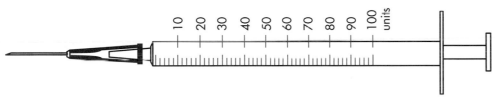

9. Ordered: Humulin Regular 20 units and Humulin Lente 40 units SC every AM $\frac{1}{2}$ ac. How many total units will you give? What is the duration?

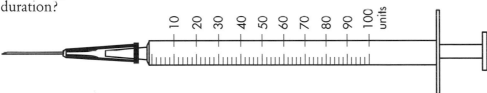

10. Ordered: Humulin Regular insulin 30 units and Humulin NPH 30 units qAM ac. How many total units will you give? When will this peak? What is the duration?

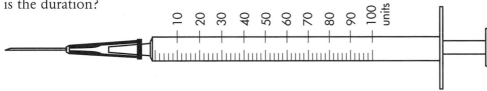

● SLIDING SCALE CALCULATIONS

Insulin administered according to a sliding scale is predicated on the type of diabetes, insulin resistance, weight, age, renal status, and activity level. Blood glucose levels indicate how much insulin to give. Blood glucose readings may be taken several times a day to determine daily insulin requirements. Sliding scales can vary greatly as they are individualized.

EXAMPLE   Ordered: Regular insulin q6h to follow the sliding scale.

Sliding Scale   Blood glucose level

0–100	No Coverage
100–150	2 units
151–200	4 units
201–250	6 units
251–300	8 units

For a blood glucose above 425, give 15 units regular insulin stat and call physician. Repeat blood glucose measurement 4 hr after it peaks.

At 1700 hr, the patient's blood glucose level was 280 mg/dl. How much insulin should be given? Shade the amount in the syringe.

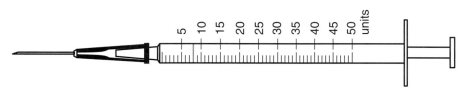

The MAR in Figure 9-12 is a typical example of how insulin is recorded.

Normal Blood Glucose M 75-110 F 65-105

JOHN DOE

BLOOD GLUCOSE FLOW SHEET—Bedside Monitoring Blood Glucose (BMBG)
****** Document all scheduled and sliding scale insulins on this sheet ******

Time → Date	Breakfast (BMBG)						Lunch (BMBG)						Dinner (BMBG)						HS (BMBG)						Total Daily Dose
Date	Time	BG Insulin	Time	BG TX	Init.		Time	BG Insulin	Time	BG TX	Init.		Time	BG Insulin	Time	BG TX	Init.		Time	BG Insulin	Time	BG TX	Init.		TDD
12/4/02	0700	247					1130	112					1700	140			AR		2100	180			AR		34 Unit
	0700	104 / 6R	0715	84	AR		1140	2R			AR		1700	10 N / 2R			AR		2105	4R					
12/5/02	0700	60	0720	10 N			1130	120			AR		1730	160			AF		2100	96			JB		26 Unit
	0700	3 Gluc Tabs					1145	2R					1740	10 N / 4R						0					
12/6/02	0715	114				JB		1130	106	1530	47		JB		1545	84	1700	26	AR		2100	140			JB		26 Unit
	0730	10 N / 2R						1135	2R	1530	3 Gluc Tabs				1715	0	1715	10 N			2110	2R				

In tials	Signature
AR	Ariel Rider RN
JB	Joren Barton LPN

Insulin Type	Onset	Peak	Effective Duration
H = Rapid acting - Humanlog/Novolog (lispo, aspart)	within 10-20 min	0.5-1.5 hours	3-4 hours
R = Short Acting - Regular	0.5-1 hour	2-3 hours	3-6 hours
N = Intermed Acting - NPH	2-4 hours	6-10 hours	10-16 hours
L = Intermed Acting - Lente	3-4 hours	6-12 hours	12-18 hours
U = Long Acting - Ultralente	6-10 hours	10-16 hours	18-20 hours
G = Long Acting - Glargine (Lantus)	2 hours	Peakless	24 hours
70/30 = 70% N/30% R	0.5-1 hour	Dual	14-18 hours
50/50 = 50% N/50% R	0.5-1 hour	Dual	14-18 hours

A = **abdomen** is the preferred site for all injections unless otherwise indicated. If another site is used, please document.

FIGURE 9-12 Insulin is given SC according to the blood glucose levels. The sliding scale on page 224 is used to determine the amount of insulin to give. (*From Scottsdale Healthcare, Scottsdale, AZ.*)

● INTRAVENOUS INSULIN

During acute phases of illness, regular insulin is given by the IV route to ensure a controlled supply of medication that will vary depending on laboratory monitoring. A piggyback infusion is always administered with an IV controlled infusion device. Discard the first 2 to 3 mL of combined infusion through IV tubing to prevent the insulin from binding to the tubing.

◐◀◀◀◀◀◀◀◀RULE   Begin the problem with known amount of medication in the total solution.

The pharmacy standard insulin drip: 100 units Human Regular in 100 mL of NS.

EXAMPLE   Ordered: Regular human insulin 5 units/hr IV drip. Pharmacy has delivered 100 mL 0.9% NS with 100 U of regular human insulin.
- How many mL/hr will infuse 5 U/hr?
- How many hours will the IV infuse?

	Know	*Want to Know*	**PROOF**
Step 1:	100 units : 100 mL :: 5 units : x mL		$100 \times 5 = 500$
	$100x = 100 \times 5 = 500$		$100 \times 5 = 500$
	$100x = 500$		
	$x = 5$ mL/hr = 5 units of insulin		

	Have	*Want to Have*	**PROOF** $20 \times 5 = 100$
Step 2:	5 mL : 1 hr :: 100 mL : x hr		$1 \times 100 = 100$
	$5x = 100$		
	$x = 20$ hr		

CLINICAL ALERT!

Only clear regular insulin can be used intravenously. Discard if cloudy (Figure 9-13).

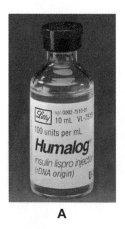 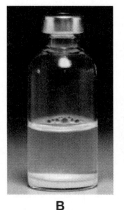 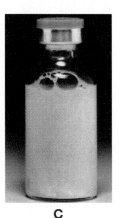 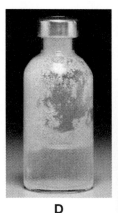

| A | B | C | D |

FIGURE 9-13 A, Regular or Humalog insulin should always look clear. **B,** Insulin at the bottom of the bottle; do not use if insulin stays on the bottom of the bottle after gentle rolling. **C,** Clumps of insulin; do not use if there are clumps of insulin in the liquid or on the bottom of the vial. **D,** Bottle appears frosted; do not use if particles of insulin on the bottom or sides of the bottle give a frosty appearance. *(From Eli Lilly and Company, Indianapolis, IN.)*

ANSWERS ON PAGE 382

WORKSHEET
9D   **IV Insulin Calculations**

Answer questions 1 through 3 using Figure 9-14.

1. The patient's BMBG level is 310 mg/dL at 0820 hr.
   a. At what rate will you set the IV infusion device?
   b. At 0920 hr the BMBG is 270 mg/dL. What will be the rate for the IV infusion device?

2. The patient's blood glucose level is 235 mg/dL. At 0400 hr.
   a. At what rate will you set the infusion rate?
   b. In 1 hour, the BMBG level is 270 mg/dL. What will be the new IV rate?
   c. At 0600 hr the physician called and inquired about the BMBG level. He asked how many units of insulin the patient has received since the IV was started. What will you tell him?

3. Your patient is receiving insulin IV. The standard rate of 100 units in 100 mL of NS is sent from the pharmacy. The BMBG q1h is as follows: 350 mg/dL, 330, 270, 210, 190, 165, 145, 120, 120 mg/dL. How many total units has the patient received?

4. The pharmacy has sent 50 mL of NS with 100 units of insulin. The order is for 5 units/hr until the BMBG level is stable at 130 mg/dL.
   a. How many mL/hr will you set the IV infusion device?
   b. It took 16 hours for the BMBG level to stabilize at 130 mg/dL. How many total units of insulin did the patient receive during the 16 hours?

5. Ordered: 100 units Human regular insulin in 50 mL of NS to be infused at 3 mL/hr until the blood glucose level is stable at 120 mg/dL.
   a. How many units/hr will be delivered?
   b. If it took 8 hours for the blood glucose level to stabilize at 120 mg/dL, how many total units of insulin has the patient received?

Obtain initial Bedside Monitoring Blood Glucose (BMBG) IMMEDIATELY prior to starting insulin infusion. (Call physician if <70 or >340 mg/dL). Check serum K^+ q day or_____ .

Maintenance IV fluid (addition of dextrose and K^+ is recommended).
☐ D5 0.45 NS +___ mEq KC/L@ 50 cc/hr or _____ cc/hr.
☐ Other _____ cc/hr.

Insulin Infusion—Use pharmacy standard Insulin Drip: 100U Human Regular in 100 c NS (1 U − 1 cc). Begin infusion per algorithm below. Use standard column unless the "stress" or "customized" ☐ is checked below.

FIGURE 9-14
Standard Insulin Infusion Chart. *(From Scottsdale Healthcare, Scottsdale, AZ.)*

BG (mg/dL)	Std. Infusion Rate (units/hour)	☐ Stress Infusion Rate (units/hour)	☐ Customized (units/hour)
<80	0.2	0.2	_____
80-100	0.5	1.0	_____
101-140	1.0	2.0	_____
141-180	1.5	3.0	_____
181-220	2.0	4.0	_____
221-260	2.5	5.0	_____
261-300	3.0	6.0	_____
301-340	4.0	8.0	_____
>340	5.0	10.0	_____

Continued

ANSWERS ON PAGE 382

WORKSHEET 9D   IV Insulin Calculations—cont'd

For Problems 6-10, calculate the following:

- mL/hr to infuse the ordered amount via infusion device
- length of time IV is to infuse

6. Ordered: 100 U Humulin R IV at 10 units/hr. Available: 150 mL of 0.9% NS with 100 U Humulin R insulin.

7. Ordered: Humulin R in 50 mL to infuse at 8 units/hr. Available: 50 mL 0.9% NS with 50 units Humulin R insulin.

8. Ordered: Humulin R in 50 mL to infuse at 100 units/hr. Available: 50 mL 0.9% NS with 75 units Humulin R insulin.

9. Ordered: 120 units Humulin R insulin IV at 10 units/hr. Available: 100 mL of NS 0.9% with 120 units Humulin R insulin.

10. Ordered: 150 units Humulin R insulin IV at 12 units/hr. Available: 150 mL of NS 0.9% with 150 units Humulin R insulin.

Normal Blood Glucose
M 75-110 mg/dL F 65-105 mg/dL

Frequent Blood Glucose Monitoring/Insulin Drip Record

DATE → 12/5/02				
Time ↓	Glucose (mg/dL)	Intervention Insulin (U/h) or other	Ketones S/M/L/Neg	Initial
00 __ __				
01 __ __				
02 __ __				
03 __ __	IV Insulin Drip Started			
04 1 5	350	5.0		JB
05 1 5	303	4.0		JB
06 1 5	310	4.0		JB
07 1 5	270	3.0		JB
08 1 5	180	1.5		JB
09 1 5	165	1.5		JB
10 1 5	150	1.5		JB
11 __ __				
12 1 5	140	1.0		JB
13 1 5	130	1.0		JB
14 __ __				
15 1 5	135	1.0		JB
16 __ __				
17 1 5	140	1.0		JB
18 __ __	Converted to S.Q. Insulin			
19 __ __				
20 __ __				
21 __ __				
22 __ __				
23 __ __				
Insulin Total Daily Dose (TDD)				

DATE →				
Time ↓	Glucose (mg/dL)	Intervention Insulin (U/h) or other	Ketones S/M/L/Neg	Initial
00 __ __				
01 __ __				
02 __ __				
03 __ __				
04 __ __				
05 __ __				
06 __ __				
07 __ __				
08 __ __				
09 __ __				
10 __ __				
11 __ __				
12 __ __				
13 __ __				
14 __ __				
15 __ __				
16 __ __				
17 __ __				
18 __ __				
19 __ __				
20 __ __				
21 __ __				
22 __ __				
23 __ __				
Insulin Total Daily Dose (TDD)				

DATE →				
Time ↓	Glucose (mg/dL)	Intervention Insulin (U/h) or other	Ketones S/M/L/Neg	Initial
00 __ __				
01 __ __				
02 __ __				
03 __ __				
04 __ __				
05 __ __				
06 __ __				
07 __ __				
08 __ __				
09 __ __				
10 __ __				
11 __ __				
12 __ __				
13 __ __				
14 __ __				
15 __ __				
16 __ __				
17 __ __				
18 __ __				
19 __ __				
20 __ __				
21 __ __				
22 __ __				
23 __ __				
Insulin Total Daily Dose (TDD)				

Initial	Signature	Initial	Signature	Initial	Signature	Initial	Signature
JB	J Booth						

Original in Medical Chart **Copy to Pharmacy**

NOTE: IV insulin should always be used with an infusion device, never via gravity feed.

FIGURE 9-15 Diabetes Flow Sheet. *(From Scottsdale Healthcare, Scottsdale, AZ.)*

● ORAL DIABETES MEDICATIONS

Oral diabetes medications (ODMs) are used to treat persons with type 2 diabetes. They are taken alone or in combination with insulin. Blood glucose levels determine the strength of oral medication needed. ODMs are *not* insulin. Some ODMs stimulate the pancreas to produce insulin and other ODMs make more effective use of the insulin that is produced.

● INSULIN INFUSION DEVICES

Insulin infusion devices allow insulin to be delivered at a constant (basal) rate throughout the day with additional insulin boluses given before meals. The patient determines the appropriate bolus based on the premeal blood glucose level as well as the carbohydrate content of the meal. The device contains a disposable syringe connected to plastic tubing. The tubing is secured to a subcutaneous cannula, which must be changed every two to three days. Only Velosulin (Buffered Regular), Novolog, or Humalog insulin can be used in the device; therefore ketoacidosis can develop quickly if insulin infusion is interrupted. Because of this significant risk, **the device must not be stopped or disconnected without supplemental insulin coverage.**

ANSWERS ON PAGE 384

WORKSHEET

9E **Multiple-Choice Practice**

1. The IV is infusing at 10 mL/hr. You have NS 250 mL with 100 units of insulin. How many units per hour of insulin is the patient receiving?
   a. 8 units   **b.** 2 units   **c.** 10 units   **d.** 4 units

2. Using the units per hour from number 1, how many hours will it take to infuse the 100 units of insulin?
   a. 50 hr   **b.** 25 hr   **c.** 15 hr   **d.** 5 hr

3. You have 100 mL of NS with 100 units of insulin as an IVPB. The patient's BMBG level at 0600 is 300 mg/dL. Using the Standard Infusion Insulin Drip Rate chart (see Figure 9-15), at what rate per hour will you start the IV?
   a. 5 mL/hr   **b.** 4 mL/hr   **c.** 3 mL/hr   **d.** 2.5 mL/hr

4. Ordered: 30 units of insulin to be infused over 12 hr.
   Available: 50 mL NS with 30 units of insulin.
   How many units/hr will be infused?
   a. 1.5 units   **b.** 2.5 units   **c.** 5 units   **d.** 4 units

   How many mL/hr will you set the infusion device?
   a. 4 mL/hr   **b.** 12 mL/hr   **c.** 41 mL/hr   **d.** 8 mL/hr

5. Ordered: 10 units of insulin/hr IVPB.
   Available: 500 mL NS with 100 units of Regular Insulin.
   At what rate will you set the IV infusion device?
   a. 50 mL/hr   **b.** 25 mL/hr   **c.** 100 mL/hr   **d.** 5 mL/hr

6. The type of insulin that is used for infusions is
   a. Humulin NPH   **b.** Humulin Lente
   c. Humulin Regular   **d.** Humulin Ultra Lente

7. Ordered: 15 units of Lantus (glargine) SC.
   What is the length of effectiveness of the insulin?
   a. 12 hr   **b.** 4 hr   **c.** 36 hr   **d.** 24 hr

8. Ordered: Lente (L) 20 units SC at 0730.
   When will it peak?
   a. 4-5 hr   **b.** 6-12 hr   **c.** 1-3 hr   **d.** 3-4 hr

9. Lantus (glargine) is the preferred insulin because it:
   a. peaks in 15 minutes   **b.** has a duration of 16 hr
   c. is absorbed quickly   **d.** is peakless

10. Lantus (glargine) is given SC:
   a. at breakfast   **b.** at bed time   **c.** at midday   **d.** at anytime

 Refer to the Calculating Dosages, Understanding Insulin Administration sections of the enclosed CD-ROM for additional practice problems.

CRITICAL THINKING EXERCISES

Analyze the following scenario.

Mr. Johnson's blood glucose level was 350 mg/dL. The orders on his chart read: Give 10 units of Humalog stat and check the BMBG in 1 hour. The nurse gave the insulin at 1400 hr. After the change of shift, at 1430 hr, Mr. Johnson was incoherent. On checking the Diabetic Flow Sheet, the nurse found that Mr. Johnson had been given 1 mL of Humalog, which is 100 units.

Order:
Given:
Error:
Potential Injury:
Preventive Measures:

Discussion
What would be your immediate action?
How did this error occur?
How could this error have been prevented?
Do you think the nurse should have known the safe dosage range?
What were the potential injuries to the patient?

ANSWERS ON PAGE 385

CHAPTER 9 FINAL

1. Ordered: Humalog insulin 15 units stat. Available: Humalog insulin.
   - How many units will you give?
   - Which syringe will give a precise measurement?

   a.

   b.

2. The blood glucose level is 280. How many units of Regular insulin will you give SC? Use the Sliding Scale on page 224.

3. Ordered: Humulin R insulin 16 units with Humulin N insulin 30 units at 0700. Shade in the amount of regular insulin. Shade in the amount of NPH insulin.

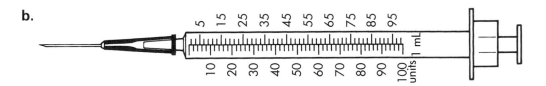

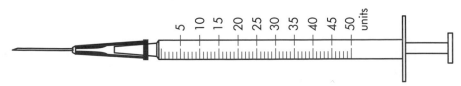

4. Ordered: Humalog 18 units ac at 0930.
  - How many units will you give?
  - Which syringe is easier to read?

a.

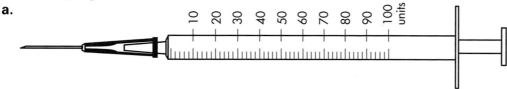

b.

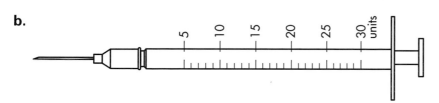

5. Ordered: Glucophage 850 mg tab and Humulin L insulin 15 units ac breakfast. How many total units will you give? Shade in the correct amount.

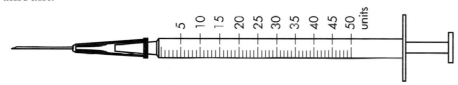

6. Ordered: 10 units/hr Humulin R insulin IV. Available: 500 mL 0.9% saline with 250 units Humulin R regular insulin.
  - How many mL/hr will deliver 10 units/hr?
  - How many hours will the IV infuse?

7. Ordered: 6 units/hr Humulin R insulin IV. Available: 10 mL vial of U-100 Humulin R insulin and 250 mL of 0.9% saline IV solution. Add 100 U Humulin R insulin (1 mL) to the 250 mL of 0.9% saline.
  - How many mL/hr will infuse 6 U of insulin?
  - How many hours will the IV infuse?

8. Ordered: 8 units/hr Humulin R insulin IV. Available: 250 mL NS with 100 units insulin.
  - How many mL/hr will infuse 8 units of insulin?
  - How many hours will the IV infuse?

9. Ordered: 7 units/hr Humulin R insulin IV. Available: 200 mL NS with 100 units Humulin R insulin.
  - How many mL/hr will infuse 7 units/hr?
  - How many hours will the IV infuse?

10. Ordered: Humulin R insulin 9 units/hr IV. Available: 500 mL NS IV solution with 100 units Humulin R insulin.
  - How many mL/hr will infuse 9 units/hr?
  - How many hours will the IV infuse?

Anticoagulants 10

OBJECTIVES

- Compare the actions of PO, SC, and IV anticoagulants.
- Measure a dose in a tuberculin syringe.
- Measure SC heparin using different concentrations.
- Calculate titrated heparin in units and mL/hr.
- Calculate the length of time to infuse.
- Calculate titrated heparin according to U/kg.
- Analyze medication errors using critical thinking.

INTRODUCTION

Various concentrations of subcutaneous (SC) Heparin, sodium, Fragmin, and Lovenox are measured with the tuberculin syringe. Titrated Heparin sodium for IV drip and titrated Fragmin are calculated for bolus and prophylactic regimens. An example of a flow chart, or MAR, is shown.

● INJECTABLE ANTICOAGULANTS

Heparin sodium injection, USP, is a drug used to interrupt the clotting process. It affects the ability of the blood to coagulate, thereby preventing clots from forming. It is used to treat deep vein thrombosis (DVT) and pulmonary embolism (PE), for cardiac surgery, during hemodialysis, myocardial infarction (MI), disseminated intravascular coagulation (DIC), and prophylactically for immobilized patients. It may be given in therapeutic doses or in small, diluted doses to maintain the patency of IV or intraarterial (IA) lines.

Because it is inactive orally, heparin sodium is administered intravenously or subcutaneously. If administered intramuscularly, the drug produces a high level of pain and may cause hematomas. The orders for heparin are highly individualized and based on the weight of the patient and coagulation values. Heparin comes in various strengths, including 1000, 5000, 10,000, 20,000, and 50,000 U/mL. Heparin also comes in 10 and 100 U/mL for IV patency flushes. The vial must be checked carefully before administration. Heparin is fast acting.

See Figure 10-1 for Heparin injection sites. Figure 10-2 is an example of how subcutaneous heparin injections are documented.

Check laboratory values for clotting times before administering heparin. Heparin therapy must not be interrupted and is incompatible with other medications.

Heparin has a half-life of 1 to 6 hours. To maintain a therapeutic level in the blood, heparin is usually given as a continuous IV during hospitalization. The heparin level is titrated on the partial thromboplastin time (PTT) levels. Heparin can be counteracted with protamine sulfate.

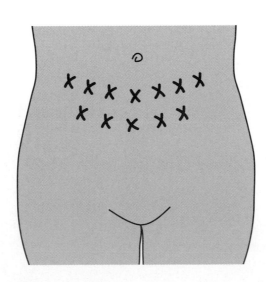

FIGURE 10-1
Subcutaneous injection sites.

M A R	**MEDICATION ADMINISTRATION RECORD**

ADM. DX   :   HT   :
DIET   :   WT   :
                                      ALLERGIES:

Start Date/Time	Stop Date/Time	RN/ LPN	Medication	0731-1530	1531-2330	2331-0730
12/13/02		NB	Heparin sodium 5,000 units sc	0800 RLQ		
		NB	Heparin sodium 5,000 units sc	1400 LLQ		
		KR	Heparin sodium 5,000 units sc	2000 RLQ		

Order Date	RN INIT.	Date/Time To Be Given	One Time Orders and Pre-Operatives Medication-Dose-Route	Actual Time Given

Site Codes			Dose Omission Code
Arm	LA	RA	A = pt absent
Deltoid	LD	RD	H = hold
Ventrogluteal	LVG	RVG	M = med absent
Gluteal	LG	RG	N = NPO
Abdomen	LUQ	RUQ	O = other
Abdomen	LLQ	RLQ	R = refused
			U = unable to tolerate

INIT	Signature	INIT	Signature
NB	Nancy Berg RN		
KR	Kay Rae RN		

FIGURE 10-2 Sample MAR. *(From Scottsdale Healthcare, Scottsdale, AZ.)*

Lovenox (enoxaparin) and Fragmin (dalteparin) (Figure 10-3) are low-molecular-weight anticoagulants. They are prescribed for the prevention and treatment of DVT and PE and also after knee and hip surgery. Lovenox and Fragmin have a longer half-life than heparin, and because of their low level of activity in the blood, there is a reduced need for PTT tests as they are more predictable with peak and duration of action.

FIGURE 10-3
Fragmin single-dose prefilled syringes.
(From Pharmacia Corporation, Peapack, NJ.)

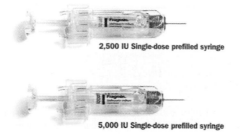

2,500 IU Single-dose prefilled syringe

5,000 IU Single-dose prefilled syringe

EXAMPLE Ordered: Lovenox 30 mg SC q12h after hip replacement. The pharmacy has sent 40 mg/0.4 mL in a prefilled syringe. How many milliliters will be administered? How many milliliters will be discarded?

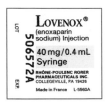

Have   *Want to Have*

40 mg : 0.4 mL :: 30 mg : x mL

$40x = 0.4 \times 30 = 12$

$40x = 12$

$\quad x = 0.3$ mL

0.1 mL will be discarded.

PROOF $40 \times 0.9 = 12$

$\qquad 0.4 \times 30 = 12$

◼ Subcutaneous Heparin Injections

EXAMPLE Ordered: Heparin 3500 units SC q6h. Available: Vial containing 5000 units/mL. How many milliliters will the patient receive? Shade in the dose on the tuberculin syringe.

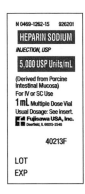

Know   *Want to Know*

5000 U : 1 mL :: 3500 U : x mL

$5000x = 3500$

$\quad x = 0.7$ mL

PROOF

$5000 \times 0.7 = 3500$

$1 \times 3500 = 3500$

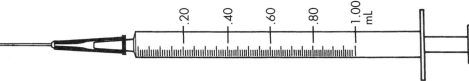

EXAMPLE Ordered: Fragmin 8000 IU SC q6h. How many milliliters will you give? Shade in the dose on the syringe.

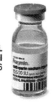

10,000 IU/mL
9.5 mL multidose vial
NDC 0013-2436-06

Know   *Want to Know*

10,000 IU : 1 mL :: 8000 IU : x mL

$10x = 1 \times 8 = 8$

$\quad x = 0.8$ mL

PROOF

$1 \times 8000 = 8000$

$10,000 \times 0.8 = 8000$

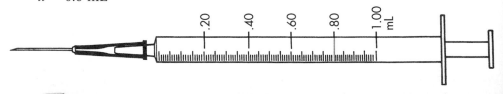

CLINICAL ALERT!

Do not massage the injection site because this increases the incidence of bleeding and hematoma development.

ANSWERS ON PAGE 386

WORKSHEET
10A   Subcutaneous Injections

Multidose vials are available in 1000, 5000, 10,000, 20,000, and 50,000 U/mL. Read labels carefully. Answer the following questions and show your proofs (carry out to nearest hundredth). Shade in dose on syringe.

1. Ordered: Heparin 7000 units SC. Available: Heparin 10,000 units/mL. How many milliliters will the patient receive?

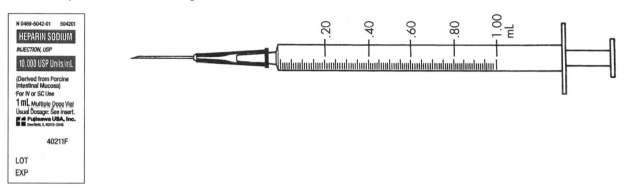

2. Ordered: Heparin 15,000 units SC q8h. Available: Heparin 20,000 units/mL. How many milliliters will the patient receive?

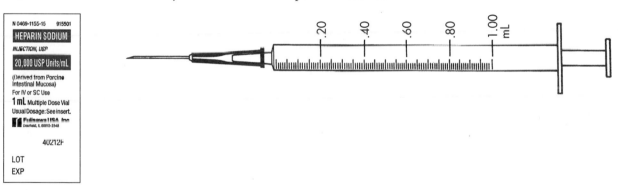

3. Ordered: Heparin 8000 units SC q8h. Available: Heparin 20,000 units/mL. How many milliliters will the patient receive?

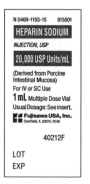

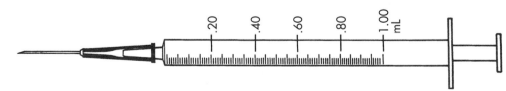

CLINICAL ALERT!

The dosage of heparin should not exceed 100 units.

Continued

ANSWERS ON PAGE 386

WORKSHEET
10A   Subcutaneous Injections—cont'd

4. Ordered: Heparin 17,000 units SC. Available: Heparin 10,000 units/mL and 20,000 units/mL. Which strength will you choose? How many milliliters will the patient receive?

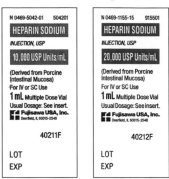

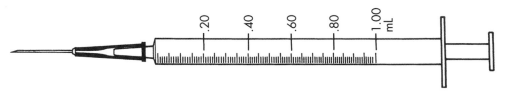

5. Ordered: Fragmin 7500 IU SC. Available: Fragmin 10,000 IU/mL. How many milliliters will the patient receive?

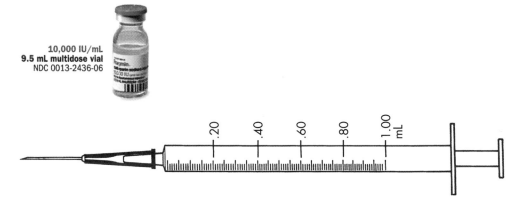

10,000 IU/mL
9.5 mL multidose vial
NDC 0013-2436-06

CLINICAL ALERT!

Check your patient's chart for allergies. Heparin is made from pork and beef.

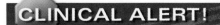

ANSWERS ON PAGE 386

WORKSHEET
10A   Subcutaneous Injections—cont'd

6. Ordered: Heparin 750 units SC q4h. Available: Heparin 1000 units/mL.
How many milliliters will the patient receive?

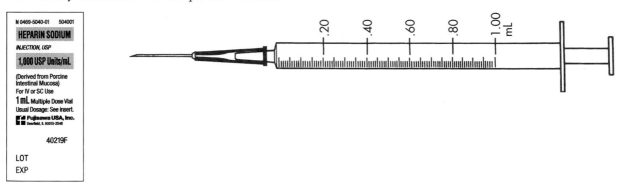

7. Ordered: Heparin 800 units SC. Available: Heparin 1000 units/mL in
multidose vial. How many milliliters will the patient receive?

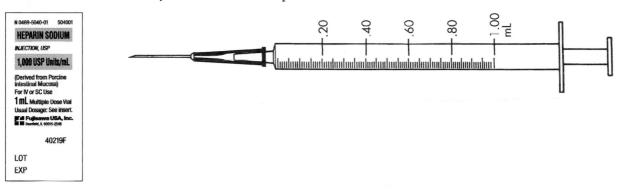

8. Ordered: Heparin 3000 units SC q8h. Available: Heparin 5000 units/mL
in a multidose vial. How many milliliters will the patient receive?

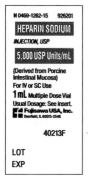

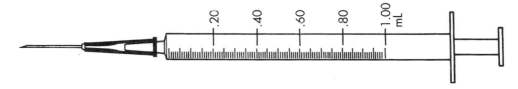

CLINICAL ALERT!

Heparin resistance has been documented in elderly patients; therefore large
doses may be ordered.

Symptoms of overdose are nosebleed, tarry stools, petechiae, and easy
bruising.

Continued

WORKSHEET
10A Subcutaneous Injections—cont'd

IV Flushes

9. Ordered: Heparin flush 5 units after each medication administration to prevent clot formation in the heparin lock. Available: Heparin 10 units/mL. How many units of medication are in the vial? How many milliliters will the patient receive?

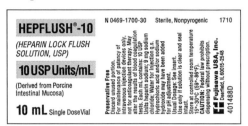

Follow hospital protocol for saline and heparin flushes after medication administration.

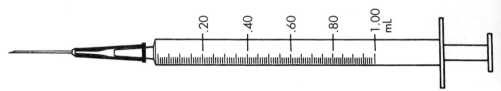

IV Flushes

10. Ordered: Heparin flush 50 units q12h for IV site patency. Available: Heparin 100 units/mL. How many milliliters will the patient receive?

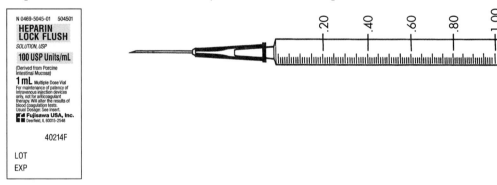

◼ IV Flushes

Heparin flushes are used to prevent clot formation in central lines and intermittent infusions. Inject heparin flush (10-100 U) or saline for injection according to hospital protocol after each medication administration or every 8 to 12 hours. Peripheral IV lines are usually flushed with isotonic saline. Heparin locks provide patient mobility.

⬡ CLINICAL ALERT!

Heparin IV flushes are available in 10 units/mL and 100 units/mL in prepared syringes and vials. Read labels carefully. Hospital protocol will determine the amount to administer.

● IV HEPARIN

When intermittent or continuous IV therapy is used, blood should be drawn for a PTT and a hematocrit level to determine the course of therapy. Therapeutic anticoagulant dosage is regulated according to the results of the PTT and the patient's weight.

Pharmacies are standardizing IV heparin preparations in concentrations of 25,000 units/500 mL and 25,000 units/250 mL. Dispensing charts indicating mL/hr and units/hr are available for each concentration. This will reduce overdosing and underdosing. Protamine sulfate is the antagonist for heparin. It is the nurse's responsibility to have protamine sulfate available.

ANSWERS ON PAGE 388

WORKSHEET 10B   IV Heparin Calculations

Answer the following questions and show your proofs (carry out to the nearest hundredth). The heparin will be administered with an infusion device.

1. Ordered: Heparin sodium 1000 units/hr IV. Available: 1 L of 0.9% saline with 20,000 units of heparin.
  a. How many mL/hr will deliver 1000 units?
  b. How many hours will it take to infuse the bag?

2. Ordered: Heparin sodium 20,000 units IV in 12 hr. Pharmacy has sent 1000 mL of 0.9% normal saline with 20,000 units heparin sodium.
  a. How many mL/hr should the IV infuse?
  b. How many units/hr will infuse?
  c. The shift reports that 250 mL has been infused. How many hours remain to infuse?

3. Ordered: Heparin 1500 units/hr IV. Pharmacy has sent 1 L 0.9% saline with 20,000 units of heparin.
  a. How many mL/hr will deliver 1500 units?
  b. How many hours will it take to infuse this bag?

4. Ordered: Heparin 10,000 units in 15 hr. Pharmacy has sent 1000 mL NS with 10,000 units of heparin. The infusion was started at 0830.
  a. How many units/hr will the patient receive?
  b. How many mL/hr will be infused?
  c. The 0700 hr shift reports that 300 mL has been infused. When will the infusion finish? How many hours remain to infuse?

5. Ordered: Heparin 1200 units/hr. Available: 500 mL NS with 10,000 units of heparin.
  a. How many mL/hr will infuse 1200 units/hr?
  b. How many hours will it take to infuse this bag?   *Continued*

ANSWERS ON PAGE 388

6. Ordered: Heparin 2000 units/hr IV. Available: 50,000 units per 1000 mL
   0.9% NS.
   a. How many mL/hr will deliver 2,000 units/hr?
   b. How many hours will it take to infuse?

7. Ordered: Heparin 1000 units/hr IV. Available: 25,000 units/500 mL.
   a. How many mL/hr will deliver 1000 units/hr?
   b. How many hours will it take to infuse?

8. Ordered: Heparin 1300 units/hr IV. Available: 500 mL with 25,000 units
   of heparin sodium.
   a. How many mL/hr will deliver 1300 units/hr?
   b. How long will it take to infuse?

9. Ordered: Heparin 1800 units/hr IV. Your patient is on fluid restrictions;
   therefore the pharmacy has sent a concentrated solution of
   25,000 units/250 mL of NS.
   a. How many mL/hr will deliver 1800 units/hr?
   b. How many hours will it take to infuse?

10. Ordered: Heparin 1000 units/hr. Your patient is on fluid restrictions. The
    pharmacy has sent 20,000 units/250 mL of NS.
    a. How many mL/hr will deliver 1000 units/hr?
    b. How many hours will it take to infuse?

● ORAL ANTICOAGULANTS

Oral anticoagulants such as warfarin (Coumadin) (Figure 10-4) and anisindione (Miradon) are used as a prophylaxis after an episode of thrombolytic complications. They inhibit the activity of vitamin K, which is required for the activation of clotting factors. Patients receiving heparin therapy are converted to oral anticoagulants while still receiving heparin. The level of oral anticoagulants in the blood is monitored with the laboratory value of the International Normalized Ratio (INR). The INR standardizes the results of the prothrombin time (PT) test. The INR should be maintained at 2 to 3 for best results depending on the illness being treated. The most common oral anticoagulant is warfarin. Other anticoagulants in use are anisindione and integrilin. Dosing for all anticoagulants is individualized. The antidote for oral anticoagulants is vitamin K, plasma, or whole blood.

FIGURE 10-4
Dose range for Coumadin.

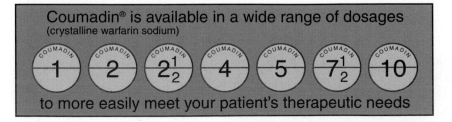

● TITRATED HEPARIN

Heparin is titrated in units/kg when administered as a continuous infusion during and after cardiac surgery, for DVT and PE, and for treatment of children. A PTT is the criterion used to titrate the dosage.

The PTT results are needed to maintain a continuous therapeutic range. A normal PTT has a varying value of 26 to 36 or 30 to 40 seconds. The value varies with laboratory test methods. To maintain a therapeutic range, the PTT value should be within $1\frac{1}{2}$ and $2\frac{1}{2}$ times the control value obtained by the institution. It is imperative that you know normal ranges for your institution. Ranges can differ depending on the type or reagent used by the laboratory. Heparin is most therapeutically effective when based on weight in kilograms. The standardized INR is used only for oral anticoagulants at this time.

ANSWERS ON PAGE 390

WORKSHEET
10C Multiple-Choice Practice

1. Ordered: Fragmin SC titrate to 120 IU/kg q12h × 5 days. The patient weighs 185 lb. How many international units of Fragmin will you administer q12h?
   a. 5800 IU   **b.** 1800 IU   **c.** 10,080 IU   **d.** 6400 IU

2. Refer to question 1. Available: 25,000 IU/mL multidose vial of Fragmin. How many milliliters of Fragmin will you give?
   a. 2.2 mL   **b.** 0.4 mL   **c.** 4.4 mL   **d.** 0.2 mL

3. Titrate Fragmin to 120 IU/kg SC. Ordered: Fragmin SC q12h titrated to kg. The patient weighs 132 lb. How many kilograms does the patient weigh?
   a. 50 kg   **b.** 120 kg   **c.** 60 kg   **d.** 45 kg
   How many international units of Fragmin will you prepare?
   a. 7000 IU   **b.** 5000 IU   **c.** 83,000 IU   **d.** 7200 IU

4. Refer to question 3. How many milliliters of Fragmin will you give? Available: 10,000 IU/mL multidose vial.
   a. 0.7 mL   **b.** 0.5 mL   **c.** 1 mL   **d.** 1.2 mL

5. The patient weighs 160 lb. Order: Administer a bolus of Heparin Sodium IV. The hospital protocol is 80 units/kg. How many units will you give?
   a. 5840 units   **b.** 6620 units   **c.** 4320 units   **d.** 2420 units

6. Ordered: IV Heparin to infuse at 18 units/kg/hr. Available: 1000 mL D5W with 20,000 units heparin. The patient weighs 175 lb. How many units per hour will the patient receive?
   a. 1220 units/hr   **b.** 880 units/hr   **c.** 1280 units/hr   **d.** 1440 units/hr
   At what rate will you set the infusion device?
   a. 110 mL/hr   **b.** 85 mL/hr   **c.** 68 mL/hr   **d.** 72 mL/hr

Continued

WORKSHEET 10C Multiple-Choice Practice—cont'd

7. Ordered: Heparin drip at 40 units/kg. Available: 25,000 units of heparin in 1000 mL of D5W. The patient weighs 75 kg. At what rate will you set the infusion device?
   a. 100 mL/hr   **b.** 120 mL/hr   **c.** 75 mL/hr   **d.** 82 mL/hr

8. Ordered: Heparin IV drip at 500 units/hr. Available: 500 mL 0.9% NS with 10,000 units of heparin. At what hourly rate will you set the infusion?
   a. 50 mL/hr   **b.** 75 mL/hr   **c.** 100 mL/hr   **d.** 25 mL/hr

9. Ordered: Fragmin SC titrated to 120 IU/kg q12h × 8 days. Begin treatment at 0800 hr. The patient weighs 220 lb. How many kg does the patient weigh?
   a. 100 kg   **b.** 120 kg   **c.** 110 kg   **d.** 60 kg
   How many IU of Fragmin will the patient receive per dose?
   a. 10,000 IU   **b.** 15,000 IU   **c.** 8,000 IU   **d.** 12,000 IU

10. Refer to question 9. Available: Fragmin 10,000 IU/mL and Fragmin 25,000 IU/mL multidose vials. Which multidose vial will you use? How many mL will you give?
    a. 1 mL   **b.** 0.75 mL   **c.** 0.48 mL   **d.** 0.66 mL

 Refer to the Calculating Dosages, Anticoagulant Calculations sections of the enclosed CD-ROM for additional practice problems.

CRITICAL THINKING EXERCISES

Mrs. Smith, 26 years old, was recuperating after abdominal surgery. The physician ordered 1000 U of heparin SC. You administer 0.5 mL dose taken from a multidose vial labeled 20,000 units/mL. Later that day the physician reduced the heparin order. He wrote: *Reduce SC heparin from 1000 U to 500 U q8h.* It is at this time that you realize that you gave Mrs. Brown 10,000 U of heparin instead of 1000 U.

- Order:
- Given:
- Error:
- Preventive measures:
- Potential injury:

Discussion:
What factors contributed to the error? How many units of heparin was the patient overdosed?

ANSWERS ON PAGE 391

CHAPTER **10** FINAL

1. Ordered: Heparin 4000 units SC for prophylaxis for cerebral thrombosis. Available: 5000 units/mL. How many milliliters will the patient receive?

2. Ordered: Heparin 2500 units q4h SC to prevent thrombi from recurring. Available: 10,000 units/mL vial. How many milliliters will the patient receive?

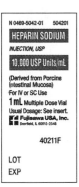

3. Ordered: Heparin 2000 units q4h for venous stasis. Available: 5000 units/mL and 10,000 units/mL. Which vial will you choose? If a tuberculin syringe is used, how many milliliters will the patient receive?

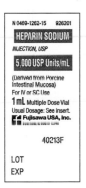 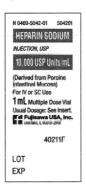

4. Ordered: Heparin 7000 units SC q8h before initiating a heparin infusion for a venous thromboembolism. Available: 5000, 10,000, and 20,000 units/mL. Which one will you choose? How many milliliters will the patient receive?

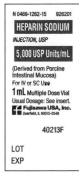 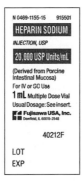 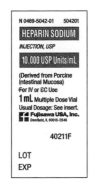

5. Ordered: Heparin 800 units SC q4h as a prophylaxis for immobility. Available: Heparin 1000 units/mL. How many milliliters will the patient receive?

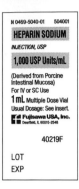

6. Ordered: 700 units/hr to infuse. Available: 20,000 units/500 mL. How many mL/hr will provide 700 units/hr? How many hours will the IV infuse?

7. Ordered: 1500 units/hr IV for hyperlipemia. Available: 25,000 units/ 500 mL. How many mL/hr will provide 1500 units/hr? How many hours will the IV infuse?

8. Ordered: Heparin 25,000 units IV in 24 hr for peripheral arterial embolization. Available: 1000 mL with 25,000 units of heparin sodium. How many mL/hr will give 25,000 units in 24 hr? How many units/hr will infuse?

9. Ordered: Heparin 35,000 units IV in 24 hr for atrial fibrillation. Available: 1000 mL 0.9% NS with 35,000 units of heparin sodium. How many mL/hr will the patient receive? How many units/hr will the patient receive?

10. Ordered: Heparin 2000 units/hr IV for pulmonary emboli. Available: Heparin 20,000 units in 1000 mL 0.9% NS. How many mL/hr will be delivered via the infusion device? How long will the IV infuse?

Children's Dosages

11

OBJECTIVES

- Calculate 24-hour pediatric drug doses and divided doses for specific weights.
- Calculate safe dose ranges in mg/kg and μg/kg and square meters.
- Calculate pediatric doses using the BSA formula.
- Calculate reconstituted pediatric drug doses and small-volume IV flow rates for children.
- Evaluate order and safe dose range calculations.
- Make a decision:

    Give medication (within therapeutic range).

    Give and clarify promptly (below therapeutic range).

    Hold *medication and clarify promptly* (overdose).
- Analyze medication errors using critical thinking.

INTRODUCTION

Medication amounts for infants and children are usually less than those for an average adult. Calculation and delivery of correct doses to a child incorporates several steps to protect the patient. With the step-by-step practice offered in this chapter, you will develop the skills, habits, and thinking processes necessary to ensure that the dose ordered is safe and to calculate accurate medication doses for at-risk patient populations.

● DOSAGES BASED ON BODY WEIGHT AND SURFACE AREA

Infants and children have special medication needs because of their smaller size, weight, and body surface area (BSA). They have varying capabilities for drug absorption, digestion, distribution, metabolism, and excretion. It is very important for the nurse to check current references for pediatric medication orders and to double-check safe dose ranges (SDR) to prevent errors and injury. Minute dosages that require scrupulous mathematics may be ordered. Pediatric and intensive care nurses use written pediatric drug guidelines and calculators to determine weights and verify SDRs.

The two methods currently used for calculating safe pediatric doses are based on (1) *body weight* in mg/kg or μg/kg and (2) *body surface area* (BSA) in square meters (m^2) using a scale called a *nomogram* (Fig. 11-1). Of the two methods, the BSA method is the most accurate and is used mostly for powerful chemotherapeutic drugs.

● THE mg/kg METHOD

The most *frequently* used calculation method for pediatric medication administration is *mg/kg*. References usually state the safe amount of drug in mg/kg for a 24-hour period to be given in one or more divided doses. You may also see *μg/kg* cited for therapeutic dosages when very small amounts of medication will be given.

● Steps to Solving mg/kg Problems

Step 1   *Estimate* the child's weight in kilograms by dividing the pounds in half; then *calculate* the weight in kilograms using 2.2 lb = 1 kg equivalency (divide pounds by 2.2). Use a calculator.
   a. If the child's weight is in pounds, convert the pounds directly to kilograms (one-step calculation).
   b. If the child's weight is in pounds and ounces, convert the ounces to the nearest tenth of a pound and *add* this to the total pounds. Then convert the total pounds to kilograms to the nearest tenth (two-step calculation). (Refer to page 251 for kilogram to pound conversions and page 26 for rounding instructions.)

Step 2   *Calculate* the SDR using a calculator and current pediatric recommendations found in the drug literature or drug handbook for this weight child in mg/kg or μg/kg.

Step 3   *Compare* and *evaluate* the 24-hour ordered amount with the recommended SDR. Be sure the comparisons are for the *same* time frame!

Step 4   If safe, *calculate* the actual dose to be administered using written ratio and proportion.

Shortcut steps

1. Weight in kg
2. SDR
3. Compare with order
4. Calculate dose if safe to give

◉◀◀◀◀◀◀◀◀◀RULES   All pediatric medication administration begins with an accurate weight (Step 1) and a calculation of the SDR (Step 2).

To convert an infant's weight from pounds to kilograms with a calculator, convert ounces to pounds (if applicable) by dividing the ounces by 16 to get part of a pound, then divide the *total pounds* (*to the nearest tenth*) by 2.2.

EXAMPLE   Ordered: EryPed (erythromycin ethylsuccinate suspension) 150 mg q6h po. The infant weighs 15 lb, 6 oz today. The literature states that the SDR is 30 to 50 mg/kg per day up to 100 mg/kg per day in four divided doses for severe infections.

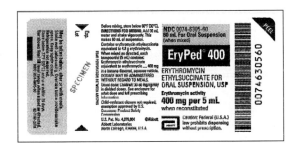

Step 1   **Estimate** the infant's weight.
a. *Pounds to kilograms:* 15 lb ÷ 2 = 7.5 kg
Calculate the actual weight.
b. **Two-step** conversion because ounces are involved.
Ounces to pounds: 6 oz ÷ 16 = 0.37 lb   Add part of pound to total pounds. The infant thus weighs 15.4 lb.
Pounds to kilograms: 15.4 lb ÷ 2.2 = 7 kg   (close to estimate)

Step 2   The **SDR** recommended for children more than 1 month of age is 30 to 100 mg/kg per day po in four divided doses.
Low-range calculation: 30 mg × 7 kg = 210 mg (low SDR)
High-range calculation: 100 mg × 7 kg = 700 mg (high SDR)

Step 3   **Evaluate:** The **SDR** recommended for this child's weight is 210 to 700 mg total q24h in four divided doses.
Ordered: 150 mg q6h   or   150 mg × 4 or 600 mg total in 24 hr

Step 4   **Decision:** Give medication. 600 mg for the day is within the SDR of 210 to 700 mg in four divided doses.

Calculate the individual dose (write out and prove).

Know	*Want to Know*	**PROOF**	**ANSWER**
400 mg : 5 mL :: 150 mg : x mL		$400 \times 1.87 = 748$	Give 1.9 mL

$$\frac{\cancel{400}}{\cancel{400}} x = \frac{750}{400} \qquad (5 \times 150)$$

$$x = 1.87 \text{ or } 1.9 \text{ mL}$$

$$5 \times 150 = 750$$

HINT ■ Review and analyze the logic of these four steps.

CLINICAL ALERT!

Avoid two potential errors when converting pounds and ounces to kilograms. First, ounces must be converted to part of a pound *before* converting total pounds to kilograms; for example, 6 oz does not convert to 0.6 lb. Second, 15.4 lb does not equal 15.4 kg.

Don't forget the second step—convert the total pounds to kilograms.

ANSWERS ON PAGE 392

WORKSHEET

11A Calculator Practice

◉◀◀◀◀◀◀◀◀◀RULE   Calculators are used in pediatric and intensive care units to determine weights and SDRs. Dividing ounces by 16 will give the pound equivalent in the first step of two-step problems. Dividing or multiplying by 2.2 will give pound and kilogram equivalents.

1. Estimate the weights, then use a calculator to convert from pounds to kilograms or kilograms to pounds. Round to the *nearest* tenth.* Double check all work.
   a. 14 lb (1 or 2 steps?)
   Estimate:
   Actual:
   b. 12 lb, 2 oz (1 or 2 steps?)
   Estimate:
   Actual:
   c. 10 lb
   Estimate:
   Actual:
   d. 14 kg
   Estimate:
   Actual:
   e. 10 kg
   Estimate:
   Actual:

2. Calculate the 24-hour total dose in milligrams.
   a. 150 mg q8h
   b. 200 mg q6h
   c. 400 μg q4h
   d. 50 mg tid
   e. 750 μg q12h

3. Calculate the unit dose.
   a. 1 g in 4 equally divided doses
   b. 750 mg divided tid
   c. 2 g in 4 to 6 equally divided doses
   d. 16 g a day in 2 to 4 divided doses
   e. 500 mg in 4 divided doses

4. Calculate the SDR in milligrams for the following weights. Note that the answers will only be in milligrams or micrograms, since x, the unknown, is a *dosage* measurement not a weight measurement. You want to know how many milligrams a day and milligrams per dose are safe for this patient. (2.2 lb = 1 kg)

SDR	WT	SDR
a. 10 mg/kg;	weight is 5 kg	_____ safe total mg/day
b. 5 to 8 mg/kg;	weight is 7.3 kg	_____ SDR for the day in mg
c. 6 to 8 mg/kg;	weight is 8 lb	_____ SDR for the day in mg
d. 3 to 6 mg/kg;	weight is 5 lb, 8 oz	_____ SDR for the day in mg
e. 200 to 400 μg/kg;	weight is 4 lb, 6 oz	_____ SDR for the day in mg

5. Ordered: Drug X, 50 mg tid.
   SDR: 2 to 3 mg/kg given in three divided doses. Child's weight is 18 kg.
   a. SDR for 24 hr
   b. SDR per dose
   c. Total ordered dose for day and per dose
   d. Evaluation and decision: Safe or unsafe to give? Why?

---

* For rounding instructions, refer to p. 26.

ANSWERS ON PAGE 393

WORKSHEET
11B

Children's Safe Dose Range (SDR) Practice

For each problem, use a calculator to determine the child's weight in kilograms to the nearest tenth, calculate the SDR, and compare it with the order. If the total dose for 24 hours is excessive, the unit dose is automatically excessive. Evaluate the order and make a decision.

1. Give medication (within SDR for unit dose and 24-hour dose).
2. Give and clarify (underdose).
3. Hold and clarify promptly (overdose).

Double check your work.

1. Weight: 25.4 lb
   SDR in literature: 10 to 30 mg/kg/day in divided doses
   Order: 100 mg tid
   a. Estimated wt in kg: **b.** Actual wt in kg:
   c. SDR for this child: **d.** Dose ordered:
   e. Evaluation and decision:

2. Weight: 33 lb
   SDR in literature: 100 to 200 µg/kg/day in divided doses
   Order: 0.5 mg tid
   a. Estimated wt in kg: **b.** Actual wt in kg:
   c. SDR for this child: **d.** Dose ordered:
   e. Evaluation and decision:

3. Weight: 20 lb
   SDR in literature: 2 to 4 mg/kg/day
   Order: 50 mg daily
   a. Estimated wt in kg: **b.** Actual wt in kg:
   c. SDR for this child: **d.** Dose ordered:
   e. Evaluation and decision:

4. Weight: 85 lb
   SDR: 10 to 15 mg/kg/day in 4 to 6 divided doses
   Order: 100 mg q6h
   a. Estimated wt in kg: **b.** Actual wt in kg:
   c. SDR for this child: **d.** Dose ordered:
   e. Evaluation and decision:

5. Weight 5 lb
   SDR: 10 to 20 µg/kg/day
   Order: 0.03 mg qid
   a. Estimated wt in kg: **b.** Actual wt in kg:
   c. SDR for this child: **d.** Dose ordered:
   e. Evaluation and decision:

THE BSA METHOD (mg/m²)

The body surface area (BSA) refers to the total area exposed to the outside environment. The estimated BSA in square meters (m^2) is derived from height and weight measurements by using a mathematical formula. It is considered the most reliable way to calculate therapeutic dosages.

This method may be used to calculate safe doses for antineoplastic drugs; new drugs; and drugs for special populations such as infants, children, frail elderly patients, and patients with cancer. It may also be used to double check medication orders for safe dosage.

Nurses are not usually expected to calculate BSA. The pharmacy provides the BSA calculations. Nurses *do* have a critical responsiblity to distinguish the difference in a medication order and dosage based in mg/**lb** or mg/**kg** of weight and an order based on mg/**m²** of BSA: 20 mg/kg versus 20 mg/m² vs 20 mg/lb.

EXAMPLE   Child weighs 33 lb (15 kg) and has a BSA of 0.55 m^2.

ORDERED: 20 mg/kg	vs	**ORDERED:** 20 mg/m²	vs	**ORDERED** 20 mg/lb
20 mg:1 kg::x mg:15 kg		20 mg:1 m²::x mg:0.55		20 mg:1 lb::x mg:33 lb
$x = 20 \times 15 = 300$ mg		$x = 20 \times 0.55 = 11$ mg		$x = 20 \times 33 = 660$ mg

As seen, the doses calculated range from 11 mg to 660 mg, and depending on the unit of measurement, reflect extremely large differences. This illustrates the need to check the details of the ordered drugs—not only all of the numbers but also the units of measurement.

The West nomogram in Figure 11-1 allows the user to plot the *estimated* square meters of BSA by using height and weight mesurements.

Although the pharmacy usually supplies BSA calculations, the nurse has the option of estimating safe doses easily and rapidly by using a mathematical formula and a calculator and entering the patient's height and weight data.

Calculating BSA (m²) Using a Mathematical Formula

There are two formulas for calculating BSA (m^2) and both use height and weight dimensions.

A. Formula using only Metric System

$$\frac{\text{Weight (kg)} \times \text{Height (cm)}}{3600}$$

B. Formula using only pounds and inches

$$\frac{\text{Weight (lb)} \times \text{Height (in)}}{3131}$$

Note the differences in the divisors. The formulas must be used exactly as shown.

Directions: Using a calculator and a weight of 20 kg and a height of 95 cm determine the BSA in square meters for a child using the metric formula

Step 1   Multiply the kilograms by centimeters first and *divide* the result by 3600 ($20 \times 95 = 900/3600 = 0.527$)

Step 2   Obtain the *square root* of 0.527 by pushing the square root button and *round* your answer to the *nearest* hundredth.

$$\frac{20 \times 95}{3600} = 0.527 \qquad \sqrt{0.527} = 0.725 = 0.73 \ m^2$$

Compare this answer with the West nomogram (see Figure 11-1). Create a straight line between 20 kg and 95 cm and read the result in the SA column on the nomogram. Take care to plot the height and weight on the metric graph—the outside columns. When reading the results (m²) columns, be sure to note the value of each calibrated line on the scale at the intersection point.

You may use either the nomogram or the formula. The formula method is more accurate, and if you have a calculator on hand, it is faster.

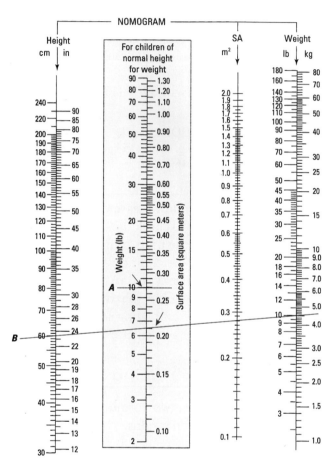

FIGURE 11-1 West nomogram for estimation of body surface area (BSA). *A,* The estimated BSA in square meters for children of normal height for weight is determined by reading the m² at the alignment point with the child's weight in pounds in the highlighted column. The red line denoted by the arrow reveals that an infant weighing 10 lb has an approximate BSA of 0.27 m². *B,* The BSA in square meters for children who are *under*weight or *over*weight* is determined by connecting the child's plotted weight in the left column and plotted height in the right column with a straight line and reading the intersection point on the SA (surface area) column as indicated by the arrow on the red line. This illustrates an estimated BSA of 0.28 m² for an infant of 60 cm height weighing 4.5 kg. The SA column reading requires that height and weight both be plotted in the same system of measurement, metric or pounds/inches. *Refer to Pediatric standard growth charts and developmental grids for normal height and weight ranges for pediatric groups. *(Nomogram modified with data from Behrman RE, Klegiman R, Jenson HB, eds: Nelson textbook of pediatrics, ed 16, Philadelphia, 2000, WB Saunders.)*

ANSWERS ON PAGE 394

WORKSHEET 11C
Comparing BSA-based (mg/m²) Dosages with mg/lb and mg/kg Orders

Use the West nomogram (Figure 11-1, *A,* p. 256), highlighted section for children of normal height and weight to obtain the BSA (m²) based on weight.

Calculate the dose to be given based on the mg/m² and dose ordered.

	WT IN lb	BSA IN m²	DOSE ORDERED	DOSE TO BE GIVEN
1.	4 lb	0.15	10 mg/m²	$10 \times 0.15 = 1.5$ mg
2.	6 lb	_____	15 mg/m²	_____
3.	10 lb	_____	5 mg/m²	_____

Calculate the dose for the same weight children in mg/lb measurements as illustrated in Problem 4.

	WT IN lb	DOSE ORDERED	DOSE TO BE GIVEN
4.	4 lb	10 mg/lb	$4 \times 10 = 40$ mg
5.	6 lb	15 mg/lb	_____
6.	10 lb	5 mg/lb	_____

Calculate the dose to be given in mg/kg measurements as illustrated in Problem 9. Divide lb by 2.2 to obtain kg.

	WT IN kg (TO NEAREST TENTH)	DOSE ORDERED	DOSE TO BE GIVEN
7.	4 lb = 1.81 kg	10 mg/kg	$10 \times 1.8 = 18$
8.	6 lb = _____ kg	2 mg/kg	

9. Using a calculator, obtain the BSA in m² for a child with a height of 60 cm and a weight of 100 kg using the appropriate BSA formula on p. 255 _____

10. Using a calculator, obtain the BSA in m² for a child with a height of 70 in and weight of 12 lb using the appropriate BSA formula on p. 255 _____

⬡ CLINICAL ALERT!

Consider that the patient safety implications when mg/m², mg/lb, and mg/kg are erroneously interchanged. This has resulted in serious errors. The nurse must understand the differences among these three terms even if the equivalents are provided and must focus on the terms of the medication order to ensure that the correct values are being used in calculation of the dose.

ANSWERS ON PAGE 394

WORKSHEET 11D

Children's Safe Dose Range (SDR) Practice

1. Weight: 14 lb
   SDR: 0.02 to 0.05 mg/kg/day
   Order: 150 μg bid
   a. Estimated wt in kg: **b.** Actual wt in kg:
   c. SDR for this child: **d.** Dose ordered:
   e. Evaluation and decision:

2. Weight: 44 lb, normal weight for height
   SDR: 5 to 8 mg/m^2* qd
   Order: 4 mg qd
   a. SDR for this child: **b.** Dose ordered:
   c. Evaluation and decision:

3. Weight: 19 lb
   SDR: 0.1 to 0.3 mg/kg/day in 2 divided doses
   Order: 2500 μg bid
   a. Estimated wt in kg: **b.** Actual wt in kg:
   c. SDR for this child: **d.** Dose ordered:
   e. Evaluation and decision:

4. Weight: 9 lb
   SDR 1 to 5 μg/kg/day
   Order: 0.01 mg qd
   a. Estimated wt in kg: **b.** Actual wt in kg:
   c. SDR for this child: **d.** Dose ordered:
   e. Evaluation and decision:

5. SDR: 1 to 2 g/day in 4 divided doses
   Order: 500 mg q6h
   a. SDR for this child: **b.** Dose ordered:
   c. Evaluation and decision:

---

*For BSA conversion, refer to West nomogram on page 256.

ANSWERS ON PAGE 395

WORKSHEET

11E   Children's Oral Medications

These medications can be given to infants with a dropper or in a pre-prepared oral medication syringe (Figure 11-2). Small amounts may be given to an infant in a nipple. You may need to prepare and administer these medications using an oral syringe (without a needle).

FIGURE 11-2
Prefilled oral syringe.

For each problem, use a calculator to determine the child's weight in kilograms or pounds if required, calculate the SDR, and compare it with the order. Evaluate the order and make a decision:

1. Give medication (within SDR for unit dose and 24-hour dose).
2. Give and clarify (underdose).
3. Hold and clarify promptly (overdose).

For decisions 1 and 2 only, calculate the medication amount to be administered using *written ratio and proportion.* Double check and prove your work. Do *not* calculate overdose orders.

1. Ordered: Tylenol (acetaminophen elixir) 160 mg po for a 4-year-old child who weighs 14 kg today. Label: 80 mg per $^1/_2$ tsp.

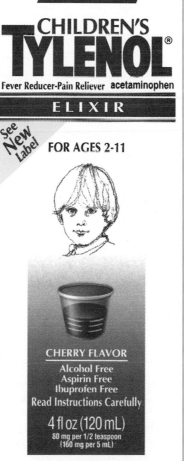

Directions:
1. Find right dose on chart below. If possible, use weight to dose; otherwise use age.
2. Only use enclosed measuring cup.
3. If needed, repeat dose every 4 hours.
4. Do not use more than 5 times a day.

WEIGHT (lb)	AGE (yr)	DOSE (tsp)
Under 24	Under 2	Consult Physician
24–35	2–3	1
36–47	4–5	1 1/2
48–59	6–8	2
60–71	9–10	2 1/2
72–95	11	3

Attention:
Specially designed for use with enclosed measuring cup. Use only enclosed measuring cup to dose this product. Do not use any other dosing device.

Inactive Ingredients: Benzoic Acid, Citric Acid, Flavors, Glycerin, Polyethylene Glycol, Propylene Glycol, Purified Water, Sodium Benzoate, Sorbitol, Sucrose, Red #33 and Red #40.

● Tylenol® products are the first choice of Pediatricians.

● Children's Tylenol® Liquids are not the same concentration as Infants' Tylenol® Drops. For accurate dosing, follow the dosing instructions on this label.

● Use only enclosed measuring cup to dose.
● Items like kitchen teaspoons may not be accurate.
● Never use spoons, droppers or cups that come with other medicines.

Store at room temperature.
See bottom panel of carton for expiration date and lot number.

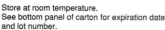

McNEIL CONSUMER PRODUCTS CO.
DIVISION OF McNEIL-PPC, INC.
FORT WASHINGTON, PA 19034 USA
© McN-PPC, Inc.'97

ORIGINAL

CHILDREN'S
TYLENOL®
Fever Reducer-Pain Reliever   acetaminophen
ELIXIR

FOR AGES 2-11

See New Label

CHERRY FLAVOR
Alcohol Free
Aspirin Free
Ibuprofen Free
Read Instructions Carefully
4 fl oz (120 mL)
80 mg per 1/2 teaspoon
(160 mg per 5 mL)

a. Estimated wt in lb:
b. Actual wt in lb:
c. SDR for this child:
d. Dose ordered:
e. Evaluation and decision:
f. Amount to be given in mL if applicable.

Continued

WORKSHEET
11E Children's Oral Medications—cont'd

2. Ordered: Erythromycin ethylsuccinate oral suspension 300 mg q6h po. The child weighs 55 lb today. The SDR is 30 to 50 mg/kg/day in 4 divided doses.

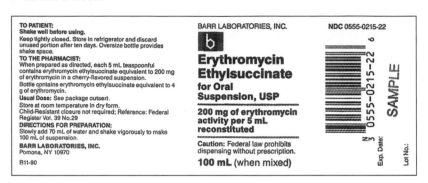

a. Estimated wt in kg:

b. Actual wt in kg:

c. SDR for this child:

d. Dose ordered:

e. Evaluation and decision:

f. Amount to be given in mL if applicable:

3. Ordered: Leucovorin calcium 5 mg q6h po. The child weighs 24 lb and has normal weight and height. The SDR according to the literature is 10 mg/m^2 q6h for 72 hr. For BSA calculation, refer to the nomogram in Figure 11-1. The BSA is determined by pounds, not kilograms.

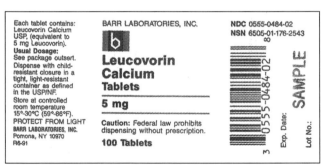

a. SDR for this child:

b. Dose ordered:

c. Evaluation and decision:

d. Amount to be given if applicable:

CLINICAL ALERT!

Differentiate elixirs and concentrated drops from oral suspensions. Elixers contain alcohol for flavoring. Suspensions contain solids which must be dispersed in the liquid by shaking or stirring. Concentrated drops contain a higher amount of drug in a smaller volume of liquid than ordinary drops.

ANSWERS ON PAGE 395

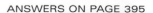

Children's Oral Medications—cont'd

4. Ordered: Tegretol (carbamazepine) oral suspension 0.25 g po tid. The SDR for maintenance for a child over 12 years of age is 400 to 800 mg/day in 3 to 4 divided doses.

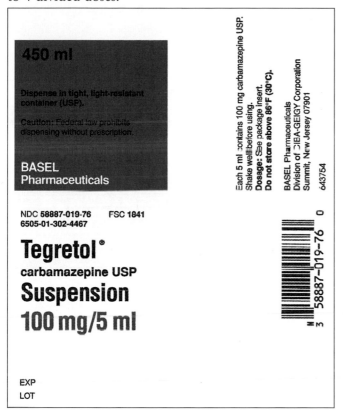

450 ml

Dispense in tight, light-resistant container (USP).

Caution: Federal law prohibits dispensing without prescription.

BASEL
Pharmaceuticals

NDC **58887-019-76**   FSC **1841**
6505-01-302-4467

Tegretol®
carbamazepine USP
Suspension
100 mg/5 ml

EXP
LOT

Each 5 ml contains 100 mg carbamazepine USP.
Shake well before using.
Dosage: See package insert.
Do not store above 86°F (30°C).

BASEL Pharmaceuticals
Division of CIBA-GEIGY Corporation
Summit, New Jersey 07901

643754

3 58887-019-76 0

a. SDR for this child:
b. Dose ordered in mg:
c. Evaluation and decision:
d. Amount to be given if applicable:

5. Ordered: Amoxil 180 mg q8h po for a child who weighs 27 lb. The SDR is 40 mg/kg/day in 3 divided doses.

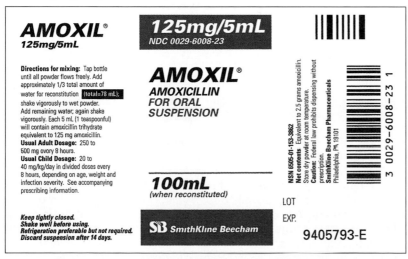

AMOXIL®
125mg/5mL

125mg/5mL
NDC 0029-6008-23

AMOXIL®
AMOXICILLIN
FOR ORAL
SUSPENSION

Directions for mixing: Tap bottle until all powder flows freely. Add approximately 1/3 total amount of water for reconstitution (total=78 mL); shake vigorously to wet powder. Add remaining water; again shake vigorously. Each 5 mL (1 teaspoonful) will contain amoxicillin trihydrate equivalent to 125 mg amoxicillin.
Usual Adult Dosage: 250 to 500 mg every 8 hours.
Usual Child Dosage: 20 to 40 mg/kg/day in divided doses every 8 hours, depending on age, weight and infection severity. See accompanying prescribing information.

Keep tightly closed.
Shake well before using.
Refrigeration preferable but not required.
Discard suspension after 14 days.

100mL
(when reconstituted)

SB SmithKline Beecham

NSN 6505-01-153-3862
Net contents Equivalent to 2.5 grams amoxicillin.
Store dry powder at room temperature.
Caution: Federal law prohibits dispensing without prescription.
SmithKline Beecham Pharmaceuticals
Philadelphia, PA 19101

3 0029-6008-23 1

LOT
EXP.
9405793-E

a. Estimated wt in kg:
b. Actual wt in kg:
c. SDR for this child:
d. Dose ordered:
e. Evaluation and decision:
f. Amount to be given in mL if applicable:

ANSWERS ON PAGE 396

Children's Subcutaneous and Intramuscular Medications

For each problem, use a calculator to determine the child's weight in kilograms to the nearest tenth, calculate the SDR, and compare it with the order. Evaluate the order and make a decision:

1. Give medication (within SDR for unit dose and 24-hour dose).
2. Give and clarify (underdose).
3. Hold and clarify promptly (overdose).

For decisions 1 and 2 only, calculate the medication amount to be administered using *written ratio and proportion.* Double check and prove your work. Do *not* calculate overdose orders.

1. Ordered: Meperidine HCl 30 mg IM preoperatively for a child who weighs 32 lb, 5 oz. The SDR is 1 to 2.2 mg/kg.
   a. Estimated wt in kg:
   b. Actual wt (1 or 2 steps?):
   c. SDR for this child:
   d. Dose ordered:
   e. Evaluation and decision:
   f. Volume to be administered if applicable:

25 DOSETTE● AMPULS — Each contains **1 mL**
NDC 0641-**1140-35**

MEPERIDINE
HCl INJECTION, USP

75 mg/mL

FOR INTRAMUSCULAR SUBCUTANEOUS OR SLOW INTRAVENOUS USE

Warning: May be habit forming.
Each mL contains meperidine hydrochloride 75 mg in Water for Injection. pH 3.5-6.0, sodium hydroxide and/or hydrochloric acid added, if needed, for pH adjustment. Sealed under nitrogen.
USUAL DOSE: See package insert.
DO NOT USE IF PRECIPITATED.
Store at controlled room temperature 15°-30° C (59°-86° F).
Caution: Federal law prohibits dispensing without prescription.
To open ampuls, ignore color line; break at constriction.
Product Code: 1140-35   B-51140d

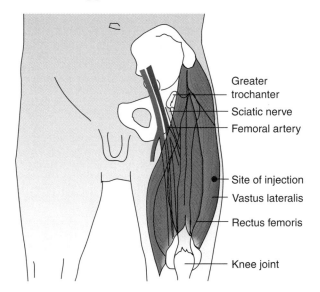

FIGURE 11-3 The mid-anterolateral thigh (vastus lateralis muscle) is the preferred site for injections for infants. *(From Lilley, LL, Aucker RS: Pharmacology and the nursing process, ed 3, St Louis, 2001, Mosby.)*

- Greater trochanter
- Sciatic nerve
- Femoral artery
- Site of injection
- Vastus lateralis
- Rectus femoris
- Knee joint

CLINICAL ALERT!

Intramuscular injections are rarely ordered on a routine basis for children because of limited sites, painful physical trauma, and psychosocial implications.

Mid-anterolateral thigh is the preferred site for injections for infants (Figure 11-3) until the child has walked for a year. The ventrogluteal muscle is a preferred site after age 7 months. Never use the deltoid muscle for young children. Needle lengths, gauge, and fluid amounts are much smaller for infants and children than for adults.*

*Refer to current pediatric clinical skills manuals.

ANSWERS ON PAGE 396

WORKSHEET 11F Children's Subcutaneous and Intramuscular Medications—cont'd

2. Ordered: Morphine sulfate (MS) 5 mg IM stat for a child who weighs 55 lb, 8 oz. The SDR is 0.1 to 0.2 mg/kg q4h.

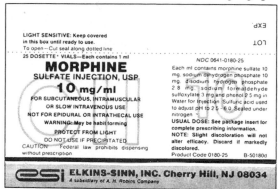

   a. Estimated wt in kg:
   b. Actual wt (1 or 2 steps?):
   c. SDR for this child:
   d. Dose ordered:
   e. Evaluation and decision:
   f. Volume to be administered if applicable:

3. Ordered: Atropine sulfate 0.2 mg SC preoperatively for a child who weighs 17 lb, 9 oz. The SDR for a child weighing 7 to 9 kg is 0.2 mg 30 to 60 min before surgery.

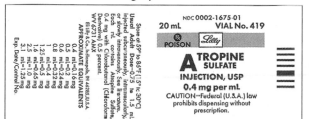

   a. Estimated wt in kg:
   b. Actual wt (1 or 2 steps?):
   c. SDR for this child:
   d. Dose ordered:
   e. Evaluation and decision:
   f. Volume to be administered if applicable:

4. Ordered: Ampicillin sodium 250 mg IM qid for a baby with septicemia weighing 7 lb. SDR is 100 to 200 mg/kg/day in divided doses q6h

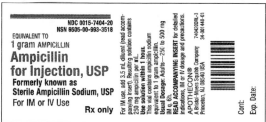

   a. Estimated wt in kg:
   b. Actual wt (1 or 2 steps?):
   c. SDR for this child:
   d. Dose ordered:
   e. Evaluation and decision:
   f. Volume to be administered if applicable:

5. Ordered: Oxacillin sodium 1500 mg IM q8h for an 11-year-old child weighing 75 lb. The SDR is 50 to 100 mg/kg/day in 4 divided doses.

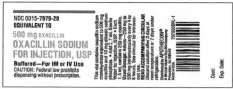

   a. Estimated wt in kg:
   b. Actual wt (1 or 2 steps?):
   c. SDR for this child:
   d. Dose ordered:
   e. Evaluation and decision:
   f. Volume to be administered if applicable:

● CHILDREN'S IV MEDICATIONS: RECONSTITUTION, DILUTION, AND FLOW RATE INFORMATION

Hospital pharmacies and pediatric drug references provide directions for dilution and rates of administration of IV medications for children. The volumes are smaller than those for adults. After determining that the ordered dose is within the SDR, the nurse may have to dilute the medication in a prescribed ratio, withdraw the ordered amount, then further dilute using a compatible IV solution and administer directly or with an infusion pump in a volume-control device. An electronic infusion pump is shown in Figure 11-4.

FIGURE 11-4
A, Electronic infusion pump with volume control device. **B,** Gravity infusion with microdrip tubing (60 gtt/mL delivered through a needle) and volume control device. Electronic infusion devices with a volume-control device are preferred for the administration of IV fluids to infants and children. If one of these is not available, microdrip (60 drop factor) tubing should be used with a volume control device to prevent fluid or drug overload. Very small volumes to be delivered IV within a short period may be administered directly through a syringe or syringe pump **(C)**. Some institutions prefer the use of the syringe pump. **C,** Freedom 60 syringe infusion pump system. *(Part C from Repro-Med Systems, Inc., Chester, NY.)*

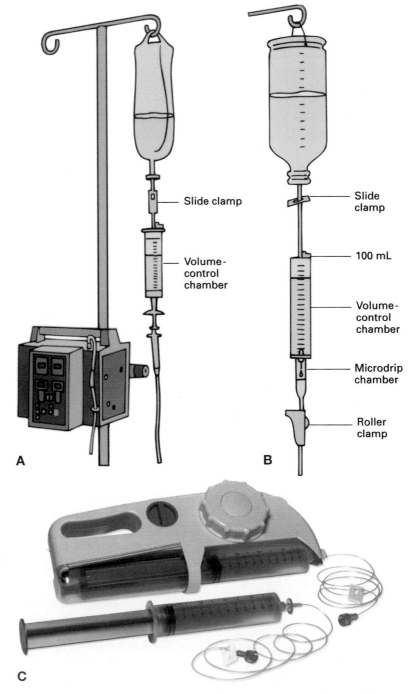

EXAMPLE   Ordered: Antibiotic 1 g q6h. Supplied: A powder form of antibiotic that requires reconstitution. Pediatric directions from pharmacy: Dilute to 100 mg/mL, withdraw ordered amount, then further dilute to 30 mL, and administer over 20 min. Refer to page 151 for intermittent infusion calculations. The label reads 2 g.

Step 1   Dilute to 100 mg/mL.

The label reads 2 g. (Change to milligrams for dilution: 2 g = 2000 mg.)

Know   *Want to Know*   **PROOF**
100 mg : 1 mL :: 2000 mg : x mL $100 \times 20 = 2000$
$\frac{100}{100}x = \frac{2000}{100}$ $1 \times 2000 = 2000$

   $x = 20$ mL

Reconstitute antibiotic with 20 mL compatible solution.*

Step 2   Withdraw ordered amount (1 g).

Know   *Want to Know*   **PROOF** $2 \times 10 = 20$ **ANSWER**
2 g : 20 mL :: 1 g : x mL $20 \times 1 = 20$ 10 mL
$2x = 20$

   $x = 10$ mL $= 1$ g

Step 3   Place the medication in a volume control device adding a compatible IV solution to 30 mL. Set the flow rate. Consult a procedure book for use of volume control devices.

Flow rate:

Know   *Want to Know*   **PROOF**   **ANSWER**
30 mL : 20 min :: x mL : 60 min $30 \times 60 = 1800$ Set rate at
$\frac{20}{20}x = \frac{1800}{20}$ $20 \times 90 = 1800$ 90 mL/hr
                                                                for 20 min
   $x = 90$ mL

◖◀◀◀◀◀◀◀RULES   To *estimate* hourly IV flow rates for amounts to be delivered in less than 60 minutes on a pump: for **10** minutes, multiply the volume by 6 because there are six 10-minute periods in an hour; for **15** minutes, multiply the volume by 4; for **20** minutes, multiply the volume by 3; and for **30** minutes, multiply the volume by 2. This will only work for 10-, 15-, 20-, 30-minute orders.

To *calculate* the setting for mL/hr on a pump for medications to be delivered in less than 1 hour, set up a ratio and proportion of milliliters to minutes. The final dilution may be made with an existing IV solution if it is compatible with the medication.

EXAMPLE   To give 10 mL in 15 min with a pump, *estimate* ($10 \times 4 = 40$ mL/hr):

Know   *Want to Know*   **PROOF**   **ANSWER**
10 mL : 15 min :: x mL : 60 min $10 \times 60 = 600$ 40 mL/hr
$\frac{15}{15}x = \frac{600}{15}$ $15 \times 40 = 600$

   $x = 40$ mL

*For information and practice reconstituting medications, refer to Chapter 5.

EXAMPLE Ordered: Antibiotic 250 mg q4h IV.

The label reads: *Mix (dilute) with 4.2 mL sterile water for injection to yield 5 mL of 100 mg per mL.*

Amount of ordered antibiotic to be withdrawn after mixing:

Know	*Want to Know*	**PROOF**	**ANSWER**
100 mg : 1 mL :: 250 mg : x mL		$100 \times 2.5 = 250$	2.5 mL
$\frac{\cancel{100}}{\cancel{100}} x = \frac{250}{100}$		$1 \times 250 = 250$	
$x = 2.5$ mL			

Directions for pediatric administration: *Further dilute to 25 mL and administer over 30 minutes.*

Total volume to be administered: 25 mL.

EXAMPLE Flow rate in volume-control device, estimate ($2 \times 25 = 50$ mL/hr):

Know	*Want to Know*	**PROOF**	**ANSWER**
25 mL : 30 min :: x mL : 60 min		$25 \times 60 = 1500$	50 mL/hr
$30x = 25 \times 60$ or 1500		$30 \times 50 = 1500$	
$x = 50$ mL			

ANSWERS ON PAGE 397

WORKSHEET 11G Children's IV Medications

For each problem, use a calculator to determine the child's weight in kilograms if required, calculate the SDR, and compare it with the order. Evaluate the order and make a decision:

1. Give medication (within SDR for unit dose 24-hour dose).
2. Give and clarify (underdose).
3. Hold and clarify promptly (overdose).

For directions 1 and 2 *only,* calculate the medication amount to be administered from the label provided. Use written ratio and proportion and prove your answer even if you use a calculator to verify. Calculate the IV pump flow rate in mL/hr if medication is to be administered for more than 5 min. Round kilograms to the nearest tenth. Prove all work.

1. Ordered: Luminal sodium 65 mg IV stat. The child's weight is 62 lb. The SDR for sedation is 1 to 3 mg/kg q24h.

   Directions: Dilute to 3 mL sterile water for injection.

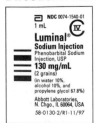

   a. Estimated wt in kg:
   b. Actual wt in kg:
   c. SDR for this child:
   d. Dose ordered:
   e. Evaluation and decision:
   f. Volume to be administered if applicable:

ANSWERS ON PAGE 397

WORKSHEET

11G Children's IV Medications—cont'd

2. Ordered: Furosemide 25 mg IV stat. The SDR is 1 mg/kg to increase gradually in 1 mg/kg increments to desired response, not to exceed 6 mg/kg. The child weighs 55 lb today.

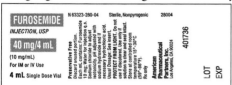

    a. Estimated wt in kg:
    b. Actual wt in kg:
    c. SDR for this child:
    d. Dose ordered:
    e. Evaluation and decision:
    f. Volume to be administered if applicable:

3. Ordered: Zinacef (cefuroxime sodium) IV 0.3 g q6h. The SDR is 50 to 100 mg/kg/day in divided doses q6-8h. To reconstitute for children in an intermittent infusion, dilute medication with 9 mL of compatible solution, then further dilute medication ordered to 20 mL of a compatible solution and administer in a volume-control device on an IV infusion pump in 30 min. The child weighs 34 lb today.

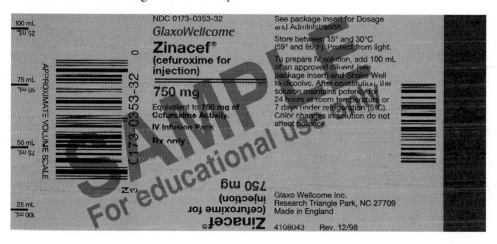

a. Estimated wt in kg: **b.** Actual wt in kg:
c. SDR for this child: **d.** Dose ordered:
e. Evaluation and decision: **f.** Ordered amount of medication in mL to
g. Flow rate on infusion pump   be withdrawn after first dilution:
    after final dilusion:

Continued

CLINICAL ALERT!

Consult pediatric IV drug references and pharmacy for pediatric IV dilutions and rates of administration. Note that liquids added to solids result in a higher total volume than just the amount of liquid added. Instructions to dilute **with** *x* *mL* result in more volume than instructions to dilute **to** *x mL*. Dilute **to** limits a total volume for the mixture. Dilute **with** is just stating the amount of liquid to be added to the solid.

WORKSHEET

11G Children's IV Medications—cont'd

4. Ordered: Nebcin (tobramycin sulfate) 60 mg IV q8h. The child weighs 56 lb today. The SDR is 3 mg/kg q8h. Directions from the pharmacy state to dilute to 50 mL and administer over 60 minutes.

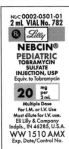

    a. Estimated wt in kg:

    b. Actual wt in kg:

    c. SDR for this child:

    d. Dose ordered:

    e. Evaluation and decision:

    f. Amount withdrawn from vial:

    g. Flow rate in mL/hr on pump if applicable:

5. Ordered: Geopen (carbenicillin disodium) 2 g IV q6h. The SDR is 50 to 500 mg/kg q24h in divided doses every 4 to 6 hr. Dilute to 200 mg/mL with compatible solution and administer at rate of 1 g/10 min. The child weighs 26 lb.

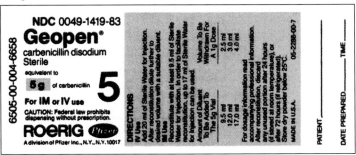

    a. Estimated wt in kg:

    b. Actual wt in kg:

    c. SDR for this child:

    d. Dose ordered:

    e. Evaluation and decision:

    f. Amount withdrawn after reconstitution:

    g. Flow rate in mL/hr if applicable:

CLINICAL ALERT!

Many of the antibiotics, particularly the cephalosporins (refer to Problem 3), have very similar names such as ceftizoxime, ceftriaxone, and cephradine. However, the uses and the SDRs are very different!

ANSWERS ON PAGE 398

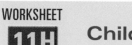

WORKSHEET
11H   Children's Dosages

For each problem, use a calculator to determine the child's weight in kilograms to the nearest tenth, calculate the SDR, and compare it with the order. If total dose for 24 hours is excessive, the unit dose is automatically excessive. Evaluate the order and make a decision:

1. Give medication (within SDR for unit dose and 24-hour dose).
2. Give and clarify (underdose).
3. Hold and clarify promptly (overdose).

Calculate doses less than 1 mL to nearest hundredth and doses more than 1 mL to nearest tenth. Double check your work and show your proof.

1. Ordered: Amoxil 100 mg tid po for a child with otitis media.
Weight: 34 lb
SDR: 20 mg/kg in 3 divided doses

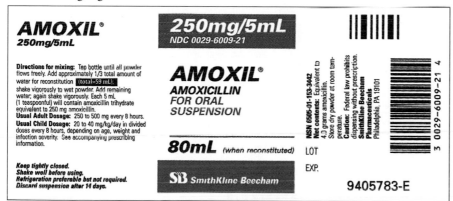

   a. Estimated wt in kg:
   b. Actual wt in kg:
   c. SDR for this child:
   d. Dose ordered:
   e. Evaluation and decision:
   f. Amount to be administered if applicable:

Continued

Children's Dosages—cont'd

2. Ordered: Lufyllin (dyphilline elixir) 75 mg bid for a child with asthma.
Weight: 70 lb
SDR: 5 mg/kg in 2 to 3 divided doses per day

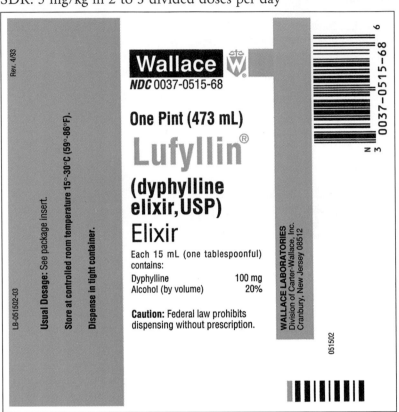

a. Estimated wt in kg:
b. Actual wt in kg:
c. SDR for this child:

d. Dose ordered:
e. Evaluation and decision:
f. Amount to be administered if applicable:

3. Ordered: Synthroid 0.1 mg qAM IV for a
6-year-old child with hypothyroidism.
Weight: 49 lb
SDR: 4 to 5 mcg/kg/day po; IV $\frac{1}{2}$ of po dose
a. Estimated wt in kg:
b. Actual wt in kg:
c. SDR for this child:
d. Dose ordered:
e. Evaluation and decision:
f. Amount to be administered if applicable:

code 3P1312
NDC 0048-1014-99
SYNTHROID®
(levothyroxine sodium,
USP) for Injection

200 mcg

Sterile, nonpyrogenic.
This vial contains 200 mcg
Levothyroxine Sodium, USP, 10 mg
Mannitol, USP, 0.7 mg Tribasic
Sodium Phosphate, Anhydrous,
Sodium Hydroxide, Q.S. for pH
adjustment.
CAUTION: Federal law prohibits
dispensing without prescription.

Administer intravenously after
reconstitution with 5 mL of 0.9%
Sodium Chloride Injection, USP.
Shake vial to insure complete
mixing. Do not add to other intravenous fluids. Use immediately
after reconstitution. Discard any
unused portion.

For complete prescribing
information see attached
brochure.

Store at controlled room
temperature, 15°-30°C (59°-86°F).
Mfg. for:
Knoll Pharmaceutical Company
Mount Olive, NJ 07828 USA
By: Ben Venue Laboratories, Inc.
Bedford, Ohio 44146 USA

Knoll Pharmaceutical Company
3000 Continental Drive North
Mount Olive, New Jersey 07828-1234

BASF Pharma

ANSWERS ON PAGE 398

WORKSHEET

11H   Children's Dosages—cont'd

4. Ordered: Meperidine HCl 35 mg IM preoperatively.
Weight: 66 lb
SDR: 1 to 2.2 mg/kg

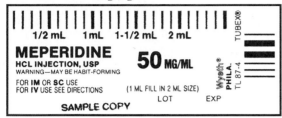

a. Estimated wt in kg:
b. Actual wt in kg:
c. SDR for this child:
d. Dose ordered:
e. Evaluation and decision:
f. Amount to be administered if applicable:

5. Ordered: Deltasone (prednisone) 30 mg/day po for a child with acute asthma.
Weight: 13.6 kg BSA = 0.6 m^2
SDR: 40 mg/m^2 day po

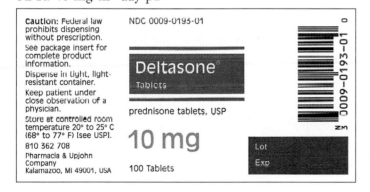

a. Estimated wt in lb:
b. Actual wt in lb:
c. SDR for this child:
d. Dose ordered:
e. Evaluation and decision:
f. Amount to be administered if applicable:

Continued

ANSWERS ON PAGE 398

WORKSHEET
11H   Children's Dosages—cont'd

6. Ordered: Ampicillin sodium 250 mg IV q6h for a child with a kidney infection.
Weight: 22 lb
SDR: 50 to 100 mg/kg/day in 4 divided doses

Directions: Dilute 1 g vial in at least 10 mL of sterile water for injection before further dilutions. Further dilute to 20 mg/mL in D5W. Final concentration should never exceed 30 mg/mL.

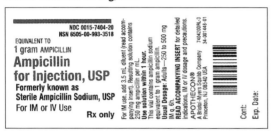

a. Estimated wt in kg:
b. Actual wt in kg:
c. SDR for this child:
d. Dose ordered:
e. Evaluation and decision:
f. Amount to be administered if applicable:

7. Ordered: Potassium chloride (KCl) 0.9 mEq to be added to each IV q8h.
Weight: 6 lb
SDR: Up to 3 mEq/kg/24 hr

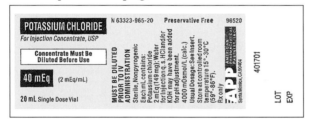

a. Estimated wt in kg:
b. Actual wt in kg:
c. SDR for this child:
d. Dose ordered:
e. Evaluation and decision:
f. Dose to be added to IV:

8. Ordered: Rocephin (ceftriaxone sodium) 600 mg IV q12h for a child with a *Shigella* infection.
Weight: 31 lb
SDR: Up to 100 mg/kg/day in 2 divided doses

Directions: Add 9.6 mL sterile water for injection to equal 100 mg/mL. Further dilute to 30 mL with compatible solution over 30 min.

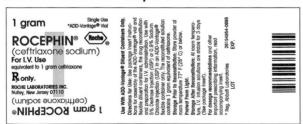

a. Estimated wt in kg:
b. Actual wt in kg:
c. SDR for this child:
d. Dose ordered:
e. Evaluation and decision:
f. Dose to be administered after reconstitution if applicable:
g. Flow rate in Volutrol:

ANSWERS ON PAGE 398

WORKSHEET

11H   Children's Dosages—cont'd

9. Ordered: Acetaminophen drops 20 mg po q4h for a 3-month-old infant.
Physician has verified dosage and infant concentrated drop preparation.

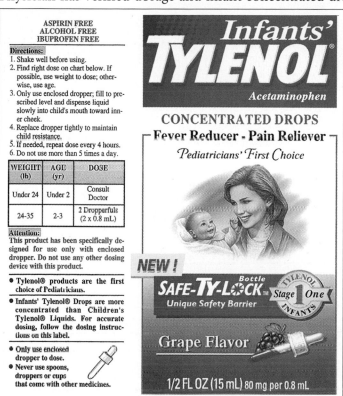

a. Dose to be administered:

b. Measuring device to be used:

10. Ordered: Amoxil oral suspension 120 mg po q8h.
Weight: 26.4 lb.
SDR: 20 to 40 mg/kg/day

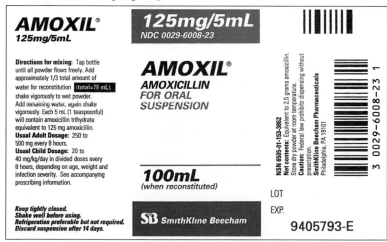

a. Estimated wt in kg:

c. SDR for this child:

e. Evaluation and decision:

b. Actual wt in kg:

d. Dose ordered:

f. Dose to be administered:

ANSWERS ON PAGE 400

WORKSHEET
111 **Multiple-Choice Practice**

For the following problems, estimate kilograms, then calculate kilograms to *nearest* tenth when a pound to kilogram conversion is needed and estimate answers before solving each step.

1. Ordered: 20 mg/kg of Drug X for a child weighing 50 lb. How many milligrams of the drug will you administer to the child?
   a. 400 mg
   b. 454 mg
   c. 500 mg
   d. 1000 mg

2. Ordered: methotrexate sodium 30 mg/m^2 daily maintenance for a child with leukemia. The child's BSA is 1.20 m^2. How much medication will you administer?
   a. 1.20 mg
   b. 30 mg
   c. 36 mg
   d. 30.12 mg

3. Ordered: 1.5 tsp of acetaminophen suspension liquid for a child with fever. How many milliliters will you administer?
   a. 5 mL
   b. 7.5 mL
   c. 8 mL
   d. 10 mL

4. Ordered: 30 mg of Drug X for a child weighing 25 lb. SDR is 2 to 5 mg/kg. Using the nursing process, what decision will you make regarding this medication order?
   a. Hold the order. It is an overdose.
   b. Give the medication but call the physician for clarification because it is an underdose.
   c. Give the medication because the order is within SDR.
   d. Consult with a supervisor about this order. It is unclear.

5. Ordered: V-Cillin K 125 mg daily for a child weighing 5.5 lb. The literature states: 40 mg/kg day in divided doses. Label states: 125 mg per 5 mL. Your decision:
   a. Give the medication. The order is safe.
   b. Hold the medication. Consult with a colleague.
   c. Give the medication and clarify with the physician at next visit.
   d. Hold the medication and clarify with the physician by telephone.

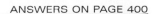

WORKSHEET
11I Multiple-Choice Practice—cont'd

6. Ordered: Garamycin 50 mg IV q8h for a child weighing 55 lb. The SDR is 2 to 2.5 mg/kg q8h. Your decision:
   a. Give the medication. The order is within safe limits.
   b. Hold the medication. Consult with physician. The order is an overdose.
   c. Give the medication and consult with the physician. The order is an underdose.
   d. Call the pharmacy and clarify the order.

7. Ordered: Phenytoin oral suspension 15 mg bid po for a 6-kg child with seizures. The SDR is 5 mg/kg in 2 to 3 divided doses. Label reads: Dilantin pediatric suspension 30 mg/5 mL. Your decision:
   a. Hold and clarify the order with the physician. It is an overdose.
   b. The order is safe. Give 2.5 mL.
   c. Clarify the order with an experienced supervisor.
   d. The order is safe. Give 5 mL.

8. Ordered: Synthroid 0.5 mg qAM IV for a child with hypothyroidism. Label reads: Synthroid 200 µg/10 mL. What is the amount to be administered?
   a. 2.0 mL
   b. 2.5 mL
   c. 20 mL
   d. 25 mL

9. Ordered: Meperidine 30 mg IM preoperatively for a child weighing 58 lb. SDR is 1 to 2.2 mg/kg. Label states: Meperidine HCl injection 25 mg/mL. What is your decision?
   a. The order is unsafe. Hold and contact physician.
   b. The order is an underdose. Give and contact physician.
   c. The order is safe. Give 0.83 mL.
   d. The order is safe. Give 1.2 mL.

10. Ordered: Ampicillin suspension 250 mg po q8h. Weight is 30 lb. SDR is 25 to 50 mg/kg/day po in 4 divided doses. The label reads: 125 mg/5 mL. What is your decision?
    a. The order is safe. Give 10 mL.
    b. The order is an overdose. Hold and contact physician.
    c. The order is an underdose. Give and contact physician.
    d. Give 5 mL and contact the physician.

Refer to Introducing Drug Measures, Measuring Dosages sections of the enclosed CD-ROM for additional practice problems.

CRITICAL THINKING EXERCISES

Baby Louise is in your unit with a diagnosis of congestive heart failure secondary to a congenital heart defect. She weighs 8.4 kg at age 18 months. Her orders include lanoxin 0.05 mg po bid and furosemide 2 mg/kg po stat. The orders include temporary fluid restriction to 500 mL per 24-hr period.

On hand is digoxin elixir 50 μg/mL. Given this AM by the night nurse: 5 mL.

On hand is furosemide oral solution 10 mg/mL. Given this AM by the reporting nurse: 2 mL.

During report, the nurse tells you that the intake exceeded 500 mL for the past 24 hours by 120 mL because the baby wouldn't take the medicine without a lot of juice. Is there a problem with mathematics? What error in concepts of arithmetic rounding might have led to one of the problems? Which knowledge bases are insufficient?

Medication error(s) and possible causes:

Fluid intake error:

Potential Injury/ies:

Nursing actions:

Recommendations for the nurse and for patient safety if you were on a hospital committee studying these incidents:

ANSWERS ON PAGE 403

CHAPTER 11 FINAL

Use a calculator to determine the child's weight in kilograms (to the nearest tenth) and the SDR for each child. Evaluate the order and make a decision.

1. **Give medication (within SDR for unit dose and 24-hour dose).**
2. **Give and clarify (underdose).**
3. **Hold and clarify promptly (overdose).**

If the order is to be carried out, use written ratio and proportion to calculate doses, and show your proof.*

1. Ordered: Cephalexin 200 mg oral suspension qid po for Johnny who has a streptococcal infection of the throat and a history of allergy to penicillin. The SDR is 25 to 50 mg/kg/day in 4 divided doses. The child weighs 42 lb today.

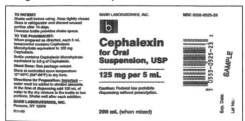

   a. Estimated wt in kg:
   b. Actual wt in kg:
   c. SDR for this child:
   d. Dose ordered:
   e. Evaluation and decision:
   f. Dose to be administered if applicable:

---

*Calculate amounts *less* than 1 mL to the nearest hundredth and greater than 1 mL to the nearest tenth. Calculate flow rates in mL/hr because an IV infusion pump will be used.

2. Johnny's mother returns to the office with him 3 days after the initial visit because he has a generalized pruritic rash. His practitioner changes his antibiotic order to erythromycin oral suspension 175 mg qid po. The SDR is 30 to 50 mg/kg/day divided q6h. Johnny still weighs 42 lb.

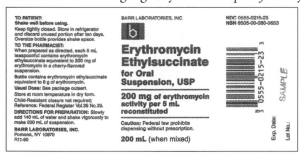

a. Actual wt in kg:
b. SDR for this child:
c. Dose ordered:
d. Evaluation and decision:
e. Dose to be administered:

3. Also ordered for Johnny's pruritis is Benadryl Allergy Liquid (diphenhydramine HCl) 25 mg tid hs × 3 days. Johnny is 6 years old. Read the label and make your decision.

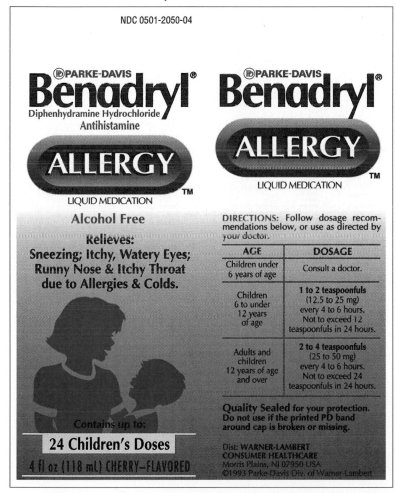

a. Safe daily dose maximum for this child:
b. Dose ordered for 24 hr:
c. Evaluation and decision:
d. Dose to be administered:

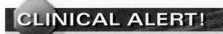

CLINICAL ALERT!

Approximately 15% or 1 in 6 persons with an allergy to penicillin will have an allergy to the cephalosporins.

4. Ordered for Johnny's 8-year-old sister is dicloxacillin sodium capsules 500 mg q6h. The SDR is 12.5 to 25 mg/kg/day in divided doses q6h for a maximum of 4 g/day. His sister weighs 32 kg. Read the label and make your evaluation and decision.

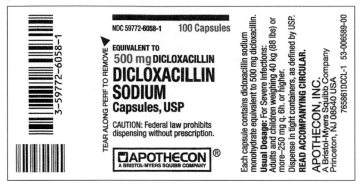

   a. SDR for this child:

   b. Dose ordered:

   c. Evaluation and decision:

   d. Dose to be administered if applicable:

5. Karen, age 3, is admitted to the hospital with a compound fracture of the femur incurred during an automobile accident. Ordered: Atropine sulfate 0.3 mg preop IM. The SDR for children weighing 12 to 16 kg is 0.3 mg 30 to 60 min before surgery. Karen weighs 35 lb.

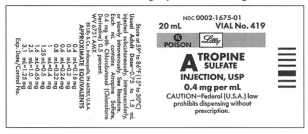

   a. Estimated wt in kg:

   b. Actual wt in kg:

   c. SDR for this child:

   d. Dose ordered:

   e. Evaluation and decision:

   f. Dose to be administered if applicable:

6. Ordered postoperatively for Karen is Amoxil oral suspension 0.5 tid po. The SDR is 20 to 40 mg per kg in three divided doses. Karen weighs 35 lb.

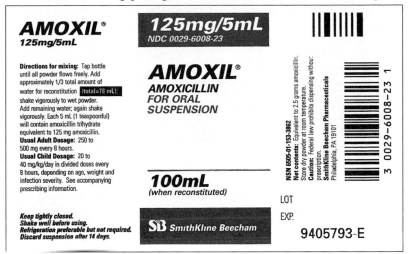

a. Estimated wt in kg:
b. Actual wt in kg:
c. SDR for this child:
d. Dose ordered:
e. Evaluation and decision:
f. Dose to be administered if applicable:

7. Also ordered for Karen postoperatively is Nebcin (tobramycin sulfate) 35 mg tid IV. The SDR is 6 to 7.5 mg/kg day in 3 divided doses. The directions from pharmacy state to dilute in 1 mg/mL and administer over 30 min on an IV infusion pump.

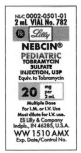

a. Actual wt in kg:
b. SDR for this child:
c. Dose ordered:
d. Evaluation and decision:
e. Dose after reconstitution if applicable:
f. IV flow rate on pump:

8. Morphine sulfate 5 mg IV q4h prn pain × 48 hr is ordered for Karen. The SDR is 0.05 to 0.1 mg/kg q4h for direct IV. Directions state to dilute with 5 mL of sterile water or sterile saline for injection and administer over 5 min.

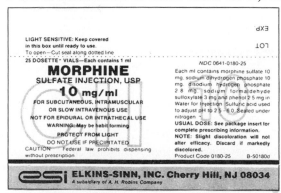

a. Actual wt in kg:
b. SDR for this child:
c. Dose ordered:
d. Evaluation and decision:
e. Dose before dilution:

9. Ordered: Leucovorin calcium 0.01 g q6h po for a child with toxic effects from an antineoplastic agent. The child weighs 70 lb and has normal height for weight. The SDR for children is up to 10 mg/m² q6h for 72 hr. Use the West nomogram* to determine the BSA for this child's weight.
  a. BSA in m²:
  b. SDR for this child:
  c. Dose ordered:
  d. Evaluation and decision:
  e. Amount to be given if applicable:

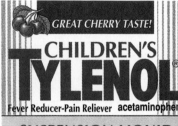

Each tablet contains:
Leucovorin Calcium USP,
(equivalent to 5 mg
Leucovorin).
Usual Dosage:
See package outsert.
PROTECT FROM LIGHT.
Dispense with child-
resistant closure in a
tight, light-resistant
container as defined
in the USP/NF.
Store at controlled
room temperature
15°-30° C (59°-86° F).
BARR LABORATORIES, INC.
Pomona, NY 10970
R7-91

BARR LABORATORIES, INC.

Leucovorin Calcium Tablets
5 mg

NDC 0555-0484-01
NSN 6505-01-230-3140

Caution: Federal law prohibits dispensing without prescription.

30 Tablets

SAMPLE

10. Ordered: Tylenol suspension liquid 240 mg for a 3-year-old child with a fever who weighs 18 kg. The SDR for a child weighing 24 to 35 lb is 1 tsp, and 1½ tsp for a child weighing 36 to 47 lb.
  a. Estimated wt in lb:
  b. Wt in lb:
  c. SDR for this child:
  d. Dose ordered:
  e. Evaluation and decision:
  f. Dose to be administered if applicable:
  g. Measuring device to be used:

Directions:
1. Shake well before using.
2. Find right dose on chart below. If possible, use weight to dose; otherwise use age.
3. Only use enclosed measuring cup.
4. If needed, repeat dose every 4 hours.
5. Do not use more than 5 times a day.

WEIGHT (lb)	AGE (yr)	DOSE (tsp)
Under 24	Under 2	Consult Physician
24–35	2–3	1
36–47	4–5	1 1/2
48–59	6–8	2
60–71	9–10	2 1/2
72–95	11	3

Attention:
Specially designed for use with enclosed measuring cup. Use only enclosed measuring cup to dose this product. Do not use any other dosing device.

Inactive Ingredients: Butylparaben, Cellulose, Citric Acid, Corn Syrup, Flavors, Glycerin, Propylene Glycol, Purified Water, Sodium Benzoate, Sorbitol, Xanthan Gum and FD&C Red #40.

● Tylenol® products are the first choice of Pediatricians.

● Children's Tylenol® Liquids are not the same concentration as Infants' Tylenol® Drops. For accurate dosing, follow the dosing instructions on this label.

● Use only enclosed measuring cup to dose.
● Items like kitchen teaspoons may not be accurate.
● Never use spoons, droppers or cups that come with other medicines.

Store at room temperature.
See bottom panel of carton for expiration date and lot number.

McNEIL
McNEIL CONSUMER PRODUCTS CO.
DIVISION OF McNEIL-PPC, INC.
FORT WASHINGTON, PA 19034 USA
U.S. Patent No. 5,272,137
© McN-PPC, Inc.'97

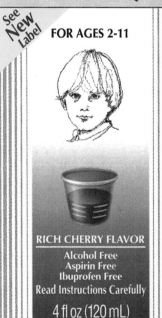

GREAT CHERRY TASTE!

CHILDREN'S TYLENOL®
Fever Reducer-Pain Reliever acetaminophen

SUSPENSION LIQUID

See New Label

FOR AGES 2-11

RICH CHERRY FLAVOR
Alcohol Free
Aspirin Free
Ibuprofen Free
Read Instructions Carefully

4 fl oz (120 mL)
80 mg per 1/2 teaspoon
(160 mg per 5 mL)

*For the West nomogram, refer to page 256.

CLINICAL ALERT!

Beware of medication orders for "T" and "t" and "tsp"; for example, 1 T qid or 1 tsp qid. Teaspoon and tablespoon abbreviations can easily be confused. Do not use household utensils.

Also, dosage strength may vary per teaspoon among infant, child, and adult preparations and may also vary among manufacturers. Call the physician and clarify the specific strength desired in milligrams or milliequivalents.

Dimensional Analysis 12

INTRODUCTION

In this chapter you will learn how to calculate clinical medication doses using dimensional analysis. Dimensional analysis is a fractionalized method for setting up medication calculation problems. There are four worksheets, ranging from simple to complex. The setups include: conversions from one metric measurement to another, IM injections, SC insulin and heparin injections, IV gravity and infusion device calculation problems, and safe dose ranges.

● DIMENSIONAL ANALYSIS

The dimensional analysis process is similar to the ratio and proportion method. The setup is in fraction form. The entire medical calculation can be written on one line with all of the information given. Always start with the outcome, or what it is that you are solving for. That becomes your unknown quantity. The unknown becomes the X factor. The X factor always goes on the left so that you don't forget what you want the outcome to be.

◀◀◀◀◀◀◀◀RULE   All symbols in the equation must cancel out **except the X factor symbol on the left**.

EXAMPLE   Convert g to mg.

800 mg = ? g

 REMEMBER ● **Put the symbol that you are solving for on the left. All matching symbols must be canceled, and the remaining symbol will be the X symbol.**

Know   *Want to Know*

$Xg = 1 \, g/1000 \, mg \times 800 \, mg/1 = 800/1000 = 0.8 \, g$

Both mg symbols were able to be canceled and the remaining symbol was g. In order for the mg symbols to be canceled out, one had to be in the numerator, and one, in the denominator.

EXAMPLE   Convert lb to kg.

155 lb = ? kg

The unknown is kg, which goes on the left.

Know   *Want to Know*

$X \, kg = 1 \, kg/2.2 \, lb \times 155 \, lb/1 = 70.5 \, kg$

Note that the lb symbols are in the numerator and the denominator and are therefore able to be canceled out, leaving the kg symbol remaining.

This example will use the conversion factor to determine how many mL to give.

EXAMPLE   Ordered: Ampicillin 300 mg IM q8h

Available: Ampicillin 1 g/2 mL
How many milliliters will you give?

| *Know* | *Conversion (know)* | *Want to Know* |

X mL = 2 mL/1 g × 1 g/1000 mg × 300 mg/1 = 600/1000 = 0.6 mL

Note that the mg and the g cancel out and the remaining symbol is mL.

Can you see the similarity to the ratio and proportion method?

ANSWERS ON PAGE 404

WORKSHEET 12A   Basic Calculations

1. Ordered: Pfizerpen 800 mg IM.
   Available: Pfizerpen One Million Units. After reconstitution with 1.8 mL
   of sterile water, each milliliter will contain 500 mg.
   How many milliliters will you give?

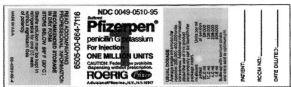

2. Ordered: Cimetidine tablets 0.8 g qid.
   Available: 400 mg/tab.
   How many tablets will you give?

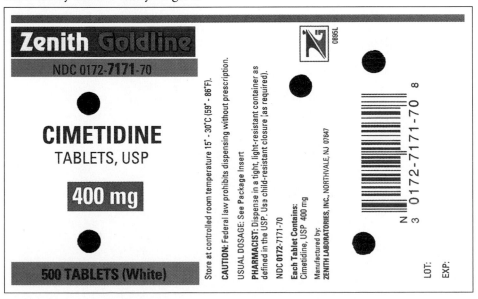

Continued

ANSWERS ON PAGE 404

WORKSHEET

12A   **Basic Calculations—cont'd**

3. The IV is infusing at 125 mL/hr. The drop factor is 20 gtt/mL.
How many drops per minute will you regulate the IV?

4. Ordered: 35 mg Demerol IM q4h prn for pain.
Available: Demerol 50 mg/mL.
How many milliliters will you give?

5. Ordered: Erythromycin sulfate 250 mg po q6h.
Available: After reconstitution, there will be 200 mg/5 mL.
How many milliliters will you give?

TO PATIENT:
Shake well before using.
Keep tightly closed. Store in refrigerator
and discard unused portion after ten days.
Oversize bottle provides shake space.

TO THE PHARMACIST:
When prepared as directed, each 5 mL
teaspoonful contains erythromycin
ethylsuccinate equivalent to 200 mg of
erythromycin in a cherry-flavored
suspension.
Bottle contains erythromycin ethylsuccinate
equivalent to 8 g of erythromycin.
Usual Dose: See package outsert.
Store at room temperature in dry form.
Child-Resistant closure not required;
Reference: Federal Register Vol.39 No.29.
DIRECTIONS FOR PREPARATION: Slowly
add 140 mL of water and shake vigorously to
make 200 mL of suspension.
BARR LABORATORIES, INC.
Pomona, NY 10970
R11-90

BARR LABORATORIES, INC.

Erythromycin Ethylsuccinate
for Oral Suspension, USP

200 mg of erythromycin activity per 5 mL reconstituted

Caution: Federal law prohibits
dispensing without prescription.

200 mL (when mixed)

NDC 0555-0215-23
NSN 6505-00-080-0653

0555-0215-23 3

SAMPLE

Exp. Date:

Lot No.:

6. Ordered: 750 mg Lorabid po q12h.
Available: Lorabid 200 mg/5 mL.
How many milliliters will you give?

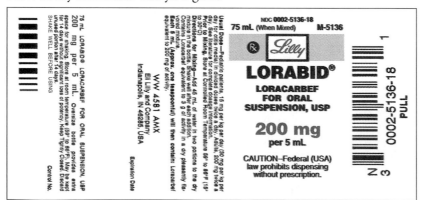

7. Ordered: 1260 mL of parenteral nutrition.
How many liters is this?

ANSWERS ON PAGE 404

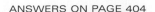

WORKSHEET

12A Basic Calculations—cont'd

8. Ordered: Solu-Cortef 300 mg IM q8h.
   Available: Solu-Cortef 250 mg/2 mL.
   How many milliliters will you give?

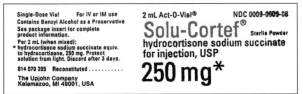

9. Ordered: Ampicillin 400 mg IM q6h.
   Available: Ampicillin for injection 1 g. After reconstitution, each
   milliliter contains 250 mg.
   How many milliliters will you give?

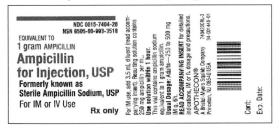

10. Ordered: Cefadyl 700 mg IM q6h.
    Available: 1 g. Each 1.2 mL = 500 mg.
    How many milliliters will you give?

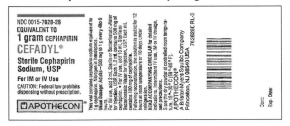

ANSWERS ON PAGE 405

WORKSHEET
12B　　IV Calculations

This worksheet will give you practice in calculating the IV rate for units/hr, mL/hr, mg/hr, mEq/hr, and hours to infuse.

◉◄◄◄◄◄◄◄◄◄RULE　　Always start the equation with what you want to find out or X. Then put in the remainder of the information given to you in a sequence in which the numerator and denominator can cancel out and the X will be the only symbol not crossed out in the equation.

EXAMPLE　　Ordered: 500 mL Ringer's lactate to infuse at 112 mL/hr. How long will it take the IV to infuse?

X hr = 1 hr/112 mL × 500 mL/1 = 500/112 = 4.46 = 4 hr 27 min

The mL cancels out and the remaining symbol is the hr.

1. Ordered: 20,000 units of heparin sodium in 1000 mL of 0.9% saline.
   Infuse at 1000 units/hr.
   How many mL/hr will you set the IV infusion device?

2. Refer to the answer from number 1 to answer this question.
   How many units per hour will be infused?

3. Ordered: Dopamine 400 mg in 500 mL to infuse at 60 mL/hr.
   How many milligrams will infuse per hour?

4. Order: Pitocin 30 units in 1000 mL of normal saline (NS). Infuse at
   2 units/hr.
   How many mL/hr will you set the IV infusion device?

5. Ordered: 50 units of Humulin Regular to infuse in 24 hr. The pharmacy
   has sent 1000 mL of 0.45% sodium chloride with 50 units of Humulin
   Regular insulin.
   a. How many mL/hr will you set the IV infusion device?
   b. How many units/hr will be infused?

6. Ordered: 30 units of Humulin Regular insulin IV to infuse in 12 hours.
   Available: 250 mL of 0.9% sodium chloride with 30 units of Humulin
   Regular insulin.
   a. How many mL/hr will you set the IV infusion device?
   b. How many units/hr will be infused?

7. Ordered: 300 mg aminophylline IV in 250 mL of 0.9% sodium chloride
   to infuse in 8 hours.
   a. How many milliliters will infuse in 1 hr?
   b. How many mg/hr will be infused?

8. Ordered: 1000 mL lactated Ringer's with 20 mEq of KCl IV to infuse in
   12 hr.
   a. How many mL/hr will you set the IV infusion device?
   b. How many milliequivalents will infuse per hour?

ANSWERS ON PAGE 405

WORKSHEET

12B   IV Calculations—cont'd

9. Ordered: 1000 mL of D5W to infuse IV at 20 gtt/min. The drop factor is 15 gtt/mL.
   How many hours will it take to infuse 1000 mL?

10. Ordered: 1000 mL D5W IV to infuse at 120 mL/hr.
    How many hours will it take to infuse?

ANSWERS ON PAGE 406

WORKSHEET

12C   IV Calculations Continued

This worksheet will give you practice in calculating units/hr, drops/min, μg/min, and mL/hr, and safe dose ranges (SDRs).

EXAMPLE   Ordered: Cephalexin 150 mg oral suspension qid.
Available: Cephalexin 125 mg/5 mL. The SDR is 25 to 50 mg/kg/day in 4 divided doses. The child weighs 38 lb.

a. What is the low dose range for one day?

$$\text{x mg/kg/day} = \frac{1 \text{ kg}}{2.2 \text{ lb}} \times \frac{38 \text{ lb}}{1} \times \frac{25 \text{ mg}}{1 \text{ kg}} = \frac{950}{2.2} = 431.8 = 432 \text{ mg/kg/day}$$

Know .... Want to Know

b. What is the high dose range for one day?

$$\text{x mg/kg/day} = \frac{1 \text{ kg}}{2.2 \text{ lb}} \times \frac{38 \text{ lb}}{1} \times \frac{50 \text{ mg}}{1 \text{ kg}} = \frac{1900}{2.2} = 863.6 = 864 \text{ mg/kg/day}$$

Know .... Want to Know

c. Is this a safe dose?

$$\text{x mg} = \frac{150 \text{ mg}}{1 \text{ dose}} \times \frac{4 \text{ doses}}{1} = 600 \text{ mg/day}$$

Have .... Want to Have

d. How many milliliters will you give per dose?

$$\text{x mL/dose} = \frac{5 \text{ mL}}{125 \text{ mg}} \times \frac{150 \text{ mg}}{1} = \frac{750}{125} = 6 \text{ mL}$$

Have .... Want to Have

1. Ordered: Nitroprusside sodium 30 mg in 250 mL Ringer's lactate solution.
   Available: 250 mL Ringer's lactate solution with 30 mg Nipride. The directions read: Infuse at 3 μg/min. The patient weighs 190 lb. The IV tubing is microdrip.
   a. How many μg/min will be infused?
   b. Use the answer from a. to calculate how many mL/hr will deliver the required μg/min.
   c. How many gtt/min will be infused?

Continued

ANSWERS ON PAGE 406

WORKSHEET

12C IV Calculations Continued—cont'd

2. Ordered: Dobutamine 200 mg in 250 mL to infuse at 5 μg/kg/min. The patient weighs 110 kg.
   a. How many μg/min will the patient receive?
   b. How many mL/hr will you set the infusion device?

3. Ordered: Dopamine HCl 800 mg in 500 mL in D5W to infuse at 6 μg/kg/min. The patient weighs 160 lbs. The drop factor is microdrip.
   a. How many μg/min will the patient receive?
   b. How many mL/hr will you set the IV rate?

4. Ordered: 10,000 units heparin in 1000 mL 0.9% sodium chloride to infuse in 12 hr.
   a. How many mL/hr will you set the infusion device?
   b. How many units/hr will the patient receive?

5. A peripheral parenteral nutrition solution of 1350 mL is infusing at 112 mL/hr.
   How many hours will it take to infuse?

6. Ordered: 1000 mL of 0.9% sodium chloride with 50 mEq of potassium is to be infused over 4 hours. The drop factor of the tubing is 20 gtt/mL.
   How many gtt/min will be delivered?

7. Ordered: 500 mL 0.9% normal saline to be infused in 90 min. The drop factor is 12 gtt/mL.
   How many gtt/min will be delivered?

8. Ordered: 500 mL D5W to infuse in 2 hr by gravity flow. The drop factor is 10.
   How many gtt/min will you regulate the IV?

9. Ordered: 2000 mL IV fluids to infuse in 24 hr.
   How many mL/hr will infuse?

10. Ordered: 1000 mL D5W to infuse in 6 hr.
   How many mL/hr will you set the IV infusion device?

ANSWERS ON PAGE 407

WORKSHEET
12D Multiple-Choice Practice

This worksheet combines various types of calculations and is presented in a multiple choice format.

1. Calculate the safe dose for a child weighing 5 kg. The safe dosage is 10 mg/kg.
   a. 0.2 mg   **b.** 0.5 mg   **c.** 50 mg   **d.** 2 mg
   The order is for a one-time dose of 25 mg. Is this a safe dose?
   a. Yes   **b.** No

2. The medication label reads 6 to 8 mg/kg. The baby weighs 8 lb. How many kilograms does the baby weigh?
   a. 4.5 kg   **b.** 16 kg   **c.** 6.6 kg   **d.** 3.6 kg

   Calculate the low end of the dose range.
   a. 24 mg   **b.** 22 mg   **c.** 36 mg   **d.** 12 mg

   Calculate the high end of the dose range.
   a. 29 mg   **b.** 26 mg   **c.** 32 mg   **d.** 35 mg

3. Ordered: Tylenol elixer 240 mg for a 5-year-old child who weighs 16 kg.
   Available: 80 mg/2.5 mL.
   How many milliliters will you give?
   a. 6.5 mL   **b.** 5 mL   **c.** 4 mL   **d.** 7.5 mL

4. Ordered: 600 mg of Cefadyl IM q6h.
   Available: Cefadyl 1g. Each mL contains 0.5 g.
   How many milliliters will you give?
   a. 2.5 mL   **b.** 1.2 mL   **c.** 2.2 mL   **d.** 1.5 mL

5. Ordered: 1330 mL of a parenteral nutrition solution to infuse at 112 mL/hr.
   How many hours will the IV infuse?
   a. 10 hr 10 min **b.** 9 hr 36 min **c.** 11 hr 52 min **d.** 12 hr 11 min

   If the infusion was started at 2000 hr, what time will it finish?
   a. 0800 hr   **b.** 0600 hr   **c.** 1800 hr   **d.** 0400 hr

6. Ordered: Heparin 50,000 units in 1000 mL of NS to infuse in 12 hr.
   How many mL/hr will you set the infusion device?
   a. 83 mL/hr   **b.** 100 mL/hr   **c.** 33 mL/hr   **d.** 10 mL/hr

   How many units per minute will infuse?
   a. 24 units/min   **b.** 110 units/min
   c. 56 units/min   **d.** 69 units/min

Continued

ANSWERS ON PAGE 407

WORKSHEET

12D Multiple-Choice Practice—cont'd

7. Ordered: Erythromycin oral suspension 200 mg q4h. The child weighs 40 lb.
   Available: Erythromycin oral suspension 200 mg/5 mL.
   The SDR is 30 to 50 mg/kg/day in 4 divided doses.
   How many kilograms does the child weigh?
   a. 18 kg   **b.** 16.8 kg   **c.** 20 kg   **d.** 22 kg

   What is the low dosage for this child?
   a. 300 mg   **b.** 400 mg   **c.** 540 mg   **d.** 450 mg

   What is the high dosage for this child?
   a. 1000 mg   **b.** 650 mg   **c.** 900 mg   **d.** 700 mg

8. Ordered: 40 units Humulin Regular insulin IV in 500 mL 0.9% sodium chloride to infuse at 3 units/hr.
   How many mL/hr will deliver 3 units/hr?
   a. 32 mL/hr   **b.** 18 mL/hr   **c.** 28 mL/hr   **d.** 38 mL/hr

9. Ordered: Heparin 20,000 units in 500 mL D5W to infuse at 0.5 units/kg/min. The patient weighs 195 lb. The drop factor is microdrip.
   How many kilograms does the patient weigh?
   a. 100 kg   **b.** 95 kg   **c.** 78 kg   **d.** 89 kg

   How many units per minute will infuse?
   a. 22 units/min   **b.** 45 units/min
   c. 78 units/min   **d.** 18 units/min

   How many mL/hr will you set the infusion device?
   a. 54 mL/hr   **b.** 42 mL/hr   **c.** 68 mL/hr   **d.** 108 mL/hr

10. Ordered: 1000 mL Ringer's lactate solution with 60,000 units of heparin to infuse 5000 units per hour.
    How many mL/hr will you set the infusion device?
    a. 44 mL/hr   **b.** 83 mL/hr   **c.** 92 mL/hr   **d.** 100 mL/hr

 Refer to the Calculating Dosages, Introduction section on the enclosed CD-ROM for additional practice problems.

ANSWERS ON PAGE 408

CHAPTER **12** FINAL

1. Ordered: 750 mg IM q8h.
    Available: Keflin 1 g/mL.
    How many milliliters will you give?

2. Ordered: 400 mg IM q12h.
    Available: 0.5 g/2 mL.
    How many milliliters will you give?

3. Ordered: 100 mg IM q12h.
    Available: 0.075 g/mL.
    How many milliliters will you give?

4. Ordered: 100 mg Biaxin po q8h.
    Available: Biaxin 125 mg/5 mL oral suspension.
    a. How many milliliters per dose will you give?
    b. How many milligrams will the patient receive in 24 hr?

5. Ordered: Erythromycin 250 mg tablets qid × 10 days.
    Available: 500 mg scored tablets.
    How many tablets are needed for 10 days?

6. Ordered: An IV bolus of heparin.
    The hospital protocol for heparin states 80 units/kg.
    The patient weights 70 kg.
    How many units of heparin will the patient receive?

7. Ordered: 200 mL of 0.45% sodium chloride to infuse in 4 hours.
    The drop factor is 15.
    How many drops per minute will you set the gravity pump?

8. Ordered: Penicillin 600,000 units in 200 mL IVPB to infuse in 2 hr.
    The drop factor is 20.
    How many drops per minute will infuse?

9. Ordered: 100 mL IVPB with gentamycin 80 mg to infuse in 40 min.
    The IV tubing is microdrip.
    How many gtt/min will you regulate the IV?

10. Ordered: Norcuron 0.5 mg tid.
    The label reads: 100 to 200 μg/kg/day.
    The child weighs 25 lb.
    a. How many kilograms does the child weigh?
    b. What is the low end of the dose range for this child?
    c. What is the high end of the dose range for this child?
    d. Is the ordered medication within the safe dose range?

Multiple-Choice Final

1. Ordered Naloxone HCl 600 µg. Give:

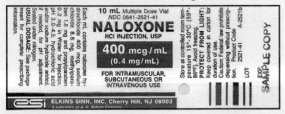

   a. 0.8 mL

   b. 1.1 mL

   c. 1.3 mL

   d. 1.5 mL

2. Ordered: Synthroid 0.1 mg po. Give:

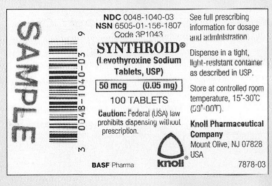

   a. $\frac{1}{2}$ tab

   b. 1.5 tab

   c. 2 tab

   d. 3 tab

3. Ordered: Meperidine 10 mg. Give:

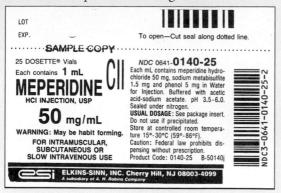

a. 0.2 mL

b. 0.4 mL

c. 0.5 mL

d. 1.25 mL

4. Ordered: Digoxin 0.25 mg po daily. Give:

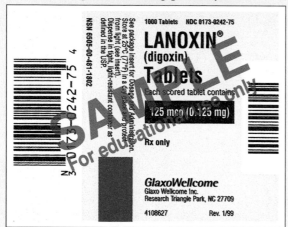

a. $\frac{1}{2}$ tab

b. 1 tab

c. 2 tab

d. 3 tab

5. Ordered: 500 mg Claforan IM q8h. Available: Claforan (cefotaxime sodium) 1 g IM or IV. Follow the preparation directions. Give 500 mg with the least volume.

STRENGTH	DILUENT	WITHDRAWABLE VOLUME	APPROX. CONCENTRATION
1 g vial (IM)	3.0 mL	3.4 mL	300 mg/mL
2 g vial (IM)	5.0 mL	6.0 mL	330 mg/mL
1 g vial (IV)	10.0 mL	10.4 mL	95 mg/mL
2 g vial (IV)	10.0 mL	11.0 mL	180 mg/mL

How many milliliters will you give the patient?

a. 2.0 mL

b. 1.5 mL

c. 2.5 mL

d. 3.0 mL

6. Ordered: Atropine Sulfate 0.6 mg IV for bradycardia. Give:

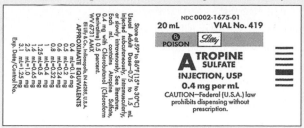

  a. 0.8 mL

  b. 1.2 mL

  c. 1.5 mL

  d. 2.2 mL

7. The pharmacy standard insulin drip is 100 units of Human Regular in 100 mL of normal saline. 1 unit = 1 mL. Your patient's blood glucose level is 222 mg/dL. How many units/hr should the patient receive? Use the following chart to determine the correct insulin rate for the IV:

BLOOD GLUCOSE (BG)/dL	STANDARD RATE/UNITS/HR
101-140	1.0
141-180	1.5
181-220	2.0
221-260	2.5
261-300	3.0

  a. 1.5 units/hr

  b. 2.5 units/hr

  c. 3.0 units/hr

  d. 2.0 units/hr

At what rate will you set the IV infusion device?

  a. 3 mL/hr

  b. 4 mL/hr

  c. 2 mL/hr

  d. 2.5 mL/hr

8. Ordered: Ampicillin 1 g IV bid. Available: Ampicillin 1 g for IV use. Direction: Add 4.5 mL of sodium chloride diluent to yield 5 mL. Dilute in 50 mL of normal saline and infuse in 15 minutes. On hand you have a microdrip infusion set. How many mL/hr will you set the IV?

  a. 200 mL/hr

  b. 100 mL/hr

  c. 60 mL/hr

  d. 20 mL/hr

9. Ordered: Rocephin 1 g q8h IV. Available: ceftrioxone sodium (Rocephin) 1 g for IM or IV use. Directions for IV use: Reconstitute with 5 mL of normal saline (NS) solution. Mix well. Further dilute in 100 mL of NS and infuse in 20 to 40 minutes. What is the maximum rate in milliliters per hour you could set the infusion device?
   a. 100 mL/hr
   b. 200 mL/hr
   c. 300 mL/hr
   d. 400 mL/hr

10. The IV is infusing at 30 gtt/min. The drop factor is 20 gtt/mL. The IV label reads 500 mL 5%. Dextrose and 0.45% Sodium Chloride. The IV had been infusing for $1^1/_2$ hours when you came on duty. How much longer does the IV have to infuse?
    a. 4 hr
    b. 50 min
    c. 3 hr
    d. $3^1/_2$ hr

11. The patient has a TPN solution with 8.5% amino acids in 375 mL. The total volume (TV) is 1500 mL. How many grams of protein will the patient receive? Use the following formula for calculating the amino acids.

    Step 1 % $\times$ mL = g/L

    Step 2 g/L $\times$ TV = g/bag
    a. 8.5 g/bag
    b. 47.8 g/bag
    c. 478 g/bag
    d. 31.8 g/bag

12. Ordered: Humulin R insulin 15 units/hr IV. Available: 250 mL of sodium chloride 0.9% with 100 units of Humulin R insulin. How many mL/hr will you need to set the infusion device?
    a. 56 mL/hr
    b. 33 mL/hr
    c. 38 mL/hr
    d. 58 mL/hr

    How many hours will it take to infuse the 250 mL?
    a. 5 hr 30 min
    b. 8 hr
    c. 9 hr 40 min
    d. 6 hr 36 min

13. Ordered: Fragmin 18,000 units SC for deep venous thrombosis (DVT). Available: A 9.5 mL multidose vial of Fragmin. The label reads: 1 mL = 10,000 units. How many milliliters will you give?
   a. 1.8 mL
   b. 2 mL
   c. 1.5 mL
   d. 1.2 mL

14. Ordered: Methotrexate 3.3 mg/m^2 po daily for a child with lymphocytic leukemia. Child's weight is 30 lb, which is normal weight for height. Using the appropriate column in the West nomogram on p. 256, calculate the dose.
   a. 12 mg
   b. 15 mg
   c. 18 mg
   d. 20 mg

15. Ordered: Dobutrex HCl to be infused at 2 µg/kg/min in a solution of 500 mL/D5W. Patient's weight: 110 lb. How many mL/hr will you set the IV infusion device?

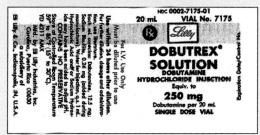

   a. 6 mL/hr
   b. 8 mL/hr
   c. 10 mL/hr
   d. 12 mL/hr

16. Ordered: Heparin sodium 10,000 units IV in 15 hr. Available: Pharmacy has sent 1000 mL of normal saline solution with 10,000 units of heparin sodium. How many mL/hr will you set the IV infusion device?
   a. 67 mL/hr
   b. 125 mL/hr
   c. 83 mL/hr
   d. 100 mL/hr

If the IV described above was started at 2000 hr on 10/21, when should it be finished?
   a. 10/22 at 0900 hr
   b. 10/23 at 0200 hr
   c. 10/23 at 1000 hr
   d. 10/22 at 1100 hr

17. Ordered: Lincocin 0.3 g IM for a patient with pneumonia. Given: Lincocin 10 mL IM. Examine the label below and select the correct analysis:

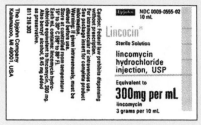

a. The nurse administered the correct dose.
b. An underdose of 1/3 the ordered dose was given.
c. The order needed to be clarified with the physician.
d. An overdose of 10 times the ordered dose was given.

18. Ordered: Morphine sulfate 5 mg IV push for a patient in severe pain. Directions: Dilute *to* 5 mL of NS or sterile water for injection and administer over 5 minutes. Identify the correct total dose and mL/minute to inject.

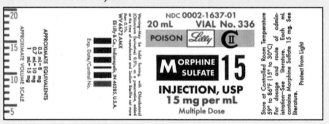

a. Administer 5 mL at 1 mL/min
b. Administer 5 mL at 0.4 mL/min
c. Administer 6 mL at 0.4 mL/min
d. Administer 8 mL at 0.03 mL/min

19. Ordered: Tobramycin sulfate 60 mg tid IV for a 40 lb child. Safe dose range (SDR): 6 to 7.5 mg/kg/day in 3 divided doses. Your decision:

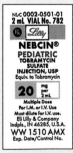

a. Give 60 mg. The order is within the safe dose range.
b. Give 60 mg but contact physician for clarification. The order is an underdose.
c. Hold. Contact the physician promptly and clarify. The order is an overdose.
d. Hold. The order is unclear.

20. Ordered: Geopen 1 g IM q8h. Available: Geopen (carbenicillin disodium) 5 g for IM or IV use. Directions for IM use: Use sterile water for injection as diluent. The medication displaces 3 mL. If you reconstitute the Geopen using 12 mL of sterile water for injection, how many doses of 1 g will you have?

ADD DILUENT	VOLUME TO BE WITHDRAWN FOR 1 g DOSE
9.5 mL	2.5 mL
12.0 mL	3.0 mL
17.0 mL	4.0 mL

a. 2 doses
b. 4 doses
c. 5 doses
d. 3 doses

If the first dose was given at 0700 hr on 10/20, what will be the date and time that the last dose from the vial will be given?

a. 10/22 at 0700 hr
b. 10/22 at 2000 hr
c. 10/21 at 2400 hr
d. 10/21 at 1500 hr

Comprehensive Final

Estimate answers, and then solve the following problems. Prove your answers.

1. Ordered: Zantac 0.6 g po for a patient with duodenal ulcers. How many tablets will be administered?

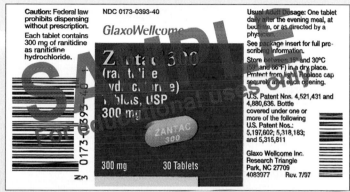

2. Ordered: Isoniazid 0.1 g po for a patient with tuberculosis. How many tablets will be administered?

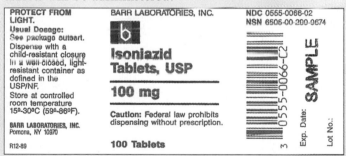

3. Ordered: Prozac liquid 30 mg po for a patient with anxiety. How many milliliters will be administered?

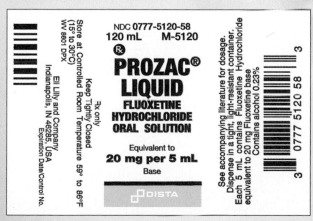

4. Ordered: Tofranil-PM 0.15 g hs for a patient with depression. How many capsules will be administered?

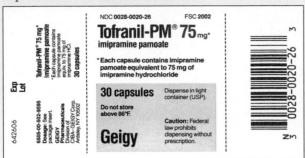

5. Ordered: Atropine sulfate 0.5 mg IV for apical pulse 40 beats/min or below. On hand is atropine sulfate 0.4 mg/mL. How many milliliters will you give?

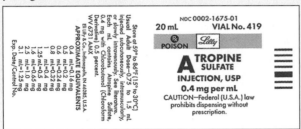

6. Ordered: Leucovorin calcium 0.01 g po for a child who has delayed excretion of methotrexate. The SDR is 10 mg/m². The child's weight is 70 lb. Refer to the West nomogram for the child's body surface area in square meters. How many milligrams are needed? How many tablets will you prepare?

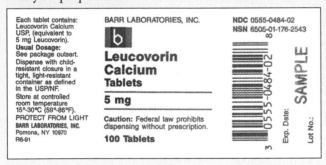

7. Ordered: Dopamine 5 μg/kg/min. The dopamine is infusing at
30 mL/hr on an infusion device with an IV container of 200 mg/250 mL
D5W. The patient weighs 176 lb. How many mg/hr are infusing? How
many μg/hr are infusing? How many μg/kg/min are infusing? Is the
flow rate correct?

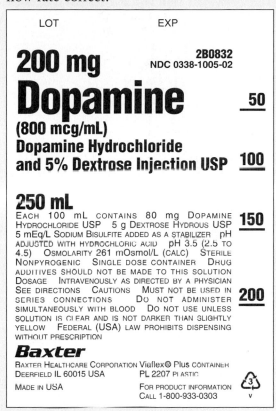

8. Ordered: Meperidine HCl 75 mg q4h prn, last administered according to
the MAR at 0400 hr.
Given: Demerol 75 mg at 0800 hr by Nurse A.
Given: Demerol 75 mg at 0845 hr by Nurse B, a busy staff nurse who
covered Nurse A's patient during Nurse A's break.
Error:
Current Actions:
What are some ways this error might have been prevented?

9. Ordered: Thorazine 2 mg IV push. Directions: Dilute each 25 mg (1 mL)
with 24 mL of NS for IV injection. Each mL will contain 1 mg. Give at
slow rate of 1 mg/min.

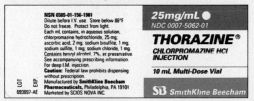

   a. Total milliliters to be injected:
   b. Total time in *seconds* to be injected:
   c. Seconds to be injected per calibration:
   d. mL/min to be injected for how many minutes:

10. Ordered: Furosemide 3 mg IV q8h for a child with edema weighing 9 lb.

SDR: 0.5 to 1 mg/kg/dose

Directions: may be given undiluted.

  a. Estimated weight in kilograms:

  b. Actual weight in kilograms:

  c. SDR for this child:

  d. Dose ordered:

  e. Evaluation and decision:

  f. If safe, calculate dose using label below:

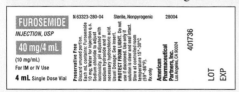

11. Calculate the grams per bag of amino acids, dextrose, and lipids the patient will receive. Use the following formula on the TPN label below.

STEP 1   % × mL = g/L   STEP 2   g/L × TV/L = g/bag

TPN Label

Amino Acid 5.5% in 300 mL
Dextrose 10% in 250 mL
Lipids 10% in 125 mL
Total volume 1158 mL

12. Using the answers from problem number 11, how many kilocalories will the patient receive?

13. Your patient's blood glucose (BG) level at 0600 hr is 176 mg/dL. According to the titration schedule, how many international units of Lantus will the patient receive? Shade in the amount on the insulin syringe.

Effective Diabetes Management

Logical titration schedule helps
achieve tight control, with low
incidence of severe hypoglycemia

Self-monitored FPG (mg/dL) for 2 consecutive days with no episodes of severe hypoglycemia or PG ≤72 mg/dL	Increase in insulin dose (IU/day)
100-120 mg/dL	2
120-140 mg/dL	4
140-180 mg/dL	6
≥180 mg/dL	8

Treat-to-Target FPG ≤100 mg/dL

Small decreases (2-4 IU/day per adjustment) in dose are allowed in the instance of self-monitored plasma glucose below 56 mg/dL or in the occurrence of a severe hypoglycemic episode.

14. Ordered: Fragmin Injection 8000 IU SC q12h before surgery.
Available: A multidose vial of Fragmin (dalteparin sodium injection).
The label reads: 1 mL = 10,000 IU.
How many milliliters will you give? Shade in the amount on the syringe.

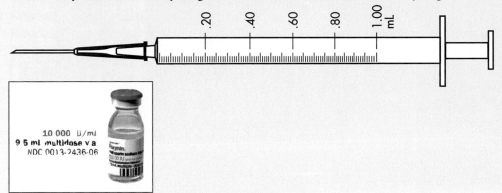

15. Ordered: Heparin Sodium 1000 units/hr IV in 1000 mL NS. The
pharmacy has sent 1000 mL of 0.9% sodium chloride with 20,000 units
heparin sodium.
At what rate will you set the infusion device?
How long will it take to infuse the 20,000 units?

LOT   EXP

2B1324
NDC 0338-0049-04
DIN 00060208

1

2

0.9% Sodium
Chloride
Injection USP

3

Heparin Sodium 20,000 units

4

1000 mL

EACH 100 mL CONTAINS   900 mg SODIUM CHLORIDE USP
pH 5.0 (4.5 TO 7.0) mEq/L SODIUM 154 CHLORIDE 154
OSMOLARITY   308 mOsmol/L (CALC)   STERILE
NONPYROGENIC   SINGLE DOSE CONTAINER   ADDITIVES MAY BE
INCOMPATIBLE   CONSULT WITH PHARMACIST IF AVAILABLE   WHEN
INTRODUCING ADDITIVES USE ASEPTIC TECHNIQUE   MIX
THOROUGHLY   DO NOT STORE   DOSAGE   INTRAVENOUSLY AS
DIRECTED BY A PHYSICIAN   SEE DIRECTIONS   CAUTIONS
SQUEEZE AND INSPECT INNER BAG WHICH MAINTAINS PRODUCT
STERILITY   DISCARD IF LEAKS ARE FOUND   MUST NOT BE USED
IN SERIES CONNECTIONS   DO NOT USE UNLESS SOLUTION IS
CLEAR   FEDERAL (USA) LAW PROHIBITS DISPENSING WITHOUT
PRESCRIPTION   STORE UNIT IN MOISTURE BARRIER OVERWRAP AT
ROOM TEMPERATURE (25°C/77°F) UNTIL READY TO USE   AVOID
EXCESSIVE HEAT   SEE INSERT

5

6

7

Baxter

BAXTER HEALTHCARE CORPORATION
DEERFIELD IL 60015 USA

MADE IN USA
DISTRIBUTED IN CANADA BY
BAXTER CORPORATION
TORONTO ONTARIO CANADA

Viaflex® CONTAINER
PL 146® PLASTIC

FOR PRODUCT INFORMATION
CALL 1-800-933-0303

8

9

16. Ordered: Gentamicin 60 mg in 50 mL, IVPB. Infuse in 40 minutes.
How many milliliters/hr will you set the infusion device?
How many gtt/min will be infused with a microdrip set?

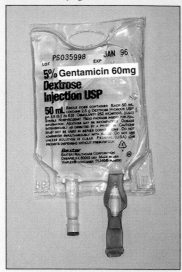

17. Ordered: Pfizerpen 400,000 units IM q8h.
Available: Penicillin G Potassium (Pfizerpen) five million units for reconstitution.
Follow the directions on the label to answer the questions.
If you add 18.2 mL of diluent, how many units per milliliter will you have?
How many milliliters will yield 400,000 units?
If you add 8.2 mL of diluent, how many units per milliliter will you have?
How many milliliters will yield 400,000 units?

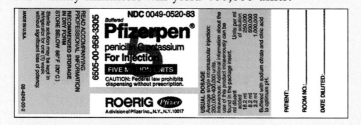

18. Ordered: Humulin R insulin 50 units in 500 mL of 0.9% NS IV to
infuse at 7 units/hr. At what rate will you set the IV pump?

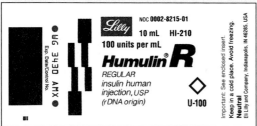

19. Ordered: Cefadyl 1 g IM q6h for cellulitis. How much diluent will you
add? Shade in the syringe. How many vials will be used in 24 hr?
How many mL will you give per dose?

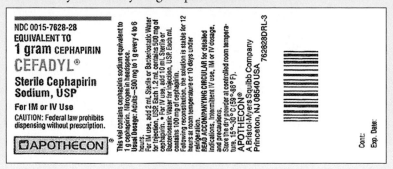

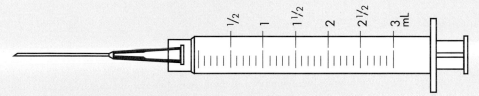

20. Ordered: 2000 mL D5LR to be infused in 24 hr. The drop factor is 15.
How many gtt/min will be infused via gravity infusion?
How many mL/hr on a pump?

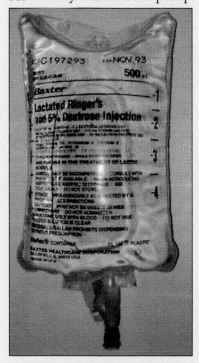

Answer Key

General Mathematics Self-Assessment (PAGE 1)

1. $5\frac{1}{2}$
2. $5\frac{1}{7}$
3. $\frac{56}{9}$
4. $\frac{19}{2}$
5. 66
6. 45
7. $1\frac{1}{30}$
8. $6\frac{19}{24}$
9. $\frac{13}{28}$
10. $4\frac{7}{8}$
11. $\frac{1}{12}$
12. $\frac{1}{3}$
13. $\frac{5}{6}$
14. $\frac{9}{20}$
15. $\frac{1}{50}$
16. $\frac{4}{19}$
17. 0.14
18. 3.016
19. 4.905
20. 28.708
21. 2.96
22. 0.8241
23. 0.0036
24. 1.5
25. 10.055
26. 98.095
27. 0.534
28. 9.125
29. 9.45
30. 84.2
31. $\frac{7}{10}$
32. $\frac{492}{1000}$
33. 0.17 and $\frac{17}{100}$
34. 0.125 and 12.5%
35. $\frac{11}{1000}$ and 1.4%
36. 0.6
37. 0.9
38. 0.87
39. 3
40. 4

1 General Mathematics

1A (PAGE 5)

1. 1
2. 3
3. $3\frac{1}{4}$
4. $1\frac{5}{9}$
5. $5\frac{2}{3}$
6. 4
7. $1\frac{3}{4}$
8. $1\frac{7}{8}$
9. 3
10. $6\frac{5}{6}$

1B (PAGE 5)

1. $\frac{6}{5}$
2. $\frac{5}{4}$
3. $\frac{35}{8}$
4. $\frac{43}{12}$
5. $\frac{68}{5}$
6. $\frac{49}{3}$

7. $\frac{23}{6}$

8. $\frac{21}{8}$

9. $\frac{63}{6}$

10. $\frac{377}{3}$

1C (PAGE 9)

1.
$$\frac{1}{5}$$
$$+\frac{2}{5}$$
$$\overline{\frac{3}{5}}$$

2.
$$\frac{3}{5} = \frac{9}{15}$$
$$+\frac{2}{3} = \frac{10}{15}$$
$$\overline{\frac{19}{15} = 1\frac{4}{15}}$$

3.
$$6\frac{1}{6} = 6\frac{4}{24}$$
$$+9\frac{5}{8} = 9\frac{15}{24}$$
$$\overline{15\frac{19}{24}}$$

4.
$$2\frac{1}{4} = 2\frac{2}{8}$$
$$+3\frac{1}{8} = 3\frac{1}{8}$$
$$\overline{5\frac{3}{8}}$$

5.
$$1\frac{3}{8} = 1\frac{15}{40}$$
$$+9\frac{9}{10} = 9\frac{36}{40}$$
$$\overline{10\frac{51}{40} = 11\frac{11}{40}}$$

6.
$$\frac{1}{8} = \frac{9}{72}$$
$$\frac{1}{4} = \frac{18}{72}$$
$$+\frac{2}{9} = \frac{16}{72}$$
$$\overline{\frac{43}{72}}$$

7.
$$\frac{7}{9} = \frac{70}{90}$$
$$\frac{4}{5} = \frac{72}{90}$$
$$+\frac{9}{10} = \frac{81}{90}$$
$$\overline{\frac{223}{90} = 2\frac{43}{90}}$$

8.
$$3\frac{1}{4}$$
$$+9\frac{3}{4}$$
$$\overline{12\frac{4}{4} = 13}$$

9.
$$8\frac{2}{5} = 8\frac{4}{10}$$
$$14\frac{7}{10} = 14\frac{7}{10}$$
$$+9\frac{9}{10} = 9\frac{9}{10}$$
$$\overline{31\frac{20}{10} = 33}$$

10.
$$2\frac{1}{3} = 2\frac{2}{6}$$
$$+4\frac{1}{6} = 4\frac{1}{6}$$
$$\overline{6\frac{3}{6} = 6\frac{1}{2}}$$

1D (PAGE 11)

1.
$$\frac{4}{5} = \frac{8}{10}$$
$$-\frac{1}{2} = \frac{5}{10}$$
$$\overline{\frac{3}{10}}$$

2.
$$\frac{27}{32}$$
$$-\frac{18}{32}$$
$$\overline{\frac{9}{32}}$$

3.
$$21\frac{7}{16} = 20\frac{23}{16}$$
$$-7\frac{12}{16} = 7\frac{12}{16}$$
$$\overline{13\frac{11}{16}}$$

4.
$$7\frac{16}{24} = 7\frac{16}{24}$$
$$-3\frac{1}{8} = 3\frac{3}{24}$$
$$\overline{4\frac{13}{24}}$$

(Must borrow from whole number.)

5. $6\frac{3}{10} = 6\frac{3}{10}$

$\underline{\quad -\ 2\frac{1}{5} = 2\frac{2}{10}\quad}$

$\qquad\qquad 4\frac{1}{10}$

6. $\qquad \frac{7}{8} = \frac{21}{24}$

$\qquad \underline{-\ \frac{2}{3} = \frac{16}{24}}$

$\qquad\qquad \frac{5}{24}$

7. $\qquad 3\frac{5}{8}$

$\quad \underline{-\ 1\frac{3}{8}\quad}$

$\qquad 2\frac{2}{8} = 2\frac{1}{4}$

8. $\quad 5\frac{3}{7} = 4\frac{10}{7}$

$\quad \underline{-\ 1\frac{6}{7} = 1\frac{6}{7}}$

$\qquad\qquad 3\frac{4}{7}$

(Must borrow from whole number.)

9. $\qquad 7 = 6\frac{4}{4}$

$\quad \underline{-\ 1\frac{3}{4} = 1\frac{3}{4}}$

$\qquad\qquad 5\frac{1}{4}$

10. $\quad 2\frac{7}{8} = 2\frac{7}{8}$

$\qquad \underline{-\ \frac{3}{4} = \ \frac{6}{8}}$

$\qquad\qquad 2\frac{1}{8}$

(Must borrow from whole number.)

1E (PAGE 12)

1. $\frac{1}{3} \times \frac{2}{4} = \frac{2}{12} = \frac{1}{6}$

2. $\frac{1}{5} \times \frac{1}{3} = \frac{1}{15}$

3. $1\frac{3}{4} \times 3\frac{1}{7} = \frac{\overset{1}{\cancel{7}}}{4} \times \frac{22}{\underset{1}{\cancel{7}}} = \frac{22}{4} = 22 \div 4 = 5\frac{1}{2}$

4. $4 \times 3\frac{1}{8} = 4 \times \frac{25}{8} = \frac{100}{8} = 12\frac{1}{2}$

5. $\frac{2}{4} \times 2\frac{1}{6} = \frac{\overset{1}{\cancel{2}}}{4} \times \frac{13}{\underset{3}{\cancel{6}}} = \frac{13}{12} = 1\frac{1}{12}$

6. $5\frac{1}{2} \times 3\frac{1}{8} = \frac{11}{2} \times \frac{25}{8} = \frac{275}{16} = 275 \div 16 = 17\frac{3}{16}$

7. $\frac{3}{4} \times \frac{5}{8} = \frac{15}{32}$

8. $\frac{5}{6} \times 1\frac{9}{16} = \frac{5}{6} \times \frac{25}{16} = \frac{125}{96} = 125 \div 96 = 1\frac{29}{96}$

9. $\frac{5}{100} \times 900 = \frac{5}{\underset{1}{\cancel{100}}} \times \frac{\overset{9}{\cancel{900}}}{1} = 45$

10. $2\frac{1}{10} \times 4\frac{1}{3} = \frac{\overset{7}{\cancel{21}}}{10} \times \frac{13}{\underset{1}{\cancel{3}}} = \frac{91}{10} = 9\frac{1}{10}$

1F (PAGE 13)

1. $\frac{2}{5} \div \frac{5}{8} = \frac{2}{5} \times \frac{8}{5} = \frac{16}{25}$

2. $\frac{1}{3} \div \frac{1}{2} = \frac{1}{3} \times \frac{2}{1} = \frac{2}{3}$

3. $\frac{3}{4} \div \frac{1}{8} = \frac{3}{\cancel{4}} \times \frac{\overset{2}{\cancel{8}}}{1} = 6$

4. $\frac{1}{16} \div \frac{1}{4} = \frac{1}{\underset{4}{\cancel{16}}} \times \frac{\overset{1}{\cancel{4}}}{1} = \frac{1}{4}$

5. $8\frac{3}{4} \div 15 = \frac{\overset{7}{\cancel{35}}}{4} \times \frac{1}{\underset{3}{\cancel{15}}} = \frac{7}{12}$

6. $\frac{3}{4} \div 6 = \frac{\overset{1}{\cancel{3}}}{4} \times \frac{1}{\underset{2}{\cancel{6}}} = \frac{1}{8}$

7. $2 \div \frac{1}{5} = \frac{2}{1} \times \frac{5}{1} = 10$

8. $3\frac{3}{8} \div 4\frac{1}{2} = \frac{27}{8} \div \frac{9}{2} = \frac{\overset{3}{\cancel{27}}}{\underset{4}{\cancel{8}}} \times \frac{\overset{1}{\cancel{2}}}{\underset{1}{\cancel{9}}} = \frac{3}{4}$

9. $\frac{3}{5} \div \frac{3}{8} = \frac{\overset{1}{\cancel{3}}}{5} \times \frac{8}{\underset{1}{\cancel{3}}} = \frac{8}{5} = 1\frac{3}{5}$

10. $4 \div 2\frac{1}{8} = \frac{4}{1} \times \frac{8}{17} = \frac{32}{17} = 1\frac{15}{17}$

1G (PAGE 14)

1. $\frac{1}{3}$ **2.** $\frac{1}{150}$ **3.** $\frac{1}{250}$

4. $\frac{1}{8}$ **5.** $\frac{1}{200}$ **6.** Less

7. Less   **8.** Less   **9.** More

10. Less

1H (PAGE 16)

1. Eight hundredths
2. Ninety-two thousandths
3. Seventeen ten-thousandths
4. One hundred and one hundredth
5. Six ten-thousandths
6. Three thousand two hundred eighty-seven and four hundred sixty-seven thousandths
7. 0.36
8. 0.003
9. 0.0008
10. 2.017
11. 0.05
12. 4.1
13. 24.2
14. 15.01
15. 9.0002
16. 3.008
17. 100.018
18. 18.15
19. 0.055
20. 34.1

1I (PAGE 17)

Smaller:

1. 0.2   **2.** 0.14
3. 0.68   **4.** 2.07
5. 1.29   **6.** 0.37
7. 0.512   **8.** 0.094
9. 0.005   **10.** 1.088

Larger:

11. 1.99   **12.** 0.7
13. 0.58   **14.** 0.25
15. 0.10   **16.** 2.74
17. 0.31   **18.** 25.14
19. 0.25   **20.** 0.75

1J (PAGE 18)

1.
```
   0.8
 + 0.5
   1.3
```

2.
```
   5.01
 + 2.999
   8.009
```

3.
```
   3.27
   0.06
 + 2.
   5.33
```

4.
```
    15.6
     0.19
 + 200.
   215.79
```

5.
```
   210.79
     2.
 + 68.4
   281.19
```

6.
```
    88.6
   576.46
 + 79.
   744.06
```

7.
```
     6.77
   102.
 + 88.3
   197.07
```

8.
```
   79.4
   68.44
 + 3.
   150.84
```

9.
```
    10.56
 + 356.4
   366.96
```

10.
```
    99.7
 + 293.23
   392.93
```

1K (PAGE 19)

1.
```
    98.4
 - 66.50
   31.90
```

2.
```
    21.78
 - 19.88
    1.90
```

3.
```
   0.450
 - 0.367
   0.083
```

4.
```
   108.56
 -   5.40
   103.16
```

5.
```
   266.44
 -   0.56
   265.88
```

6.
```
   7.066
 - 0.200
   6.866
```

7.
```
   34.678
 -  0.502
   34.176
```

8.
```
   78.567
 -  6.77
   71.797
```

9.
```
   1.723
 - 0.683
   1.040
```

10.
```
   0.8100
 - 0.6701
   0.1399
```

1L (PAGE 20)

1.
```
     3.14
 ×  0.002
   0.00628
```

You do not have to multiply zeros. Count 5 decimal places in from the right, adding zeros where needed.

2.
$$
\begin{array}{r}
95.26 \\
\times\ 1.125 \\
\hline
47630 \\
19052 \\
9526 \\
9526 \\
\hline
107.16750
\end{array}
$$
Count 5 decimal places in from the right.

3.
$$
\begin{array}{r}
0.5 \\
\times\ 100 \\
\hline
50.0
\end{array}
$$
Count 1 decimal place in from the right.

4.
$$
\begin{array}{r}
2.14 \\
\times\ 0.03 \\
\hline
0.0642
\end{array}
$$
Count 4 decimal places in from the right, adding zeros as needed.

5.
$$
\begin{array}{r}
36.8 \\
\times\ 70.1 \\
\hline
368 \\
2576 \\
\hline
2579.68
\end{array}
$$

6.
$$
\begin{array}{r}
200 \\
\times\ 0.2 \\
\hline
40.0
\end{array}
$$

7.
$$
\begin{array}{r}
90.1 \\
\times\ 88 \\
\hline
7208 \\
7208 \\
\hline
7928.8
\end{array}
$$

8.
$$
\begin{array}{r}
2.76 \\
\times\ 0.003 \\
\hline
0.00828
\end{array}
$$

9.
$$
\begin{array}{r}
54.5 \\
\times\ 21 \\
\hline
545 \\
1090 \\
\hline
1144.5
\end{array}
$$

10.
$$
\begin{array}{r}
203.7 \\
\times\ 28 \\
\hline
16296 \\
4074 \\
\hline
5703.6
\end{array}
$$

1M (PAGE 22)

1. $60\overline{)1.35}$

2. $4\overline{)2.013}$

3. $20\overline{)15.6}$

4. $75\overline{)35.}$

5. $19\overline{)10.14}$

6. $304\overline{)95.14}$

7. $7\overline{)60.5}$

8. $15\overline{)25.14}$

9. $25\overline{)35.9}$

10. $100\overline{)75.}$

11. $8.4\ \overline{)1.3\ 5}$

12. $0.25\overline{)3.57}$

13. $0.1\overline{).5\ 0}$

14. $94.5\ \overline{)0.0\ 29}$

15. $4.8\ \overline{)2.0\ 4}$

16. $0.52\overline{)120.00}$

17. $60.2\ \overline{)50.9\ 23}$

18. $0.75\overline{)0.50}$

19. 4.3$\overline{)2.1}$

20. 0.50$\overline{)0.25}$

21.
$$\begin{array}{r} 2.2 \\ 10\overline{)22.0} \\ 20\downarrow \\ \hline 2\ 0 \\ 2\ 0 \\ \hline \end{array}$$

22.
$$\begin{array}{r} 5.1 \\ 50\overline{)255.0} \\ 250\downarrow \\ \hline 5\ 0 \\ 5\ 0 \\ \hline \end{array}$$

23.
$$\begin{array}{r} 0.66 \\ 75\overline{)50.00} \\ 45\ 0\downarrow \\ \hline 5\ 00 \\ 4\ 50 \\ \hline \end{array}$$

24.
$$\begin{array}{r} 0.33 \\ 30\overline{)10.00} \\ 9\ 0\downarrow \\ \hline 1\ 00 \\ 90 \\ \hline \end{array}$$

25.
$$\begin{array}{r} 4.8 \\ 2.5\overline{)12.0\ 0} \\ 10\ 0\downarrow \\ \hline 2\ 0\ 0 \\ 2\ 0\ 0 \\ \hline \end{array}$$

1N (PAGE 23)

1.
$$\begin{array}{r} 3.3 \\ 48\overline{)158.4} \\ 144 \\ \hline 14\ 4 \\ 14\ 4 \\ \hline \end{array}$$

PROOF
$$\begin{array}{r} 48 \\ \times\ 3.3 \\ \hline 14\ 4 \\ 144 \\ \hline 158.4 \\ \end{array}$$

2.
$$\begin{array}{r} 3\ 3.333 \\ 6.0\overline{)200.0\ 000} \\ 180 \\ \hline 20\ 0 \\ 18\ 0 \\ \hline 2\ 00 \\ 1\ 80 \\ \hline 2\ 00 \\ 1\ 80 \\ \hline 200 \\ 180 \\ \hline \end{array}$$

PROOF
$$\begin{array}{r} 33.333 \\ \times\ \ \ \ 60 \\ \hline 1999.980 \\ \end{array}$$

3.
$$\begin{array}{r} 2.51 \\ 6\overline{)15.06} \\ 12 \\ \hline 3\ 0 \\ 3\ 0 \\ \hline 06 \\ 6 \\ \hline \end{array}$$

PROOF
$$\begin{array}{r} 2.51 \\ \times\ \ \ 6 \\ \hline 15.06 \\ \end{array}$$

4.
$$\begin{array}{r} 91.264 \\ 0.87\overline{)79.40\ 000} \\ 78\ 30 \\ \hline 1\ 10 \\ 87 \\ \hline 23\ 0 \\ 17\ 4 \\ \hline 5\ 60 \\ 5\ 22 \\ \hline 380 \\ 348 \\ \hline \end{array}$$

PROOF
$$\begin{array}{r} 91.264 \\ \times\ 87 \\ \hline 638\ 848 \\ 7301\ 12 \\ \hline 7939.968 \\ \end{array}$$

5.
```
        860.
0.78)670.80
     624
      46 8
      46 8
```

PROOF
PROOF
```
   860
 ×  78
  6880
  6020
 67080
```

6.
```
        32.345
2.43)78.60 000
     72 9
      5 70
      4 86
        84 0
        72 9
        11 10
         9 72
         1 380
         1 215
```

PROOF
```
   32.345
 ×   243
   97 035
 1293 80
 6469 0
 7859.835
```

7.
```
       3.265
8.2 )26.7 800
    24 6
     2 1 8
     1 6 4
       5 40
       4 92
         480
         410
```

PROOF
```
   3.265
 ×   82
  6 530
 261 20
 267.730
```

8.
```
        46.107
5.78)266.50 000
     231 2
      35 30
      34 68
        62 0
        57 8
         4 200
         4 046
```

PROOF
```
   46.107
 ×   578
  368 856
 3227 49
 23053 5
 26649.846
```

9.
```
       1.661
6.5 )10.8 000
     6 5
     4 3 0
     3 9 0
       4 00
       3 90
         100
          65
```

PROOF
```
   1.661
 ×   65
  8305
  9966
 107.965
```

10.
```
      7.653
10)76.530
   70
    6 5
    6 0
     53
     50
     30
     30
```

PROOF
```
   7.653
 ×   10
  76.530
```

10 (PAGE 24)

1. $\frac{4}{10} = \frac{2}{5}$

2. $\frac{8}{10} = \frac{4}{5}$

3. $\frac{25}{100} = \frac{1}{4}$

4. $4\frac{08}{100} = 4\frac{2}{25}$

5. $1\frac{32}{100} = 1\frac{8}{25}$

6. $\frac{5}{10} = \frac{1}{2}$

7. $\frac{75}{100} = \frac{3}{4}$

8. $\frac{2}{10} = \frac{1}{5}$

9. $\frac{65}{100} = \frac{13}{20}$

10. $\frac{7}{10}$

1P (PAGE 25)

1. $\begin{array}{r} 0.19 \\ 100{\overline{\smash{\big)}\,19.00}} \\ \underline{10\ 0} \\ 9\ 00 \\ \underline{9\ 00} \end{array}$

2. $\begin{array}{r} 1.285 \\ 7{\overline{\smash{\big)}\,9.00}} \\ \underline{7} \\ 2\ 0 \\ \underline{1\ 4} \\ 60 \\ \underline{56} \\ 40 \\ \underline{35} \end{array}$

3. $5\frac{9}{16} = 5 \times 16 + 9 = \frac{89}{16}$

$\begin{array}{r} 5.562 \\ 16{\overline{\smash{\big)}\,89.000}} \\ \underline{80} \\ 9\ 0 \\ \underline{8\ 0} \\ 1\ 00 \\ \underline{96} \\ 40 \\ \underline{32} \end{array}$

4. $\begin{array}{r} 0.2 \\ 5{\overline{\smash{\big)}\,1.0}} \\ \underline{1\ 0} \end{array}$

5. $\begin{array}{r} 0.666 \\ 3{\overline{\smash{\big)}\,2.000}} \\ \underline{1\ 8} \\ 20 \\ \underline{18} \\ 20 \\ \underline{18} \end{array}$

6. $\begin{array}{r} 0.5 \\ 2{\overline{\smash{\big)}\,1.0}} \\ \underline{1\ 0} \end{array}$

7. $\begin{array}{r} 0.083 \\ 12{\overline{\smash{\big)}\,1.000}} \\ \underline{96} \\ 40 \\ \underline{36} \end{array}$

8. $\begin{array}{r} 0.75 \\ 8{\overline{\smash{\big)}\,6.00}} \\ \underline{5\ 6} \\ 40 \\ \underline{40} \end{array}$

9. $\begin{array}{r} 0.075 \\ 200{\overline{\smash{\big)}\,15.000}} \\ \underline{14\ 00} \\ 1\ 000 \\ \underline{1\ 000} \end{array}$

10. $\begin{array}{r} 2.5 \\ 8{\overline{\smash{\big)}\,20.0}} \\ \underline{16} \\ 4\ 0 \\ \underline{4\ 0} \end{array}$

1Q (PAGE 27)

	NEAREST WHOLE NUMBER	NEAREST TENTH	NEAREST HUNDREDTH
1. 93.489	93	93.5	93.49
2. 25.430	25	25.4	25.43
3. 38.10	38	38.1	38.10
4. 57.8888	58	57.9	57.89
5. 0.0092	0	0	0.01
6. 3.144	3	3.1	3.14
7. 8.999	9	9.0	9.00
8. 77.788	78	77.8	77.79
9. 12.959	13	13.0	12.96
10. 5.7703	6	5.8	5.77

1R (PAGE 27)

	NEAREST WHOLE NUMBER	NEAREST TENTH	NEAREST HUNDREDTH
1. $25.3 \times 4.2 =$	106	106.3	106.26
2. $9.3 \times 2.86 =$	27	26.6	26.60
3. $4.5 \times 7.57 =$	34	34.1	34.07
4. $1.3 \times 9.69 =$	13	12.6	12.60
5. $2.4 \times 5.88 =$	14	14.1	14.11
6. $8 \div 5 =$	2	1.6	1.60
7. $4.1 \div 3 =$	1	1.4	1.37
8. $5 \div 1.2 =$	4	4.2	4.17
9. $9 \div 2.2 =$	4	4.1	4.09
10. $10.2 \div 3$	3	3.4	3.40

1S (PAGE 29)

1. Decimal: 0.5
   Percentage: 50%
2. Fraction: $\frac{2}{3}$
   Decimal: 0.67
3. Fraction: $\frac{13}{200}$
   Decimal: 0.065
4. Decimal: 0.083
   Percentage: 8.33%
5. Decimal: 0.003
   Percentage: 0.3%
6. Fraction: $\frac{1}{10}$
   Percentage: 10%
7. Fraction: $\frac{250}{100} = \frac{5}{2}$
   Decimal: 2.5
8. Fraction: $\frac{7}{20}$
   Percentage: 35%
9. Decimal: 0.8
   Percentage: 80%
10. Fraction: $\frac{78}{100} = \frac{39}{50}$
    Decimal: 0.78

1T (PAGE 30)

1.
```
    240
  × 1.14
    960
    240
    240
 273.60
```

2.
```
   1500
 × 0.02
  30.00
```

3. $\frac{1/2}{100} = \frac{1}{2} \div \frac{100}{1} = \frac{1}{2} \times \frac{1}{100} = \frac{1}{200} = 200\overline{)1.000}$ $\begin{array}{r} 0.005 \\ \hline \end{array}$

```
   9328
 × 0.005
 46.640
```

4. $\frac{1/3}{100} = \frac{1}{3} \div \frac{100}{1} = \frac{1}{3} \times \frac{1}{100} = \frac{1}{300} = 300\overline{)1.000}$ $\begin{array}{r} 0.003 \\ \hline 900 \\ \hline 100 \end{array}$

```
    930
 × 0.003
  2.790
```

5.
```
     50
  × 0.28
    400
    100
  14.00
```

6.
```
    200
 × 0.09
  18.00
```

7.
```
    400
 × 1.20
   8000
    400
 480.00
```

8.
```
 105.80
 × 0.05
 5.2900
```

9.
```
    520
 × 0.10
  52.00
```

10.
```
  40.80
 × 0.03
 1.2240
```

1U (PAGE 31)

1. **b.** $\frac{41}{7} = 5\frac{6}{7}$ The other responses can be eliminated quickly because only b offers 5 as the whole number

2. **b.** $6 \times 3 + 5 = \frac{23}{6}$

3. **d.** $5 \times 8 = 40$

4. **a.** $5\frac{1}{8} + 1\frac{2}{8} + 4\frac{4}{8} = 10\frac{7}{8}$

5. **c.** $6\frac{9}{12} - 5\frac{4}{12} = 1\frac{5}{12}$

6. **b.** $\frac{10}{48} = \frac{5}{24}$

7. **b.** $\frac{1}{6} \times \frac{2}{1} = \frac{2}{6} = \frac{1}{3}$

8. **d.** $\frac{5}{6} \times \frac{3}{1} = \frac{15}{6} = 2\frac{1}{2}$

9. **a**

10. **a.** $0.4100 - 0.2538 = 0.1562$

11. **c**

12. **d**

13. **d**

14. **b**

15. **c.** $0.0625 \times 9328 = 583$

16. **a**

17. **a.** 0.4

18. **c.** $\frac{1}{6} = 0.166$ or 0.17

19. **a**

20. **b.** $\frac{4}{100} = 0.04$

Chapter 1 Final: General Mathematics (PAGE 32)

1. $6\frac{6}{7}$

2. $5\frac{4}{6} = 5\frac{2}{3}$

3. $\frac{68}{5}$

4. $\frac{23}{6}$

5. 20

6. 40

7. $\frac{19}{36}$

8. $10\frac{7}{8}$

9. $\frac{5}{24}$

10. 1

11. $\frac{1}{15}$

12. $\frac{10}{48} = \frac{5}{24}$

13. $\frac{24}{4} = 6$

14. $\frac{3}{4}$

15. $\frac{1}{250}$

16. $\frac{1}{3}$

17. 0.36

18. 2.017

19. 8.009

20. 60.97

21. 3.824

22. 0.1562

23. 0.000010

24. 3.5

25. 3.300

26. 91.264

27. 1.1875

28. 8.0625

29. 12.48

30. 583

31. $\frac{2}{5}$

32. $\frac{57}{200}$

	FRACTION	DECIMAL TO NEAREST TENTH	DECIMAL TO NEAREST HUNDREDTH	PERCENTAGE
33.	$\frac{1}{3}$	0.3	0.33	$33\frac{1}{3}\%$
34.	$\frac{4}{100} = \left(\frac{1}{25}\right)$	0	0.04	4%
35.	$\frac{2}{5}$	0.4	0.40	40%
36.	$\frac{22}{100} = \left(\frac{11}{50}\right)$	0.2	0.22	22%
37.	$\frac{3}{8}$	0.4	0.38	$37\frac{1}{2}\%$
38.	$\frac{10}{100} = \left(\frac{1}{10}\right)$	0.1	0.10	10%
39.	$\frac{1}{12}$	0.1	0.08	$8\frac{1}{3}\%$
40.	$\frac{1}{200}$	0	0.01	$\frac{1}{2}\%$
41.	$\frac{5}{16}$	0.3	0.31	31%
42.	$\frac{15}{100} = \left(\frac{3}{20}\right)$	0.2	0.15	15%
43.	$\frac{1}{4}$	0.3	0.25	25%
44.	$\frac{12}{100} = \left(\frac{3}{25}\right)$	0.1	0.12	12%
45.	$\frac{7}{9}$	0.8	0.78	78%
46.	$\frac{80}{100} = \left(\frac{4}{5}\right)$	0.8	0.80	80%
47.	$\frac{1}{6}$	0.2	0.17	$16\frac{2}{3}\%$
48.	$\frac{33}{100}$	0.3	0.33	33%
49.	$\frac{1}{250}$	0	0	$\frac{2}{5}\%$
50.	$\frac{75}{100} = \left(\frac{3}{4}\right)$	0.8	0.75	75%

2 Ratio and Proportion

2A (PAGE 36)

1. $\frac{3}{6} = \frac{1}{2}$

2. $\frac{6}{8} = \frac{3}{4}$

3. $\frac{2}{500} = \frac{1}{250}$

4. $\frac{6}{1000} = \frac{3}{500}$

5. $\frac{43}{86} = \frac{1}{2}$

6. $\frac{2}{13}$

7. $\frac{7}{49} = \frac{1}{7}$

8. $\frac{1}{10}$

9. $\frac{1}{150}$

10. $\frac{4}{100} = \frac{1}{25}$

2B (PAGE 38)

1. $9 : x :: 5 : 300$

$5x = 9 \times 300$

$5x = 2700$

$\dfrac{\cancel{5}}{\cancel{5}}x = \dfrac{2700}{5} = 2700 \div 5$

$\quad x = 540$

PROOF

$540 \times 5 = 2700$

$9 \times 300 = 2700$

2. $\dfrac{1}{2} : x :: 1 : 8$

$1x = \dfrac{1}{2} \times 8$

$\dfrac{\cancel{x}}{\cancel{x}}x = \dfrac{1}{2} \times \dfrac{8}{1}$

$\quad x = 4$

PROOF

$4 \times 1 = 4$

$\dfrac{1}{2} \times 8 = 4$

3. $9 : 27 :: 300 : x$

$9x = 27 \times 300 = 8100$

$\dfrac{\cancel{9}}{\cancel{9}}x = \dfrac{8100}{9} = 8100 \div 9$

$\quad x = 900$

PROOF

$27 \times 300 = 8100$

$9 \times 900 = 8100$

4. $\dfrac{1}{4} : 500 :: x : 1000$

$500x = \dfrac{1}{4} \times 1000$

$500x = \dfrac{1}{4} \times \dfrac{1000}{1} = 250$

$\dfrac{\cancel{500}}{\cancel{500}}x = \dfrac{250}{500} = 250 \div 500$

$\quad x = 0.5$

PROOF

$500 \times 0.5 = 250$

$\dfrac{1}{4} \times 100 = 250$

5. $36 : 12 :: \dfrac{1}{100} : x$

$36x = 12 \times \dfrac{1}{100}$

$36x = \dfrac{12}{1} \times \dfrac{1}{100} = \dfrac{3}{25}$

$\dfrac{\cancel{36}}{\cancel{36}}x = \dfrac{^{3}/25}{36} = \dfrac{3}{25} \div 36 = \dfrac{\cancel{3}}{25} \times \dfrac{1}{\underset{12}{\cancel{36}}}$

$\quad x = \dfrac{1}{300}$

PROOF

$36 \times \dfrac{1}{300} = \dfrac{3}{25}$

$12 \times \dfrac{1}{100} = \dfrac{3}{25}$

6. $6 : 24 :: 0.75 : x$

$6x = 24 \times 0.75 = 18$

$6x = 18$

$\dfrac{\cancel{6}}{\cancel{6}}x = \dfrac{18}{6} = 18 \div 6$

$\quad x = 3$

PROOF

$24 \times 0.75 = 18$

$6 \times 3 = 18$

7. $x : 600 :: 4 : 120$

$120x = 4 \times 600 = 2400$

$\dfrac{\cancel{120}}{\cancel{120}}x = \dfrac{2400}{120} = 2400 \div 120$

$\quad x = 20$

PROOF

$600 \times 4 = 2400$

$20 \times 120 = 2400$

8. $0.7 : 70 :: x : 1000$

$70x = 0.7 \times 1000 = 700$

$\dfrac{\cancel{70}}{\cancel{70}}x = \dfrac{700}{70} = 700 \div 70$

$\quad x = 10$

PROOF

$70 \times 10 = 700$

$0.7 \times 1000 = 700$

9. $\frac{1}{1000} : \frac{1}{100} :: x : 60$

$\quad \frac{1}{100}x = \frac{1}{1000} \times 60$

$\quad \frac{1}{100}x = \frac{1}{1000} \times \frac{60}{1} = \frac{1}{50} \times \frac{3}{1} = \frac{3}{50}$

$\quad \frac{1/100}{1/100}x = \frac{3/50}{1/100} = \frac{3}{50} \div \frac{1}{100} = \frac{3}{50} \times \frac{100}{1} = \frac{300}{50}$

$\quad x = 6$

PROOF

$\quad \frac{1}{1000} \times 60 = \frac{3}{50}$

$\quad \frac{1}{100} \times 6 = \frac{3}{50}$

10. $6 : 12 :: \frac{1}{4} : x$

$\quad 6x = 12 \times \frac{1}{4} = 3$

$\quad \frac{6}{6}x = \frac{3}{6} = 3 \div 6$

$\quad x = 0.5$

PROOF

$\quad 12 \times \frac{1}{4} = 3$

$\quad 6 \times 0.5 = 3$

2C (PAGE 39)

1. $15 : 30 :: x : 12$

$\quad 30x = 15 \times 12$

$\quad 30x = 180$

$\quad \frac{30}{30}x - \frac{180}{30} - 180 : 30$

$\quad x = 6$

PROOF

$\quad 30 \times 6 = 180$

$\quad 15 \times 12 = 180$

2. $\frac{1}{200} : x :: 1 : 800$

$\quad 1x = \frac{1}{200} \times 800$

$\quad 1x = \frac{1}{200} \times \frac{800}{1} - 4$

$\quad \frac{x}{x}x = \frac{4}{1} = 4 \div 1$

$\quad x = 4$

PROOF

$\quad 4 \times 1 = 4$

$\quad \frac{1}{200} \times 800 = 4$

3. $\frac{1}{1000} : \frac{1}{100} :: x : 30$

$\quad \frac{1}{100}x = \frac{1}{1000} \times 30$

$\quad \frac{1}{100}x = \frac{1}{1000} \times \frac{30}{1} = \frac{3}{100}$

$\quad \frac{1/100}{1/100}x = \frac{3/100}{1/100} = \frac{3}{100} \div \frac{1}{100} = \frac{3}{100} \times \frac{100}{1}$

$\quad x = 3$

PROOF

$\quad \frac{1}{1000} \times 30 = \frac{3}{100}$

$\quad \frac{1}{100} \times 3 = \frac{3}{100}$

4. $6 : 12 :: 0.25 : x$

$\quad 6x = 12 \times 0.25 = 3$

$\quad \frac{6}{6}x = \frac{3}{6} = 3 \div 6$

$\quad x = 0.5$

PROOF

$\quad 12 \times 0.25 = 3$

$\quad 6 \times 0.5 = 3$

5. $300 : 5 :: x : \frac{1}{60}$

$\quad 5x = \frac{1}{60} \times 300$

$\quad 5x = \frac{1}{60} \times \frac{300}{1} = 5$

$\quad \frac{5}{5}x = \frac{5}{5} = 5 \div 5$

$\quad x = 1$

PROOF

$\quad 300 \times \frac{1}{60} = 5$

$\quad 5 \times 1 = 5$

6. $\frac{1}{150} : \frac{1}{200} :: 2 : x$

$\quad \frac{1}{150}x = \frac{1}{200} \times 2$

$\quad \frac{1}{150}x = \frac{1}{200} \times \frac{2}{1} = \frac{1}{100}$

$\quad \frac{1/150}{1/150}x = \frac{1/100}{1/150} = \frac{1}{100} \div \frac{1}{150} = \frac{1}{100} \times \frac{150}{1} = \frac{3}{2}$

$\quad x - 1\frac{1}{2}$

PROOF

$\quad \frac{1}{150} \times \frac{3}{2}\left(1\frac{1}{2}\right) = \frac{1}{100}$

$\quad \frac{1}{200} \times 2 = \frac{1}{100}$

7. $\frac{1}{2} : \frac{1}{6} :: \frac{1}{4} : x$

$\frac{1}{2}x = \frac{1}{6} \times \frac{1}{4} = \frac{1}{24}$

$\frac{\frac{1}{2}}{\frac{1}{2}}x = \frac{\frac{1}{24}}{\frac{1}{2}} = \frac{1}{24} \div \frac{1}{2} = \frac{1}{24} \times \frac{2}{1}$

$x = \frac{1}{12}$

PROOF

$\frac{1}{2} \times \frac{1}{12} = \frac{1}{24}$

$\frac{1}{6} \times \frac{1}{4} = \frac{1}{24}$

8. $7.5 : 12 :: x : 28$

$12x = 7.5 \times 28 = 210$

$\frac{12}{12}x = \frac{210}{12} = 210 \div 12$

$x = 17.5$

PROOF

$7.5 \times 28 = 210$

$12 \times 17.5 = 210$

9. $15 : x :: 1.5 : 10$

$1.5x = 15 \times 10 = 150$

$\frac{1.5}{1.5}x = \frac{150}{1.5} = 150 \div 1.5$

$x = 100$

PROOF

$15 \times 10 \times 150$

$100 \times 1.5 = 150$

10. $10 : x :: 0.4 : 12$

$0.4x = 10 \times 12 = 120$

$\frac{0.4}{0.4}x = \frac{120}{0.4} = 120 \div 0.4$

$x = 300$

PROOF

$10 \times 12 = 120$

$300 \times 0.4 = 120$

2D (PAGE 40)

1. $9 : x :: 5 : 300$

$\frac{5}{5}x = \frac{2700}{5}$

$x = 540$

PROOF

$9 \times 300 = = 2700$

$5 \times 540 = 2700$

2. $6 : 24 :: 0.75 : x$

$6x = 24 \times 0.75$

$\frac{6}{6}x = \frac{18}{6}$

$x = 3$

PROOF

$6 \times 3 = 18$

$24 \times 0.75 = 18$

3. $8 : 16 :: x : 24$

$16x = 8 \times 24$

$\frac{16}{16}x = \frac{192}{16}$

$x = 12$

PROOF

$8 \times 24 = 192$

$16 \times 12 = 192$

4. $x : 600 :: 4 : 120$

$120x = 4 \times 600$

$\frac{120}{120}x = \frac{2400}{120}$

$x = 20$

PROOF

$20 \times 120 = 2400$

$600 \times 4 = 2400$

5. $5 : 3000 :: 15 : x$

$\frac{5}{5}x = \frac{45,000}{5}$

$x = 9000$

PROOF

$5 \times 9000 = 45,000$

$3000 \times 15 = 45,000$

6. $0.7 : 70 :: x : 1000$

$\frac{70}{70}x = \frac{700}{70}$

$x = 10$

PROOF

$0.7 \times 1000 = 700$

$70 \times 10 = 700$

7. $9 : 27 :: 300 : x$

$$\frac{\cancel{9}}{\cancel{9}}x = \frac{8100}{9}$$

$$x = 900$$

PROOF

$9 \times 900 = 8100$

$27 \times 300 = 8100$

8. $6 : 12 :: \frac{1}{4} : x$

$$6x = 12 \times \frac{1}{4} = \frac{12}{4} = 3$$

$$\frac{\cancel{6}}{\cancel{6}}x = \frac{3}{6}$$

$$x = \frac{1}{2} \text{ or } 0.5$$

PROOF

$6 \times 0.5 = 3$

$12 \times \frac{1}{4} = 3$

9. $25 : x :: 75 : 3000$

$$\frac{\cancel{75}}{\cancel{75}}x = \frac{75,000}{75}$$

$$x = 1000$$

PROOF

$25 \times 3000 = 75,000$

$1000 \times 75 = 75,000$

10. $0.6 : 10 :: 0.5 : x$

$$0.6x = 10 \times 0.5 = 5$$

$$\frac{\cancel{0.6}}{\cancel{0.6}}x = \frac{5}{0.6}$$

$$x = 8.33 \text{ or } 8\frac{1}{3}$$

PROOF

$0.6 \times 8.33 = 4.998 \text{ or } 5$

$10 \times 0.5 = 5$

2E (PAGE 41)

1. *Know*   *Want to Know*

Bananas : Apples :: x Bananas : Apples

$6 : 9 :: x : 72$

$9x = 6 \times 72 = 432$

$$\frac{\cancel{9}}{\cancel{9}}x = \frac{432}{9}$$

$$x = 48 \text{ bananas}$$

PROOF

$6 : 9 :: 48 : 72$

$9 \times 48 = 432$

$6 \times 72 = 432$

2. *Know*   *Want to Know*

Scoops : Cups :: x Scoops : Cups

$7 : 8 :: x : 40$

$8x = 40 \times 7 = 280$

$$\frac{\cancel{8}}{\cancel{8}}x = \frac{280}{8}$$

$$x = 35 \text{ scoops}$$

PROOF

$7 : 8 :: 35 : 40$

$8 \times 35 = 280$

$7 \times 40 = 280$

> **REMEMBER** ● Scoops : Cups :: Scoops : Cups
> Apples : Bananas :: Apples : Bananas
> Miles : Gallons :: Miles : Gallons

You want x to stand alone. To get x to stand alone, divide by 6. Whatever you do on one side of an equation, you must do on the other.

Obtain proof by putting your answer back into the equation in place of x. Multiply the two inside numbers, and they should equal the two outside numbers.

3. *Know*   *Want to Know*
Scoops : Cups :: x Scoops : Cups
$4 : 6 :: x : 18$
$6x = 72$
$\frac{\cancel{6}}{\cancel{6}}x = \frac{72}{6}$
  $x = 12$ scoops of cocoa
PROOF
$4 : 6 :: 12 : 18$
$6 \times 12 = 72$
$4 \times 18 = 72$

4. *Know*   *Want to Know*
4 pills : 1 day :: x pills : 21 days
$x = 4 \times 21$
$x = 84$ pills
PROOF
$4 : 1 :: 84 : 21$
$4 \times 21 = 84$
$1 \times 84 = 84$

5. *Know*   *Want to Know*
Bushes : Trees :: x Bushes : Trees
$8 : 2 :: x : 36$
$2x = 8 \times 36 = 288$
$\frac{\cancel{2}}{\cancel{2}}x = \frac{288}{2}$
  $x = 144$ bushes
PROOF
$8 : 2 :: 144 : 36$
$8 \times 36 = 288$
$2 \times 144 = 288$

6. *Know*   *Want to Know*
Cups : Day :: Cups : x Days
$4 : 1 :: 84 : x$
$4x = 84$
$\frac{\cancel{4}}{\cancel{4}}x = \frac{84}{4}$
  $x = 21$ days
PROOF
$4 : 1 :: 84 : 21$
$1 \times 84 = 84$
$4 \times 21 = 84$

7. *Know*   *Want to Know*
Cups : Loaves :: Cups : x Loaves
$4 : 3 :: 24 : x$
$4x = 24 \times 3 = 72$
$\frac{\cancel{4}}{\cancel{4}}x = \frac{72}{4}$
  $x = 18$ loaves
PROOF
$4 : 3 :: 24 : 18$
$4 \times 18 = 72$
$3 \times 24 = 72$

8. *Know*   *Want to Know*
3 soda : $\frac{1}{2}$ fruit juice :: x soda : 2 fruit juice
$\frac{1}{2}x = 3 \times 2$
$\frac{\cancel{1/2}}{\cancel{1/2}}x = \frac{6}{1/2}$ $6 \div \frac{1}{2} = 6 \times \frac{2}{1}$
  $x = 12$ cups soda
PROOF
$3 : \frac{1}{2} :: 12 : 2$
$3 \times 2 = 6$
$\frac{1}{2} \times 12 = 6$

9. *Know*   *Want to Know*
4 tbsp sugar : 1 glass :: x tbsp sugar : 6 glasses
$x = 6 \times 4$
$x = 24$ tbsp sugar
PROOF
$4 : 1 :: 24 : 6$
$4 \times 6 = 24$
$1 \times 24 = 24$

10. *Know*   *Want to Know*
4 cap : 1 day :: x cap : 14 days
$x = 4 \times 14$
$x = 56$ cap
PROOF
$4 : 1 :: 56 : 14$
$4 \times 14 = 56$
$1 \times 56 = 56$

2F (PAGE 42)

1. *Know*   *Want to Know*
200 envelopes : 1 box :: 4000 envelopes : x boxes
$200x = 4000$
$\frac{200}{200}x = \frac{4000}{200}$
     $x = 20$ boxes
PROOF
$200 \times 20 = 4000$
$1 \times 4000 = 4000$

2. *Know*   *Want to Know*
10 disks : 1 package :: 300 disks : x packages
$10x = 300$
$\frac{10}{10}x = \frac{300}{10}$
     $x = 30$ packages
PROOF
$10 \times 30 = 300$
$1 \times 300 = 300$

3. *Know*   *Want to Know*
1 computer : 18 students :: x computers :
                                1280 students
$18x = 1280$
$\frac{18}{18}x = \frac{1280}{18}$
     $x = 71.1$ or 71 computers
PROOF
$1 \times 1280 = 1280$
$18 \times 71.1 = 1279.8$ or 1280

4. *Know*   *Want to Know*
3 water : 2 apples :: 24 water : x apples
$3x = 48$
$\frac{x}{3}x = \frac{48}{3}$
     $x = 16$ apples
PROOF
$3 : 2 :: 24 : 16$
$3 \times 16 = 48$
$2 \times 24 = 48$

5. *Know*   *Want to Know*
6 pens : 8 pencils :: x pens : 72 pencils
$8x = 432$
$\frac{8}{8}x = \frac{432}{8}$
     $x = 54$ pens
PROOF
$6 : 8 :: 54 : 72$
$6 \times 72 = 432$
$8 \times 54 = 432$

6. *Know*   *Want to Know*
$\frac{1}{2}$ tsp salt : 3 eggs :: x tsp salt : 30 eggs
$3x = 30 \times \frac{1}{2}$
$3x = \frac{30}{1} \times \frac{1}{2} = \frac{30}{2} = 15$
$\frac{x}{3}x = \frac{15}{3}$
     $x = 5$ tsp salt
PROOF
$\frac{1}{2} : 3 :: 5 : 30$
$3 \times 5 = 15$
$\frac{1}{2} \times 30 = 15$

7. *Know*   *Want to Know*
8 cups : 7 scoops :: 24 cups : x scoops
$8x = 7 \times 24$
$\frac{8}{8}x = \frac{168}{8}$
     $x = 21$ scoops
PROOF
$8 : 7 :: 24 : 21$
$8 \times 21 = 168$
$7 \times 24 = 168$

8. *Know*   *Want to Know*
5 carnations : 1 fern :: x carnations : 10 ferns
$x = 5 \times 10$
$x = 50$ carnations
PROOF
$5 : 1 :: 50 : 10$
$5 \times 10 = 50$
$1 \times 50 = 50$

9. *Know*   *Want to Know*
2 tbsp vinegar : 1 cup water ::
            x tbsp vinegar : 10 cups water
$x = 2 \times 10$ cups
$x = 20$ tbsp vinegar
PROOF
2 : 1 :: 20 : 10
$2 \times 10 = 20$
$1 \times 20 = 20$

10. *Know*   *Want to Know*
$\frac{1}{2}$ C milk : 3 flour :: *x* C milk : 21 flour
$3x = \frac{1}{2} \times 21$
$\frac{\cancel{3}}{\cancel{3}}x = \frac{10.5}{3}$
$x = 3.5$ cups milk
PROOF
$\frac{1}{2} \times 21 = 10.5$
$3 \times 3.5 = 10.5$

2G (PAGE 43)

1. b. *Know*   *Want to Know*
10 syringes : 1 package ::
            120 syringes : *x* packages
$\frac{\cancel{10}}{\cancel{10}}x = \frac{120}{10}$
$x = 12$ packages
PROOF
$10 \times 12 = 120$
$1 \times 120 = 120$

2. d. *Know*   *Want to Know*
4 tsp : 1 day :: 80 tsp : *x* days
$\frac{\cancel{4}}{\cancel{4}}x = \frac{80}{4}$
$x = 20$ days
PROOF
$4 \times 20 = 80$
$1 \times 80 = 80$

3. a. *Know*   *Want to Know*
10 diapers : 1 day :: 50 diapers : *x* days
$\frac{\cancel{10}}{\cancel{10}}x = \frac{50}{10}$
$x = 5$ days
PROOF
$10 \times 5 = 50$
$1 \times 50 = 50$

4. b. *Know*   *Want to Know*
5 mL : 1 dose :: 30 mL : *x* doses
$\frac{\cancel{5}}{\cancel{5}}x = \frac{30}{5}$
$x = 6$ doses
PROOF
$5 \times 6 = 30$
$1 \times 30 = 30$

5. d. *Know*   *Want to Know*
3 pills : 1 day :: *x* pills : 21 days
$x = 3 \times 21$
$x = 63$ pills
PROOF
$3 \times 21 = 63$
$1 \times 63 = 63$

6. b. *Know*   *Want to Know*
120 days : 15 depts. :: *x* days : 1 dept.
$\frac{\cancel{15}}{\cancel{15}}x = \frac{120}{15}$
$x = 8$ days
PROOF
$120 \times 1 = 120$
$15 \times 8 = 120$

7. *Know*   *Want to Know*
a. 8 patients : 1 RN :: 240 patients : *x* RNs
$\frac{\cancel{8}}{\cancel{8}}x = \frac{240}{8}$
$x = 30$ RNs
PROOF
$8 \times 30 = 240$
$1 \times 240 = 240$

8. *Know*   *Want to Know*
c. 4 oz : 1 portion :: *x* oz : 20 portions
$x = 4 \times 20$
$x = 80$ oz
PROOF
$4 \times 20 = 80$
$1 \times 80 = 80$

9. *Know*   *Want to Know*

c. $15 : 1 \text{ hr} :: \$450 : x \text{ hr}$

$\dfrac{\cancel{15}}{\cancel{15}}x = \dfrac{450}{15}$

$x = 30 \text{ hr}$

PROOF

$15 \times 30 = 450$

$1 \times 450 = 450$

10. a. *Know*   *Want to Know*

$1 \text{ NA} : 20 \text{ beds} :: x \text{ NAs} : 360 \text{ beds}$

$\dfrac{\cancel{20}}{\cancel{20}}x = \dfrac{360}{20}$

$\qquad\qquad x = 18 \text{ NAs}$

PROOF

$1 \times 360 = 360$

$20 \times 18 = 360$

Chapter 2 Final: Ratio and Proportion (PAGE 44)

1. 28 pills

2. 10 days

3. 64 oz

4. 8 inservice days

5. 8 doses

6. 12 people

7. 12 pills

8. 32 RNs

9. 12 guest speakers

10. 240 tablets

3 Patient Safety: Errors, Orders, Labels, and Records

3A (PAGE 56)

1. a. Lopressor
  b. metoprolol tartrate USP
  c. 50 mg per tab
  d. 1000 tab
  e. 50 mg : 1 tab

2. a. Rifadin
  b. rifampin
  c. 150 mg per cap
  d. 30 cap
  e. 150 mg : 1 cap

3. a. Amoxil
  b. 78 mL
  c. 125 mg/5 mL
  d. 100 mL
  e. 125 mg : 5 mL
  f. 14 days

4. a. tetracycline HCl
  b. 500 mg
  c. 100 capsules
  d. 500 mg : 1 cap

5. a. streptomycin sulfate
  b. IM only
  c. 400 mg/mL
  d. 1 g/2.5 mL
  e. Refrigerate 2° to 8° C
  f. IM use only

3B (PAGE 61)

1. Yes. Care must be taken in distinguishing this patient from other patients with the same or a similar name to avoid giving a medication to the wrong patient.

2. Yes. The patient is allergic to intravenous iodine used in some contrast media tests and to products that contain aspirin. There are many.

3. One 24-hour day

4. Digoxin was withheld as denoted by a circle and the code "R."

5. Topical

6. Promethazine, a stat order

7. Meperidine; Left arm denoted by "C."

8. 05/09/03 at 0700

9. 05/07/03 at 2000; 8 PM

10. Having both the initials and the nurse's signature identifies the nurse who administered the medication more clearly. More than one staff member may have the same initials or some initials may be illegible.

3C (PAGE 65)

1. b. Correct identification of patient is always the first priority.

2. a. b, c, and d would all be appropriate after the patient was assessed.

3. a. b is the total dose in the vial, c is the total volume after reconstitution, and d is the ordered dose.

4. d. a, b, and c are inappropriate actions.

5. b. Refer to the international/military time clock on page 59.

6. a. b, c, and d are false statements.

7. d. A solid foundation in medication mathematics, logic, estimation of a reasonable dose as applicable during calculations, and use of reliable references and pharmacy for safe doses are more protective measures than memorized formulas for complex calculations.

8. d. The right route is usually the one that is ordered but not in this case. There is a conflict and common sense dictates that the nurse must clarify. The patient is NPO and there must be a written order to be able to give a medication by mouth. Some medications are totally unsuitable for nasogastric tube administration and some just clog the tube.

9. d. The nurse took measures to correctly identify the intended patient but Tylenol and Tylenol #2 are two different medications. Two tablets of plain Tylenol were given instead of 1 tablet of Tylenol #2, which is Tylenol with a narcotic added.

10. b. Giving a medication after the expiration date, whether automatically established by the agency or written by the physician, is illegal. All other actions are appropriate.

4 Metric Calculations

4A (PAGE 72)

1. 1000 mg	**2.** 2000 mg	**3.** 1500 mg
4. 500 mg	**5.** 50 μg	**6.** 250 mg
7. 50 mg	**8.** 100 mg	**9.** 1100 mg
10. 300 mg	**11.** 0.025 g	**12.** 5000 μg
13. 3 g	**14.** 1.5 g	**15.** 15 g
16. 0.010 g	**17.** 0.1 mg	**18.** 0.0005 g
19. 0.0075 g	**20.** 0.02015 g	

4B (PAGE 76)

1. *Know*   *Want to Know*

1000 mg : 1 g :: 200 mg : x g

$$\frac{\cancel{1000}}{\cancel{1000}}x = \frac{200}{1000}$$

$$x = 0.2 \text{ g}$$

PROOF

$1000 \times 0.2 = 200$

$1 \times 200 = 200$

2. *Know*   *Want to Know*

1000 mg : 1 g :: 4 mg : x g

$$\frac{\cancel{1000}}{\cancel{1000}}x = \frac{4}{1000}$$

$$x = 0.004 \text{ g}$$

PROOF

$1000 \times 0.004 = 4$

$1 \times 4 = 4$

3. *Know*   *Want to Know*

1000 mg : 1 g :: 0.3 mg : x g

$$\frac{\cancel{1000}}{\cancel{1000}}x = \frac{0.3}{1000}$$

$$x = 0.0003 \text{ g}$$

PROOF

$1000 \times 0.0003 = 0.3$

$1 \times 0.3 = 0.3$

4. *Know*   *Want to Know*

1000 mg : 1 g :: 25 mg : x g

$$\frac{\cancel{1000}}{\cancel{1000}}x = \frac{1 \times 25}{1000}$$

$$x = 0.025 \text{ g}$$

PROOF

$1000 \times 0.025 = 25$

$1 \times 25 = 25$

5. *Know*   *Want to Know*

1000 mg : 1 g :: 15 mg : x g

$$\frac{\cancel{1000}}{\cancel{1000}}x = \frac{15}{1000}$$

$$x = 0.015 \text{ g}$$

PROOF

$1000 \times 0.015 = 15$

$1 \times 15 = 15$

6. *Know*   *Want to Know*

1 g : 1000 mg :: 0.01 g : x mg

$x = 1000 \times 0.01$

$x = 10$ mg

PROOF

$1 \times 10 = 10$

$1000 \times 0.01 = 10$

7. *Know*   *Want to Know*

1 g : 1000 mg :: 4.6 g : x mg

$x = 1000 \times 4.6$

$x = 4600$ mg

PROOF

$1 \times 4600 = 4600$

$1000 \times 4.6 = 4600$

8. *Know*   *Want to Know*

1 g : 1000 mg :: 0.03 g : x mg

$x = 1000 \times 0.03$

$x = 30$ mg

PROOF

$1 \times 30 = 30$

$1000 \times 0.03 = 30$

9. *Know*   *Want to Know*
1 g : 1000 mg :: 0.5 g : x mg
$x = 1000 \times 0.5$
$x = 500$ mg
PROOF
$1 \times 500 = 500$
$1000 \times 0.5 = 500$

10. *Know*   *Want to Know*
1 g : 1000 mg :: 2.5 g : x mg
$x = 1000 \times 2.5$
$x = 2500$ mg
PROOF
$1 \times 2500 = 2500$
$1000 \times 2.5 = 2500$

11. *Know*   *Want to Know*
1000 μg : 1 mg :: 150 μg : x mg
$\frac{\cancel{1000}}{\cancel{1000}} x = \frac{\cancel{150}}{1000}$
$x = 0.15$ mg
PROOF
$1000 \times 0.15 = 150$
$1 \times 150 = 150$

12. *Know*   *Want to Know*
1000 μg : 1 mg :: 3000 μg : x mg
$\frac{\cancel{1000}}{\cancel{1000}} x = \frac{\cancel{3000}}{\cancel{1000}}$
$x = 3$ mg
PROOF
$1000 \times 3 = 3000$
$1 \times 3000 = 3000$

13. *Know*   *Want to Know*
1000 μg : 1 mg :: 50 μg : x mg
$\frac{\cancel{1000}}{\cancel{1000}} x = \frac{\cancel{50}}{1000}$
$x = 0.05$ mg
PROOF
$1000 \times 0.05 = 50$
$1 \times 50 = 50$

14. *Know*   *Want to Know*
1000 μg : 1 mg :: 2500 μg : x mg
$\frac{\cancel{1000}}{\cancel{1000}} x = \frac{\cancel{2500}}{\cancel{1000}}$
$x = 2.5$ mg
PROOF
$1000 \times 2.5 = 2500$
$1 \times 2500 = 2500$

15. *Know*   *Want to Know*
1000 μg : 1 mg :: 500 μg : x mg
$\frac{\cancel{1000}}{\cancel{1000}} x = \frac{\cancel{500}}{\cancel{1000}}$
$x = 0.5$ mg
PROOF
$1000 \times 0.5 \text{ mg} = 500$
$1 \times 500 = 500$

16. *Know*   *Want to Know*
1 mg : 1000 μg :: 20 mg : x μg
$x = 1000 \times 20$
$x = 20,000$ μg
PROOF
$1 \times 20,000 = 20,000$
$1000 \times 20 = 20,000$

17. *Know*   *Want to Know*
1 mg : 1000 μg :: 200 mg : x μg
$x = 1000 \times 200$
$x = 200,000$ μg
PROOF
$1 \times 200,000 = 200,000$
$1000 \times 200 = 200,000$

18. *Know*   *Want to Know*
1 mg : 1000 μg :: 5 mg : x μg
$x = 1000 \times 5$
$x = 5000$ μg
PROOF
$1 \times 5000 = 5000$
$1000 \times 5 = 5000$

19. *Know*   *Want to Know*
1 mg : 1000 μg :: 0.1 mg : x μg
$x = 1000 \times 0.1$
$x = 100$ μg
PROOF
$1 \times 100 = 100$
$1000 \times 0.1 = 100$

20. *Know*   *Want to Know*
1 mg : 1000 μg :: 0.04 mg : x μg
$x = 1000 \times 0.04$
$x = 40$ μg
PROOF
$1 \times 40 = 40$
$1000 \times 0.04 = 40$

21. *Know*   *Want to Know*
1 kg : 1000 g :: 5.5 kg : x g
$x = 1000 \times 5.5$
$x = 5500$ g
PROOF
$1 \times 5500 = 5500$
$1000 \times 5.5 = 5500$

22. *Know*   *Want to Know*
1 kg : 1000 g :: 12 kg : x g
$x = 1000 \times 12$
$x = 12{,}000$ g
PROOF
$1 \times 12{,}000 = 12{,}000$
$1000 \times 12 = 12{,}000$

23. *Know*   *Want to Know*
1 kg : 1000 g :: 3 kg : x g
$x = 1000 \times 3$
$x = 3000$ g
PROOF
$1 \times 3000 = 3000$
$1000 \times 3 = 3000$

24. *Know*   *Want to Know*
1 kg : 1000 g :: 1.3 kg : x g
$x = 1000 \times 1.3$
$x = 1300$ g
PROOF
$1 \times 1300 = 1300$
$1000 \times 1.3 = 1300$

25. *Know*   *Want to Know*
1 kg : 1000 g :: 0.5 kg : x g
$x = 1000 \times 0.5$
$x = 500$ g
PROOF
$1 \times 500 = 500$
$1000 \times 0.5 = 500$

26. *Know*   *Want to Know*
1 L : 1000 mL :: 0.5 L : x mL
$x = 1000 \times 0.5$
$x = 500$ mL
PROOF
$1 \times 500 = 500$
$1000 \times 0.5 = 500$

27. *Know*   *Want to Know*
1 L : 1000 mL :: 1.3 L : x mL
$x = 1000 \times 1.3$
$x = 1300$ mL
PROOF
$1 \times 1300 = 1300$
$1000 \times 1.3 = 1300$

28. *Know*   *Want to Know*
1 L : 1000 mL :: 1.5 L : x mL
$x = 1000 \times 1.5$
$x = 1500$ mL
PROOF
$1 \times 1500 = 1500$
$1000 \times 1.5 = 1500$

29. *Know*   *Want to Know*
1 L : 1000 mL :: 3 L : x mL
$x = 1000 \times 3$
$x = 3000$ mL
PROOF
$1 \times 3000 = 3000$
$1000 \times 3 = 3000$

30. *Know*   *Want to Know*
1 L : 1000 mL :: 2.8 L : x mL
$x = 1000 \times 2.8$
$x = 2800$ mL
PROOF
$1 \times 2800 = 2800$
$1000 \times 2.8 = 2800$

4C (PAGE 77)

1. a. 300 mg/capsule **b.** 30 capsules

2. a. 75 mcg (μg) **b.** 0.175 mg

3. a. 10 USP* units/mL **b.** 10 mL

4. a. 250,000 units/mL **b.** 200,000 to **c.** 5 million units
400,000 units

5. a. 2 mEq/mL **b.** 40 mEq/20 mL

6. a. 100 units/mL **b.** 10 mL

7. a. 125 μg **b.** 0.125 mg

8. 1000 mL

9. 4 mEq/L

10. 30 mg

---

*USP refers to the *United States Pharmacopoeia*, a national listing of drugs.

4D (PAGE 80)

1. *Know*   *Want to Know*
0.2 mg : 1 cap :: 0.2 mg : x cap
$$\frac{0.2}{0.2}x = \frac{0.2}{0.2}$$
$$x = 1 \text{ cap}$$
PROOF
$0.2 \times 1 = 0.2$
$1 \times 0.2 = 0.2$

2. *Know*   *Want to Know*
200 mg : 5 mL :: 300 mg : x mL
$$\frac{200}{200}x = \frac{5 \times 300}{200} \text{ or } \frac{1500}{200}$$
$$x = 7.5 \text{ mL}$$
PROOF
$200 \times 7.5 = 1500$
$5 \times 300 = 1500$

You would use a syringe to withdraw the medication to the exact amount and then transfer it to the cup.

3. *Know*   *Want to Know*
0.125 mg : 1 tab :: 0.0625 mg : x tab
$$\frac{0.125}{0.125}x = \frac{0.0625}{0.125}$$
$$x = 0.5 \text{ or } \frac{1}{2} \text{ tab}$$
PROOF
$0.125 \times 0.5 = 0.0625$
$1 \times 0.0625 = 0.0625$

4. *Know*   *Want to Know*
175 μg : 1 tab :: 350 μg : x tab
$$\frac{175}{175}x = \frac{350}{175}$$
$$x = 2 \text{ tab}$$
PROOF
$175 \times 2 = 350$
$1 \times 350 = 350$

5. *Know*   *Want to Know*
80 mg : 0.8 mL :: 40 mg : x mL
$$\frac{80}{80}x = \frac{32}{80}$$
$$x = 0.4 \text{ mL}$$
PROOF
$80 \times 0.4 = 32$
$0.8 \times 40 = 32$

4E (PAGE 83)

1. *Know*   *Want to Know*
15 mg : 1 tab :: 30 mg : x tab

$$\frac{\cancel{15}}{\cancel{15}}x = \frac{30}{15}$$

$x = 2$ tab

PROOF
$15 \times 2 = 30$
$1 \times 30 = 30$

2. *Know*   *Want to Know*
0.125 mg : 1 tab :: 0.25 mg : x tab

$$\frac{\cancel{0.125}}{\cancel{0.125}}x = \frac{0.25}{0.125}$$

$x = 2$ tab

PROOF
$0.125 \times 2 = 0.25$
$1 \times 0.25 = 0.25$

3. *Know*   *Want to Know*
300 mg : 1 tab :: 450 mg : x tab

$$\frac{\cancel{300}}{\cancel{300}}x = \frac{\cancel{450}}{\cancel{300}}$$

$x = 1.5$ tab

PROOF
$300 \times 1.5 = 450$
$1 \times 450 = 450$

4. *Know*   *Want to Know*
0.1 mg : 1 tab :: 0.2 mg : x tab

$$\frac{\cancel{0.1}}{\cancel{0.1}}x = \frac{0.2}{0.1}$$

$x = 2$ tab

PROOF
$0.1 \times 2 = 0.2$
$1 \times 0.2 = 0.2$

5. *Know*   *Want to Know*
8 mEq : 5 mL :: 20 mEq : x mL

$$\frac{\cancel{8}}{\cancel{8}}x = \frac{100}{8}$$

$x = 12.5$ mL

PROOF
$8 \times 12.5 = 100$
$5 \times 20 = 100$

6. *Know*   *Want to Know*
0.01 mg : 1 tab :: 0.02 mg : x tab

$$\frac{\cancel{0.01}}{\cancel{0.01}}x = \frac{0.02}{0.01}$$

$x = 2$ tab

PROOF
$0.01 \times 2 = 0.02$
$1 \times 0.02 = 0.02$

7. *Know*   *Want to Know*
50 mg : 1 tab :: 75 mg : x tab

$$\frac{\cancel{50}}{\cancel{50}}x = \frac{75}{50}$$

$x = 1.5$ tab

PROOF
$50 \times 1.5 = 75$
$1 \times 75 = 75$

8. *Know*   *Want to Know*
10 mg : 1 tab :: 5 mg : x tab

$$\frac{\cancel{10}}{\cancel{10}}x = \frac{5}{10}$$

$x = 0.5$ tab

PROOF
$10 \times 0.5 = 5$
$1 \times 5 = 5$

9. *Know*   *Want to Know*
400 mg : 1 tab :: 800 mg : x tab
$400\, x = 800$

$x = 2$ tab

PROOF
$400 \times 2 = 800$
$1 \times 800 = 800$

10. *Know*   *Want to Know*
150 mg : 1 tab :: 450 mg : x tab

$$\frac{\cancel{150}}{\cancel{150}}x = \frac{\cancel{450}}{\cancel{150}}$$

$x = 3$ tab

PROOF
$150 \times 3 = 450$
$1 \times 450 = 450$

4F (PAGE 85)

1. Step 1:
Know   Want to Know
1000 mg : 1 g :: x mg : 0.5 g
$x = 1000 \times 0.5$
$x = 500$ mg
PROOF
$1000 \times 0.5 = 500$
$1 \times 500 = 500$

Step 2:
Know   Want to Know
500 mg : 1 tab :: 500 mg : x tab
$\frac{500}{500}x = \frac{500}{500}$
    $x = 1$ tab
PROOF
$500 \times 1 = 500$
$1 \times 500 = 500$

3. Step 1:
Know   Want to Know
1000 mg : 1 g :: x mg : 1 g
$x = 1000$ mg
PROOF
$1000 \times 1 = 1000$
$1 \times 1000 = 1000$

Step 2:
Know   Want to Know
500 mg : 1 tab :: 1000 mg : x tab
$\frac{500}{500}x = \frac{1000}{500}$
    $x = 2$ tabs
PROOF
$500 \times 2 = 1000$
$1 \times 1000 = 1000$

5. Step 1:
Know   Want to Know
1000 mg : 1 g :: x mg : 0.6 g
$x = 1000 \times 0.6$
$x = 600$ mg
PROOF
$1000 \times 0.6 = 600$
$1 \times 600 = 600$

Step 2:
Know   Want to Know
600 mg : 1 tab :: 600 mg : x tab
$\frac{600}{600}x = \frac{600}{600}$
    $x = 1$ tab
PROOF
$600 \times 1 = 600$
$1 \times 600 = 600$

2. Step 1:
Know   Want to Know
1000 mg : 1 g :: x mg : 0.3 g
$x = 1000 \times 0.3$
$x = 300$ mg
PROOF
$1000 \times 0.3 = 300$
$1 \times 300 = 300$

Step 2:
Know   Want to Know
300 mg : 1 cap :: 300 mg : x cap
$\frac{300}{300}x = \frac{300}{300}$
    $x = 1$ cap
PROOF
$300 \times 1 = 300$
$1 \times 300 = 300$

4. Step 1:
Know   Want to Know
1000 mg : 1 g :: x mg : 0.3 g
$x = 1000 \times 0.3$
$x = 300$ mg
PROOF
$1000 \times 0.3 = 300$
$1 \times 300 = 300$

Step 2:
Know   Want to Know
100 mg : 1 cap :: 300 mg : x cap
$\frac{100}{100}x = \frac{300}{100}$
    $x = 3$ cap
PROOF
$100 \times 3 = 300$
$1 \times 300 = 300$

4G (PAGE 87)

1. Step 1:
Know   *Want to Know*
$1000 \ \mu g : 1 \ mg :: x \ \mu g : 0.25 \ mg$
$x = 1000 \times 0.25$
$x = 250 \ \mu g$
PROOF
$1000 \times 0.25 = 250$
$1 \times 250 = 250$

Step 2:
Have   *Want to Have*
$125 \ \mu g : 1 \ tab :: 250 \ \mu g : x \ tab$
$\dfrac{\cancel{125}}{\cancel{125}} x = \dfrac{250}{125}$
$x = 2 \ tab$
PROOF
$125 \times 2 = 250$
$1 \times 250 = 250$

2. Step 1:
Know   *Want to Know*
$1000 \ mg : 1 \ g :: x \ mg : 0.01 \ g$
$x = 1000 \times 0.01$
$x = 10 \ mg$
PROOF
$1000 \times 0.01 \ g = 10$
$1 \times 10 = 10$

Step 2:
Have   *Want to Have*
$5 \ mg : 1 \ tab :: 10 \ mg : x \ tab$
$\dfrac{\cancel{5}}{\cancel{5}} x = \dfrac{10}{5}$
$x = 2 \ tab$
PROOF
$5 \times 2 = 10$
$1 \times 10 = 10$

3. Step 1:
Know   *Want to Know*
$1000 \ mg : 1 \ g :: x \ mg : 0.2 \ g$
$x = 1000 \times 0.2$
$x = 200 \ mg$
PROOF
$1000 \times 0.2 = 200$
$1 \times 200 = 200$

Step 2:
Have   *Want to Have*
$100 \ mg : 1 \ cap :: 200 \ mg : x \ cap$
$\dfrac{\cancel{100}}{\cancel{100}} x = \dfrac{\cancel{200}}{\cancel{100}}$
$x = 2 \ cap$
PROOF
$100 \times 2 = 200$
$1 \times 200 = 200$

4. Step 1:
Know   *Want to Know*
$1000 \ mg : 1 \ g :: x \ mg : 0.05 \ g$
$x = 1000 \times 0.05$
$x = 50 \ mg$
PROOF
$1000 \times 0.05 = 50$
$1 \times 50 = 50$

Step 2:
Have   *Want to Have*
$25 \ mg : 1 \ tab :: 50 \ mg : x \ tab$
$\dfrac{\cancel{25}}{\cancel{25}} x = \dfrac{50}{25}$
$x = 2 \ tab$
PROOF
$25 \times 2 = 50$
$1 \times 50 = 50$

5. Step 1:

Know   *Want to Know*

$1000 \ \mu g : 1 \ mg :: 125 \ \mu g : x \ mg$

$\dfrac{\cancel{1000}}{\cancel{1000}} x = \dfrac{125}{1000}$

$\qquad x = 0.125 \ mg$

PROOF

$1000 \times 0.125 = 125$

$1 \times 125 = 125$

Step 2:

Have   *Want to Have*

$0.125 \ mg : 1 \ tab :: 0.125 \ mg : x \ tab$

$\dfrac{\cancel{0.125}}{\cancel{0.125}} x = \dfrac{0.125}{0.125}$

$\qquad x = 1 \ tab$

PROOF

$0.125 \times 1 = 0.125$

$1 \times 0.125 = 0.125$

4H (PAGE 88)

1. Step 1:

Know   *Want to Know*

$1000 \ mg : 1 \ g :: x \ mg : 0.5 \ g$

$x = 1000 \times 0.5$

$x = 500 \ mg$

PROOF

$1000 \times 0.5 = 500$

$1 \times 500 = 500$

Step 2:

Have   *Want to Have*

$250 \ mg : 1 \ tab :: 500 \ mg : x \ tab$

$\dfrac{\cancel{250}}{\cancel{250}} x = \dfrac{\cancel{500}}{\cancel{250}}$

$\qquad x = 2 \ tab$

PROOF

$250 \times 2 = 500$

$1 \times 500 = 500$

2. Step 1:

Know   *Want to Know*

$1000 \ mg : 1 \ g :: x \ mg : 0.025 \ g$

$x = 1000 \times 0.025$

$x = 25 \ mg$

PROOF

$1000 \times 0.025 = 25$

$1 \times 25 = 25$

Step 2:

Have   *Want to Have*

$50 \ mg : 1 \ tab :: 25 \ mg : x \ tab$

$\dfrac{\cancel{50}}{\cancel{50}} x = \dfrac{25}{50}$

$\qquad x = 0.5 \ tab$

PROOF

$50 \times 0.5 = 25$

$1 \times 25 = 25$

3. Step 1:

Know *Want to Know*

1000 mg : 1 g :: 250 mg : x g

$\frac{\cancel{1000}}{\cancel{1000}}x = \frac{250}{1000}$

$x = 0.25$ g

PROOF

$1000 \times 0.25 = 250$

$1 \times 250 = 250$

Step 2:

Have *Want to Have*

0.25 g : 1 tab :: 0.25 g : x tab

$\frac{\cancel{0.25}}{\cancel{0.25}}x = \frac{0.25}{0.25}$

$x = 1$ tab

PROOF

$0.25 \times 1 = 0.25$

$1 \times 0.25 = 0.25$

5. Step 1:

Know *Want to Know*

1000 µg : 1 mg :: 5000 µg : x mg

$\frac{\cancel{1000}}{\cancel{1000}}x = \frac{\cancel{5000}}{\cancel{1000}}$

$x = 5$ mg

PROOF

$1000 \times 5 = 5000$

$1 \times 5000 = 5000$

Step 2:

Have *Want to Have*

2.5 mg : 1 tab :: 5 mg : x tab

$\frac{\cancel{2.5}}{\cancel{2.5}}x = \frac{5}{2.5}$

$x = 2$ tab

PROOF

$2.5 \times 2 = 5$

$1 \times 5 = 5$

4. Step 1:

Know *Want to Know*

1000 mg : 1 g :: x mg : 0.45 g

$x = 1000 \times 0.45$

$x = 450$ mg

PROOF

$1000 \times 0.45 = 450$

$1 \times 450 = 450$

Step 2:

Have *Want to Have*

150 mg : 1 tab :: 450 mg : x tab

$\frac{\cancel{150}}{\cancel{150}}x = \frac{\cancel{450}}{\cancel{150}}$

$x = 3$ tab

PROOF

$150 \times 3 = 450$

$1 \times 450 = 450$

4I (PAGE 90)

1. a. 3 mL
   b. tenths

2. a. 10 mL
   b. 0.2

3. a. 5 mL
   b. 0.2

4. a. 3 mL
   b. tenths

5. a. 1 mL
   b. hundredths

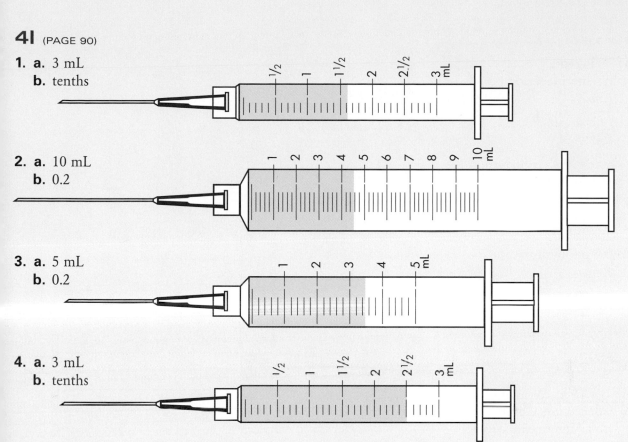

4J (PAGE 91)

1. a. 75 mg/mL
   b. 0.3 mL meperidine
   Know   *Want to Know*
   75 mg : 1 mL :: 25 mg : x mL
   $\frac{75}{75}x = \frac{25}{75}$
       $x = 0.33$ or 0.3 mL
   PROOF
   $75 \times 0.33 = 24.75$ or 25
   $1 \times 25 = 25$
   c. 50 mg/mL
   d. 0.5 mL hydroxyzine
   Know   *Want to Know*
   50 mg : 1 mL :: 25 mg : x mL
   $\frac{50}{50}x = \frac{25}{50}$
       $x = 0.5$ mL
   PROOF
   $50 \times 0.5 = 25$
   $1 \times 25 = 25$
   e. $0.3 + 0.5 = 0.8$ mL
   (total amount in syringe)

2. a. 4 mg/mL
   b. 0.8 mL hydromorphone

   Know   *Want to Know*

   4 mg : 1 mL :: 3 mg : x mL

   $\frac{4}{4}x = \frac{3}{4}$

   $x = 0.75$ or 0.8 mL
   PROOF
   $4 \times 0.75 = 3.00$
   $1 \times 3 = 3$

   c. 5 mg/mL Compazine (prochlorperazine)
   d. *Know*   *Want to Know*
   5 mg : 1 mL :: 2.5 mg : x mL
   $\frac{5}{5}x = \frac{2.5}{5}$
   $x = 0.5$ mL
   PROOF
   $5 \times 0.5 = 2.5$
   $1 \times 2.5 = 2.5$
   e. $0.8 + 0.5 = 1.3$ mL
   (total amount in syringe)

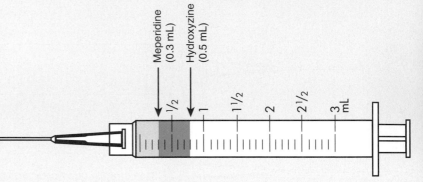

3. a. 75 mg/mL
 b. 0.7 mL meperidine
  Know   *Want to Know*
  75 mg : 1 mL :: 50 mg : x mL
  $\frac{\cancel{75}}{\cancel{75}}x = \frac{50}{75}$
     $x = 0.66$ or 0.7 mL
  PROOF
  $75 \times 0.66 = 49.5$
  $1 \times 50 = 50$
 c. 0.4 mg/mL
 d. 1.5 mL atropine sulfate
  Know   *Want to Know*
  0.4 mg : 1 mL :: 0.6 mg : x mL
  $0.4x = 0.6$
     $x = 1.5$ mL
  PROOF
  $0.4 \times 1.5 = 0.6$
  $1 \times 0.6 = 0.6$
 e. $0.7 + 1.5 = 2.2$ mL
  (total amount in syringe)

4. a. 0.5 mL hydromorphone
  Know   *Want to Know*
  4 mg : 1 mL :: 2 mg : x mL
  $\frac{\cancel{4}}{\cancel{4}}x = \frac{2}{4}$
     $x = 0.5$ mL
  PROOF
  $4 \times 0.5 = 2$
  $1 \times 2 = 2$
 b. 1.4 mL hydroxyzine
  Know   *Want to Know*
  50 mg : 1 mL :: 35 mg : x mL
  $\frac{\cancel{50}}{\cancel{50}}x = \frac{35}{50}$
     $x = 0.7$ mL
  PROOF
  $50 \times 0.7 = 35$
  $1 \times 35 = 35$
 c. $0.5 + 0.7 = 1.2$ mL
  (total amount in syringe)

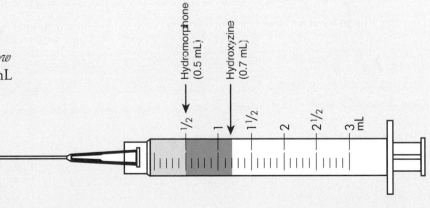

5. **a.** 0.8 mL morphine sulfate

Have   *Want to Have*

10 mg : 1 mL :: 8 mg : x mL

$\frac{10}{10}x = \frac{8}{10}$

$x = 0.8$ mL

b. 0.5 mL Vistaril

Have   *Want to Have*

50 mg : 1 mL :: 25 mg : x mL

$\frac{50}{50}x = \frac{25}{50}$

$x = 0.5$ mL

c. 0.8 + 0.5 = 1.3 mL combined in syringe

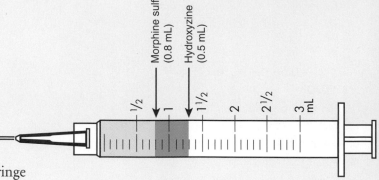

4K (PAGE 94)

1. two-step

Step 1: 1000 mg : 1 g :: x mg : 0.2 g

$x = 1000 \times 0.2$ or 200 mg

PROOF

$1000 \times 0.2 = 200$

$1 \times 200 = 200$

(more)

Step 2: 150 mg : 1 mL :: 200 mg : x mL

$\frac{150}{150}x = \frac{200}{150}$

$x = 1.3$ mL

PROOF

$150 \times 1.3 = 195$

$1 \times 200 = 200$

(rounding to 1.3 affects answer)

3. two-step

Step 1: 1000 mg : 1 g :: x mg : 0.2 g

$x = 1000 \times 0.2$ or 200 mg

PROOF

$1000 \times 0.2 = 200$

$1 \times 200 = 200$

(less)

Step 2: 250 mg : 2 mL :: 200 mg : x mL

$\frac{250}{250}x = \frac{400}{250}$

$x = 1.6$ mL

PROOF

$250 \times 1.6 = 400$

$2 \times 200 = 400$

2. two-step

Step 1: 1000 μg : 1 mg :: 500 μg : x mg

$\frac{1000}{1000}x = \frac{500}{1000}$

$x = 0.5$ mg

PROOF

$1000 \times 0.5 = 500$

$1 \times 500 = 500$

(same)

Step 2: 0.5 mg : 1 tab :: 0.5 mg : x tab

$\frac{0.5}{0.5}x = \frac{0.5}{0.5}$

$x = 1$ tab

PROOF

$0.5 \times 1 = 0.5$

$1 \times 0.5 = 0.5$

4. one-step

125 mg : 2 mL :: 75 mg : x mL

$\frac{125}{125}x = \frac{150}{125}$

$x = 1.2$ mL

PROOF

$125 \times 1.2 = 150$

$2 \times 75 = 150$

(less)

5. one-step

16 mg : 1 tab :: 32 mg : x tab

$\frac{\cancel{16}}{\cancel{16}}x = \frac{32}{16}$

$x = 2$ tab

PROOF

$16 \times 2 = 32$

$1 \times 32 = 32$

(more)

6. two-step

Step 1: 1000 mg : 1 g :: x mg : 0.8

$x = 1000 \times 0.8 = 800$ mg

PROOF

$1000 \times 0.8 = 800$

$1 \times 800 = 800$

(more)

Step 2: 400 mg : 1 tab :: 800 mg : x tab

$\frac{\cancel{400}}{\cancel{400}}x = \frac{800}{400}$

$x = 2$ tab

PROOF

$400 \times 2 = 800$

$1 \times 800 = 800$

7. one-step

300 mg : 1 mL :: 250 mg : x mL

$\frac{\cancel{300}}{\cancel{300}}x = \frac{250}{300}$

$x = 0.83$ or 0.8 mL

PROOF

$300 \times 0.8 = 240$

$1 \times 250 = 250$

(rounding 0.83 to 0.8 affects answer)

(less)

8. two-step

Step 1: 1000 mg : 1 g :: x mg : 0.3 g

$x = 1000 \times 0.3 = 300$ mg

PROOF

$1000 \times 0.3 = 300$

$1 \times 300 = 300$

(less)

Step 2: 400 mg : 1 mL :: 300 mg : x mL

$\frac{\cancel{400}}{\cancel{400}}x = \frac{300}{400}$

$x = 0.75$ or 0.8 mL

PROOF

$400 \times 0.8 = 320$

$1 \times 300 = 300$

(rounding 0.75 to 0.8 affects answer)

9. two-step

Step 1: 1000 μg : 1 mg :: 125 μg : x mg

$\frac{\cancel{1000}}{\cancel{1000}}x = \frac{125}{1000}$

$x = 0.125$ mg

PROOF

$1000 \times 0.125 = 125$

$1 \times 125 = 125$

(same)

Step 2: 0.125 mg : 1 tab :: 0.125 mg : x tab

$\frac{\cancel{0.125}}{\cancel{0.125}}x = \frac{0.125}{0.125}$

$x = 1$ tab

PROOF

$1 \times 0.125 = 0.125$

$0.125 \times 1 = 0.125$

10. one-step

175 μg : 1 tab :: 350 μg : x tab

$\frac{\cancel{175}}{\cancel{175}}x = \frac{350}{175}$

$x = 2$ tab

PROOF

$175 \times 2 = 350$

$1 \times 350 = 350$

4L (PAGE 97)

1. 0.4 mg   gr 1/150

2. 130 mg   2 grains*

3. 325 mg   5 grains†

4. 324 mg   gr 5

5. 30 mg   (1/2 gr/mL)

---

*Could also be written as grii.
†Could also be written as grv.

4M (PAGE 100)

1. **c.** one-step	2. **c.** one-step	3. **a.** one-step
4. **d.** one-step	5. **c.** two-step	6. **c.** two-step
7. **c.** two-step	8. **d.** two-step	9. **d.** one-step
10. **b.** two-step		

Chapter 4 Final: Metric Calculations (PAGE 102)

1. 2 tab
2. 1 tab
3. 2 tab
4. Give 4 tab. Clarify the order before giving because this amount exceeds the 1- to 2-unit doses usually given to patients.
5. 0.7 mL; 0.8 mL; 1.5 mL total
6. 20 mL
7. 2 cap
8. **a.** 0.5 mL   **b.** safe dose
9. 3 tab
10. 6 tab. Clarify the order before giving because this amount exceeds the 1 to 2 tablets usually given to patients.

5 Medications from Powders and Crystals

5A (PAGE 108)

1. **a.** Add 90 mL of water.
   b. Amount in bottle 100 mL.
   c. Administer 8 mL.

Know   *Want to Know*
125 mg : 5 mL :: 200 mg : x mL
125 x = 5 × 200 = 1000
  x = 8 mL

PROOF
5 × 200 = 1000
125 × 8 = 1000

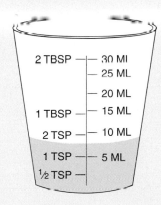

2. **a.** Add 140 mL of water.
   b. Amount in bottle: 8000 mg or 8 g.

Step 1: *Know*   *Want to Know*
    200 mg : 5 mL :: x mg : 200 mL
    5x = 200 × 200 = 40,000
    5x = 40,000
      x = 8000 mg in the bottle

PROOF
5 × 8000 = 40,000
200 × 220 = 40,000

Step 2: *Know*   *Want to Know*
    1 g : 1000 mg :: x g : 8000 mg
    x = 8 g in the bottle

PROOF
1 × 8 = 8
1 × 8 = 8

   c. Administer: 7.5 mL.

Know   *Want to Know*
200 mg : 5 mL :: 300 mg : x mL
200x = 5 × 300
   x = 7.5 mL

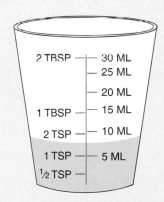

3. **a.** Add 78 mL of diluent.

b. Amount in bottle: 2500 mg.

Know   *Want to Know*
125 mg : 5 mL :: x mg : 100 mL
$5x = 125 \times 100 = 12,500$
$5x = 12,500$
  $x = 2500$ mg in bottle
PROOF
$5 \times 2500 = 12,500$
$125 \times 100 = 12,500$

c. Amount of fluid to be given per dose:
  20 mL/dose.

Know   *Want to Know*
125 mg : 5 mL :: 500 mg : x mL
$125x = 5 \times 500 = 2500$
  $x = 20$ mL/dose
PROOF
$5 \times 500 = 2500$
$125 \times 20 = 2500$

4. **a.** 30 mL of water in two portions.

b. 50 mL of Lorabid in the bottle.

c. 7.5 mL of Lorabid.

Know   *Want to Know*
100 mg : 5 mL :: 150 mg : x mL
$100x = 5 \times 150 = 75\cancel{0}$
  $x = 7.5$ mL yields 150 mg
PROOF
$100 \times 7.5 = 750$
$5 \times 150 = 750$

d. 6.6 doses per bottle

Know   *Want to Know*
7.5 mL : 1 dose :: 50 mL : x dose
$7.5x = 1 \times 50 = 50$
  $x = 6.6$
PROOF
$1 \times 50 = 50$
$7.5 \times 6.6 = 49.5 = 50$

d. Doses in bottle: 5 doses.

Know   *Want to Know*
20 mL : 1 dose :: 100 mL : x doses
$20x = 100$
  $x = 5$ doses in bottle
PROOF
$1 \times 100 = 100$
$20 \times 5 = 100$

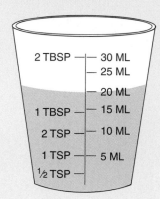

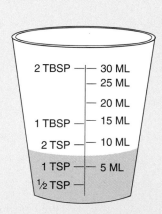

5. a. Add 20 mL of distilled water.
   b. 1000 mg Vancocin in the bottle.
   c. 6 mL of Vancocin.

Know   *Want to Know*
250 mg : 5 mL :: 300 mg : x mL
$250x = 5 \times 300 = 1500$
    $x = 6$ mL
PROOF
$5 \times 300 = 1500$
$250 \times 6 = 1500$

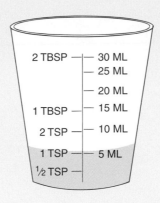

6. a. 45 mL of water in 2 portions.
   b. 75 mL of Lorabid.
   c. 5 mL = 200 mg.
   d. 15 doses in the bottle.

Know   *Want to Know*
5 mL : 1 dose :: 75 mL : x dose
$5x = 75$
   $x = 15$ doses in the bottle.
PROOF
$1 \times 75 = 75$
$5 \times 15 = 75$
   e. Effective for 14 days at room temperature.

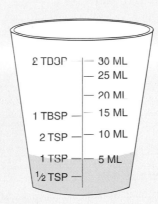

7. a. 60 mL of water in two portions.
   b. 100 mL of Lorabid.
   c. 10 mL.

Know   *Want to Know*
200 mg : 5 mL :: 400 mg : x mL
$200x = 5 \times 400 = 2000$
    $x = 10$ mL
PROOF
$5 \times 400 = 2000$
$200 \times 10 = 2000$
   d. 10 doses in the bottle.

Know   *Want to Know*
10 mL : 1 dose :: 100 mL : x dose
$10x = 1 \times 100 = 100$
   $x = 10$
PROOF
$1 \times 100 = 100$
$10 \times 10 = 100$

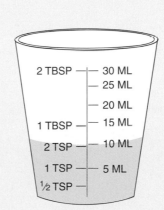

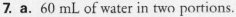

8. a. 1000 mg
   b. *Know*   *Want to Know*
   250 mg : 5 mL :: 500 mg : x mL
   $25x = 5 \times 50 = 250$
   $x = 10$ mL
   PROOF
   $5 \times 500 = 2500$
   $250 \times 10 = 2500$

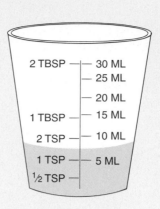

9. *Know*   *Want to Know*
   125 mg : 5 mL :: 400 mg : x mL
   $125x = 5 \times 400 = 2000$
   $x = 16$ mL
   PROOF
   $5 \times 400 = 2000$
   $125 \times 16 = 2000$

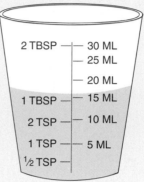

10. *Know*   *Want to Know*
   5 mL : 200 mg :: x mL : 500 mg
   $2x = 25$
   $x = 12.5$ mL
   PROOF
   $2 \times 12.5 = 25$

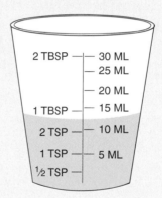

5B (PAGE 118)

1. Administer: 3 mL.

Know   *Want to Know*
1 g : 1000 mg :: x g : 500 mg
$1000x = 500$
    $x = 0.5$ g
PROOF
$1000 \times 0.5 = 500$
$1 \times 500 = 500$

Know   *Want to Know*
0.25 g : 1.5 mL :: 0.5 g : x mL
$0.25x = 1.5 \times 0.5 = 0.75$
    $x = 3$ mL
PROOF
$1.5 \times 0.5 = 0.75$
$0.25 \times 3 = 0.75$

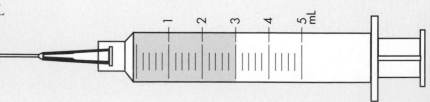

2. a. Make the 500,000 U/mL

b. Administer 0.6 mL

Know *Want to Know*

500,000 U : 1 mL :: 300,000 U : x mL

$5x = 1 \times 3 = 3$

$x = 0.6$ mL

PROOF

$1 \times 300,000 = 300,000$

$500,000 \times 0.6 = 300,000$

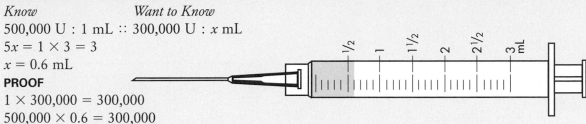

Or, you may also give another concentration, depending on the assessment of body mass.

a. Make the 200,000 U/mL.

b. Administer 1.5 mL.

Know *Want to Know*

200,000 U : 1 mL :: 300,000 U : x mL

$2x = 1 \times 3 = 3$

$x = 1.5$ mL

PROOF

$1 \times 300,000 = 300,000$

$200,000 \times 1.5 = 300,000$

Or, you may also give another concentration, depending on the assessment of body mass.

a. Make the 100,000 U/mL.

b. Administer 3 mL.

Know *Want to Know*

100,000 U : 1 mL :: 300,000 U : x mL

$1x = 1 \times 3 = 3$

$x = 3$ mL

PROOF

$1 \times 300,000 = 300,000$

$100,000 \times 3 = 300,000$

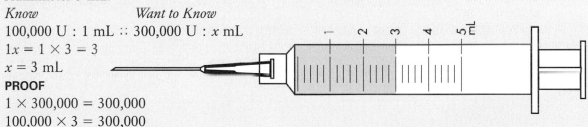

3. a. Add 1.2 mL of diluent.

b. 1 hour

c. 125 mg/mL

d. *Know* *Want to Know*

125 mg : 1 mL :: 100 mg : x mL

$125x = 100$

$x = 0.8$ mL

PROOF

$125 \times 0.8 = 100$

$100 \times 1 = 100$

4. Administer entire amount, 2.6 mL.

5. a. Add 3 mL of sterile water for injection as the diluent.
b. 280 mg/mL is the concentration
c. *Know*　　　　　　*Want to Know*
280/mg : 1 mL :: 250 mg : x mL
$280x = 250$
$x = 0.892 = 0.9$ mL
PROOF
$1 \times 250 = 250$
$0.892 \times 280 = 250$

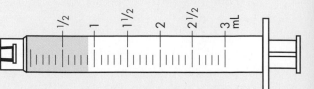

6. a. Administer 4.0 mL in first dose.
b. Divide into two equal injections.
c. Give deep intramuscularly in the right or left gluteus maximus.

7. a. Add 4.0 mL of diluent to yield 250,000 units/mL.
b. *Know*　　　　　　　*Want to Know*
250,000 units : 1 mL :: 300,000 units : x mL
$250,000x = 300,000$
$25x = 30$
$x = 1.2$ mL
PROOF
$250,000 \times 1.2 = 300,000$
$1 \times 300,000 = 300,000$

c. *Know*　　　　　　　*Want to Know*
300,000 units : 1 dose :: 1,000,000 units : x dose
$300,000x = 1,000,000$
$3x = 10$
$x = 3.3 = 3$ full doses in the vial
PROOF
$1 \times 1,000,000 = 1,000,000$
$3.3 \times 300,000 = 990,000$

8. a. Administer 4 mL.
Know　　　　　*Want to Know*
250 mg : 1 mL :: 1000 mg : x mL
$250x = 1000$
$x = 4$ mL
PROOF
$1 \times 1000 = 1000$
$250 \times 4 = 1000$

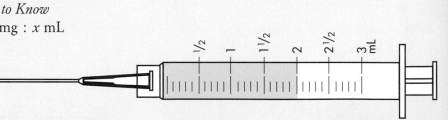

b. Give 2 mL in each site = 500 mg per injection.

9. **a.** Administer 1.7 mL

   Know   *Want to Know*

   500 mg : 1.2 mL :: 700 mg : x mL

   $5x = 1.2 \times 7$

   $5x = 8.4$

   $x = 1.68$ or 1.7 mL

   PROOF

   $5 \times 1.68 = 8.4$

   $1.2 \times 7 = 8.4$

b. Patient will receive 2800 mg/day.

   Know   *Want to Know*

   700 mg : 1 dose :: x mg : 4 doses

   $x = 4 \times 700$

   $x = 2800$ mg/day

   PROOF

   $700 \times 4 = 2800$

   $1 \times 2800 = 2800$

c. Need 2.8 or 3 vials per day

   Know   *Want to Know*

   1000 mg : 1 vial :: 2800 mg : x vials

   $10x = 280 = 2.8$ or 3 vials needed for a 24-hr period

   PROOF

   $1 \times 2800 = 2800$

   $1000 \times 2.8 = 2800$

10. **a.** Use 1.5 mL of diluent.

b. Administer 0.8 mL.

   Know   *Want to Know*

   500,000 units : 1 mL :: 400,000 units : x mL

   $5x = 1 \times 4 = 4$

   $x = 0.8$ mL

   PROOF

   $1 \times 400,000 = 400,000$

   $0.8 \times 500,000 = 400,000$

c. Use 4.0 mL of diluent.

d. *Know*   *Want to Know*

   250,000 U : 1 mL :: 400,000 U : x mL

   $250,000x = 400,000$

   $25x = 40$

   $x = 1.6$ mL

   PROOF

   $250,000 \times 1.6 = 400,000$

   $400,000 \times 1 = 400,000$

e. 2.5 doses in the vial

   Know   *Want to Know*

   400,000 units : 1 dose :: 1,000,000 units : x doses

   $4x = 10$

   $x = 2.5$ doses

   PROOF

   $1 \times 10 = 10$

   $4 \times 2.5 = 10$

5C (PAGE 124)

1. a. Add 2 mL of sterile water.
   b. Each dose will contain 1.2 mL = 500 mg.
   c. 3 vials needed in 24 hours.

Know   *Want to Know*
1 vial : 2 doses :: x vials : 6 doses
$2x = 6$
  $x = 3$ vials needed per 24 hours
PROOF
$1 \times 6 = 6$
$2 \times 3 = 6$

2. a. Add 2.7 mL of sterile water for injection.
   b. 1.5 mL/250 mg.
   c. Refrigerated, 7 days; room temperature, 3 days.
   d. 500 mg.
   e. Administer 2.7 mL.

Know   *Want to Know*
250 mg : 1.5 mL :: 450 mg : x mL
$250x = 1.5 \times 450$
$250x = 675$
   $x = 2.7$ mL
PROOF
$250 \times 2.7 = 675$
$1.5 \times 450 = 675$

3. a. Add 3.5 mL diluent.
   b. The reconstituted medication will yield 250 mg/mL.
   c. Use within 1 hr–very unstable medication.
   d. Administer 2 mL.

Know   *Want to Know*
250 mg : 1 mL :: 500 mg : x mL
$250x = 500$
   $x = 2$ mL
PROOF
$1 \times 500 = 500$
$250 \times 2 = 500$

4. a. Add 2.7 mL sterile water for injection.
   b. The reconstituted medication will yield 250 mg/1.5 mL.
   c. Refrigerated, 7 days; room temperature, 3 days.
   d. Administer 1.8 mL.

Know   *Want to Know*
250 mg : 1.5 mL :: 300 mg : x mL
$250x = 1.5 \times 300 = 450$
   $x = 1.8$ mL
PROOF
$1.5 \times 300 = 450$
$250 \times 1.8 = 450$

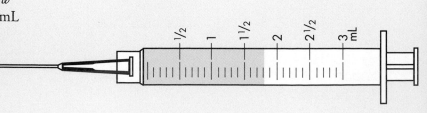

5. *Know*   *Want to Know*
  250 mg : 1 mL :: 500 mg : x mL
  250x = 500
     x = 2 mL = 500 mg
  PROOF
  500 × 1 = 500
  250 × 2 = 500
     OR

Know   *Want to Know*
  350 mg : 1 mL :: 500 mg : x mL
  350x = 1 × 500 = 500
     x = 1.428 = 1.4 mL = 500 mg
  PROOF
  1 × 500 − 500
  350 × 1.428 = 500

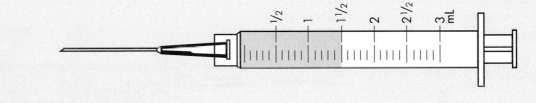

6. a. 500,000 U/mL.
   b. Add 1.6 mL diluent.
   c. Administer 1.5 mL.
   d. Refrigerated, 7 days.

Know   *Want to Know*
  500,000 U : 1 mL :: 750,000 U : x mL
  50x = 1 × 75
  50x = 75
     x = 1.5 mL
  PROOF
  50 × 1.5 − 75
  1 × 75 = 75

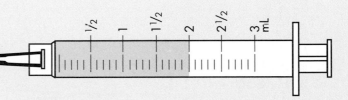

7. a. Add 2 mL of sterile water for injection.
   b. The reconstituted medication will yield 1 g/2.6 mL.
   c. Use medication promptly.
   d. 1000 mg or 1 g.
   e. Administer 2 mL.

Know   *Want to Know*
  1000 mg : 2.6 mL :: 750 mg : x mL
  1000x = 2.6 × 750 = 1950
  1000x = 1950
      x = 1.95 = 2 mL
  PROOF
  1000 × 1.95 = 1950
  2.6 × 750 = 1950

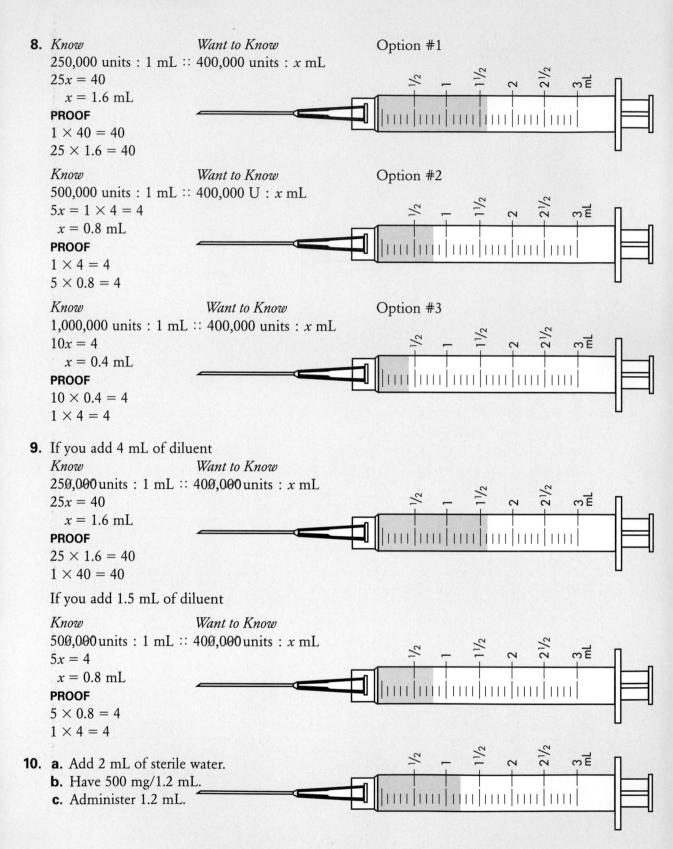

8. *Know*   *Want to Know*   Option #1
   250,000 units : 1 mL :: 400,000 units : x mL
   25x = 40
     x = 1.6 mL
   PROOF
   1 × 40 = 40
   25 × 1.6 = 40

   Know   *Want to Know*   Option #2
   500,000 units : 1 mL :: 400,000 U : x mL
   5x = 1 × 4 = 4
     x = 0.8 mL
   PROOF
   1 × 4 = 4
   5 × 0.8 = 4

   Know   *Want to Know*   Option #3
   1,000,000 units : 1 mL :: 400,000 units : x mL
   10x = 4
     x = 0.4 mL
   PROOF
   10 × 0.4 = 4
   1 × 4 = 4

9. If you add 4 mL of diluent
   Know   *Want to Know*
   250,000 units : 1 mL :: 400,000 units : x mL
   25x = 40
     x = 1.6 mL
   PROOF
   25 × 1.6 = 40
   1 × 40 = 40

   If you add 1.5 mL of diluent

   Know   *Want to Know*
   500,000 units : 1 mL :: 400,000 units : x mL
   5x = 4
     x = 0.8 mL
   PROOF
   5 × 0.8 = 4
   1 × 4 = 4

10. **a.** Add 2 mL of sterile water.
    b. Have 500 mg/1.2 mL.
    c. Administer 1.2 mL.

5D (PAGE 129)

1. c. *Know*   *Want to Know*
2.6 mL : 1000 mg :: x mL : 500 mg
$10x = 2.6 \times 5 = 13$
$x = 1.3$ mL
PROOF
$2.6 \times 500 = 1300$
$1000 \times 1.3 = 1300$

2. c. *Know*   *Want to Know*
500 mg : 1 dose :: x mg : 3 dose
$x = 500 \times 3 = 1500$
$x = 1500$ mg/24 hr
PROOF
$500 \times 3 = 1500$
$1500 \times 1 = 1500$

Know   *Want to Know*
1000 mg : 1 vial :: 1500 mg : x vial
$1000x = 1500$
$x = 1.5$ vials
PROOF
$1 \times 1500 = 1500$
$1000 \times 1.5 = 1500$ You will need to have 2 vials on hand for 24 hr.

3. d. The directions read: Add 5.7 mL sterile water for injection.
   b. *Know*   *Want to Know*
250 mg : 1.5 mL :: 500 mg : x mL.
$250x = 1.5 \times 500$ mg $= 750$
$x = 3$ mL
PROOF
$1.5 \times 500 = 750$
$250 \times 3 = 750$

4. c. Directions read: Add 1.5 mL of diluent = 500,000 units/mL
   d. *Know*   *Want to Know*
500,000 units : 1.0 mL :: 400,000 units : x mL
$500,000x = 1 \times 400,000 = 400,000$
$5x = 4$
$x = 0.8$ mL
PROOF
$0.8 \times 500,000 = 400,000$
$1 \times 400,000 = 400,000$

5. c. Add 9.0 mL of diluent = 400 mg/mL

   a. *Know*   *Want to Know*

      $400,000$ mg : 1 mL :: $500,000$ mg : x mL

      $400,000x = 1 \times 500,000 = 500,000$

      $x = 1.25 = 1.3$ mL

      PROOF

      $1 \times 500,000 = 500,000$

      $400,000 \times 1.25 = 500,000$

6. c. *Know*   *Want to Know*

      4 mL : 2000 mg :: x mL :: 1000 mg

      $2000x = 4 \times 1000 = 4000$

      $2x = 4$

      $x = 2$ mL

      PROOF

      $2000 \times 2 = 4000$

      $4 \times 1000 = 4000$

7. b. Directions read: Add 1.2 mL of diluent to yield 125 mg/mL.

   d. *Know*   *Want to Know*

      250 mg : 1 dose :: x mg : 2 doses

      $x = 250 \times 2 = 500$

      $x = 500$ mg for 2 doses

      PROOF

      $1 \times 500 = 500$

      $500 \times 1 = 500$

      Know   *Want to Know*

      125 mg : 1 vial :: 500 mg : x vials

      $125x = 1 \times 500 = 500$

      $x = 4$ vials for 24 hr

      PROOF

      $1 \times 500 = 500$

      $125 \times 4 = 500$

8. b. *Know*   *Want to Know*

      2 mL : 1 g :: x mL : 1.5 g

      $x = 2 \times 1.5 = 3$

      $x = 3$ mL

      PROOF

      $1 \times 3 = 3$

      $2 \times 1.5 = 3$

9. b. Directions read: Add 30 mL of water in 2 portions. Mix well.

   b. *Know*   *Want to Know*

      100 mg : 5 mL :: 200 mg : x mL

      $100x = 5 \times 200 = 1,000$

      $x = 10$ mL

      PROOF

      $10 \times 100 = 1000$

      $5 \times 200 = 1000$

10. d. *Know*   *Want to Know*

200 mg : 5 mL :: x mg : 200 mL

$5x = 200 \times 200 = 40,000$

$x = 8000$ mg

PROOF

$5 \times 8000 = 40,000$

$200 \times 200 = 40,000$

  c. Label reads: 200 mL = 5 mL. Give 5 mL of erythromycin.

Chapter 5 Final: Medications from Powders and Crystals (PAGE 133)

1. a. Add 9.6 mL of diluent to make 100,000 units/mL. A more concentrated solution may be caustic to the tissue.

  b. Administer 1 mL.

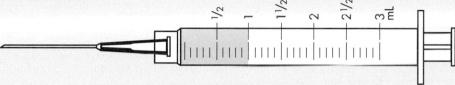

2. a. Add 2.7 mL sterile water for injection.

  b. Administer 1.5 mL.

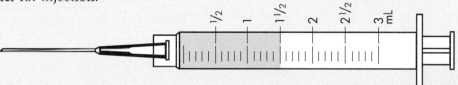

3. a. 250,000 units/mL

  b. 1.4 mL

  c. 14 doses in the vial

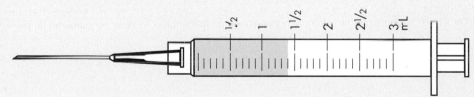

4. a. Add 2 mL of sterile water for injection.

  b. Administer 1.3 mL

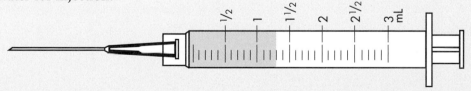

5. a. Add 3.5 mL diluent.

  b. Administer 1 mL.

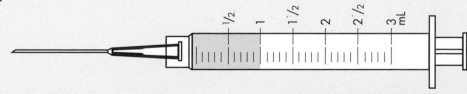

6. Administer 0.5 mL

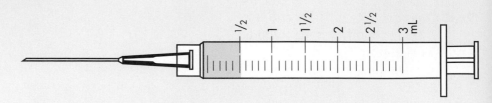

7. Administer 2.2 mL

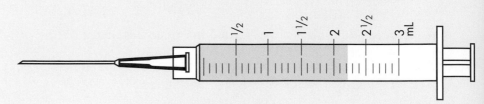

8. Add 2 mL distilled water.

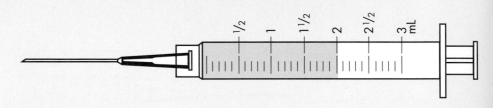

9. Administer 2 mL

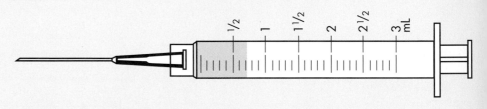

10. Administer 0.7 mL

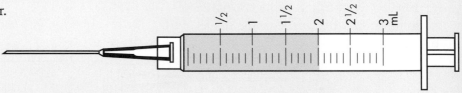

6 Basic IV Calculations

6A (PAGE 143)

$1\dfrac{TV^*}{TT \text{ in hr}} = mL/hr$

$2\dfrac{Df}{\text{Time in min}} \times V/hr = gtt/min$

1. Step 1: $\dfrac{TV}{TT} = \dfrac{1000}{8} = 125 \text{ mL/hr}$

Step 2: $\dfrac{10}{60} \times \dfrac{125 \text{ mL}}{1} = \dfrac{1}{6} \times \dfrac{125}{1} = \dfrac{125}{6} = 20.8 \text{ or } 21 \text{ gtt/min}$

2. Step 2: $\dfrac{15}{60} \times \dfrac{200}{1} = \dfrac{1}{4} \times \dfrac{200}{1} = \dfrac{200}{4} = 50 \text{ gtt/min}$

3. Step 2: $\dfrac{10}{30} \times \dfrac{100}{1} = \dfrac{1}{3} \times \dfrac{100}{1} = \dfrac{100}{3} = 33.3 \text{ or } 33 \text{ gtt/min}$

4. Step 1: $\dfrac{1500}{12} = 125 \text{ mL/hr}$

Step 2: $\dfrac{15}{60} \times \dfrac{125}{1} = \dfrac{1}{4} \times \dfrac{125}{1} = 31.25 \text{ or } 31 \text{ gtt/min}$

5. Step 2: $\dfrac{60}{60} \times \dfrac{50}{1} = \dfrac{1}{1} \times \dfrac{50}{1} = \dfrac{50}{1} = 50 \text{ gtt/min}$

6. Step 1: $\dfrac{1500}{8} = 188 \text{ mL/hr}$

Step 2: **a.** $\dfrac{10}{60} \times \dfrac{188}{1} = \dfrac{1}{6} \times \dfrac{188}{1} = \dfrac{188}{6} = 31.3 \text{ or } 31 \text{ gtt/min}$

b. $\dfrac{15}{60} = \dfrac{1}{4} \times \dfrac{188}{1} = 47 \text{ gtt/min}$

7. Step 2: $\dfrac{10}{45} \times \dfrac{75}{1} = \dfrac{750}{45} = 16.6 \text{ or } 17 \text{ gtt/min}$

8. Step 2: $\dfrac{\overset{2}{\cancel{60}}}{\underset{3}{\cancel{90}}} \times 250 = \dfrac{2}{3} \times \dfrac{250}{1} = \dfrac{500}{3} = 166.6 \text{ or } 167 \text{ gtt/min}$

9. Step 2: $\dfrac{\overset{3}{\cancel{15}}}{\underset{8}{\cancel{40}}} \times 150 = \dfrac{3}{8} \times \dfrac{150}{1} = \dfrac{450}{8} = 56.25 \text{ or } 56 \text{ gtt/min}$

10. Step 2: $\dfrac{\overset{1}{\cancel{20}}}{\underset{3}{\cancel{60}}} \times 150 = \dfrac{1}{3} \times \dfrac{150}{1} = \dfrac{150}{3} = 50 \text{ gtt/min}$

6B (PAGE 144)

$1\dfrac{TV}{TT \text{ in hr}} = mL/hr$

$2\dfrac{Df}{\text{Time}} \text{ in min} \times V/hr = gtt/min$

1. Step 1: $\dfrac{TV}{TT} = \dfrac{2000}{24} = 83.3 \text{ or } 83 \text{ mL/hr}$

2. Step 1: $\dfrac{TV}{TT} = \dfrac{1500}{8} = 187.5 \text{ or } 188 \text{ mL/hr}$

Step 2: $\dfrac{\overset{1}{\cancel{15}}}{\underset{4}{\cancel{60}}} \times \dfrac{188}{1} = 47 \text{ gtt/min}$

3. Step 1: $\frac{TV}{TT} = \frac{3000}{24} = 125$ mL/hr

Step 2: $\frac{60}{60} \times \frac{125}{1} = 1 \times 125 = 125$ gtt/min

4. Step 1: $\frac{TV}{TT} = \frac{500}{4} = 125$ mL/hr

Step 2: $\frac{\cancel{15}^{1}}{\cancel{60}_{4}} \times \frac{125}{1} = \frac{125}{4} = 31.2$ or 31 gtt/min

5. Step 1: $\frac{TV}{TT} = \frac{1000}{12} = 83.3$ or 83 mL/hr

Step 2: $\frac{\cancel{60}^{1}}{\cancel{60}_{1}} \times \frac{83}{1} = \frac{83}{1} = 83$ gtt/min

6. Start with Step 2 because we already know how many milliliters per 30 minutes.

Step 2: $\frac{\cancel{20}^{2}}{\cancel{30}_{3}} \times \frac{100}{1} = \frac{200}{3} = 67$ gtt/min

7. Step 1: $\frac{TV}{TT} = \frac{2000}{24} = 83.3$ or 83 mL/hr

Step 2: $\frac{\cancel{15}^{1}}{\cancel{60}_{4}} \times \frac{83}{1} = \frac{83}{4} = 20.75$ or 21 gtt/min

8. Step 1: $\frac{TV}{TT} = \frac{250}{10} = 25$ mL/hr

Step 2: $\frac{\cancel{60}^{1}}{\cancel{60}_{1}} \times \frac{25}{1} = 25$ gtt/min

9. Step 1: $\frac{TV}{TT} = \frac{1500}{12} = 125$ mL/hr

Step 2: $\frac{\cancel{15}^{1}}{\cancel{60}_{4}} \times \frac{125}{1} = \frac{125}{4} = 31.25$ or 31 gtt/min

10. MEMORIZE: **Step 1** $\frac{TV}{TT \text{ in hr}} = $ mL/hr

Step 2 $\frac{Df}{Time \text{ in min}} \times V/hr = $ gtt/min

6C (PAGE 145)

> ✴ **REMEMBER** • $1\dfrac{TV}{TT \text{ in hr}} = $ **mL/hr**
>
> $2\dfrac{Df}{Time \text{ in min}} \times $ **V/hr = gtt/min**

1. Step 2: $\frac{\cancel{10}}{\cancel{60}} \times 100 = \frac{100}{6} = 16.6$ or 17 gtt/min

2. Step 1: $\frac{TV}{TT} = \frac{1000}{6} = 166.6$ or 167 mL/hr

Step 2: $\frac{\cancel{15}^{1}}{\cancel{60}_{4}} \times \frac{167}{1} = \frac{167}{4} = 41.75$ or 42 gtt/min

3. Step 2: $\frac{\cancel{10}}{\cancel{30}} \times \frac{50}{1} = \frac{50}{3} = 16.6$ or 17 gtt/min

4. Step 2: $\frac{\cancel{60}^{1}}{\cancel{60}_{1}} \times \frac{100}{1} = 100$ gtt/min

5. Step 1: $\frac{TV}{TT} = \frac{2000}{12} = 166.6$ or 167 mL/hr

Step 2: $\frac{\cancel{60}^{1}}{\cancel{60}_{1}} \times \frac{167}{1} = 167$ gtt/min

6. Step 2: $\frac{15}{30} \times \frac{100}{1} = \frac{1}{2} \times \frac{100}{1} = \frac{100}{2} = 50$ gtt/min

7. Step 1: $\frac{TV}{TT} = \frac{1500}{24} = 62.5$ or 63 mL/hr

   Step 2: $\frac{10}{60} \times \frac{63}{1} = \frac{63}{6} \times 10.5 = 11$ gtt/min

8. Step 1: $\frac{TV}{TT} = \frac{500}{8} = 62.5$ or 63 mL/hr

   Step 2: $\frac{\overset{1}{\cancel{60}}}{\underset{1}{\cancel{60}}} \times \frac{63}{1} = 63$ gtt/min

9. Step 2: $\frac{\overset{1}{\cancel{15}}}{\underset{4}{\cancel{60}}} \times \frac{75}{1} = \frac{75}{4} = 18.7$ or 19 gtt/min

10. Step 2: $\frac{20}{60} \times 85 = \frac{1}{3} \times \frac{85}{1} = \frac{85}{3} = 28.3$ or 28 gtt/min

6D (PAGE 147)

1. *Know*   *Want to Know*
   5 g : 100 mL :: x g : 1000 mL
   $x = 5 \times 10 = 50$
   $x = 50$ g or mL dextrose
   PROOF
   $5 \times 1000 = 5000$
   $100 \times 50 = 5000$

   Know   *Want to Know*
   0.9 g : 100 mL :: x g : 1000 mL
   $x = 0.9 \times 10 = 9$
   $x = 9$ g of sodium chloride
   PROOF
   $0.9 \times 1000 = 900$
   $100 \times 9 = 900$

2. *Know*   *Want to Know*
   5 g : 100 mL :: x g : 500 mL
   $x = 5 \times 5 = 25$
   $x = 25$ g or mL of dextrose
   PROOF
   $5 \times 500 = 2500$
   $100 \times 25 = 2500$

   Know   *Want to Know*
   0.45 g : 100 mL :: x g : 500 mL
   $x = 0.45 \times 5 = 2.25$
   $x = 2.25$ g of sodium chloride
   PROOF
   $0.45 \times 500 = 2.25$
   $100 \times 2.25 = 225$

3. *Know*   *Want to Know*
   10 g : 100 mL :: x g : 500 mL
   $x = 10 \times 5 = 50$
   $x = 50$ g or mL of dextrose
   PROOF
   $10 \times 500 = 5000$
   $100 \times 50 = 5000$

   Know   *Want to Know*
   0.9 g : 100 mL :: x g : 500 mL
   $x = 0.9 \times 5$
   $x = 4.5$ g or mL of sodium chloride
   PROOF
   $0.9 \times 500 = 450$
   $4.5 \times 100 = 450$

4. *Know*   *Want to Know*
   0.9 g : 100 mL :: x g : 1000 mL
   $x = 0.9 \times 10 = 9$
   $x = 9$ g or mL of sodium chloride
   PROOF
   $0.9 \times 1000 = 900$
   $9 \times 100 = 900$

5. *Know*   *Want to Know*
   0.45 g : 100 mL :: x g : 500 mL
   $x = 0.45 \times 5 = 2.25$
   $x = 2.25$ g or mL of sodium chloride
   PROOF
   $0.45 \times 500 = 225$
   $100 \times 2.25 = 225$

6. *Know*   *Want to Know*
   5 g : 100 mL :: x g : 1000 mL
   $x = 5 \times 10 = 50$
   $x = 50$ g or mL of dextrose
   PROOF
   $5 \times 1000 = 500$
   $100 \times 50 = 5000$

7. *Know*   *Want to Know*
   5 g : 100 mL :: x g : 500 mL
   $x = 5 \times 5 = 25$
   $x = 25$ g or mL of dextrose
   PROOF
   $100 \times 25 = 2500$
   $5 \times 500 = 2500$

8. *Know*   *Want to Know*
600 mg : 100 mL :: x mg : 1000 mL
$x = 10 \times 600 = 6000$
$x = 6000$ mg of sodium chloride in 1000 mL
PROOF
$600 \times 1000 = 600{,}000$
$100 \times 6000 = 600{,}000$

Know   *Want to Know*
1 g : 1000 mg :: x g : 6000 mg
$x = 6 \times 1 = 6$
$x = 6$ g of sodium chloride in 1000 mL

9. *Know*   *Want to Know*
5 g : 100 mL :: x g : 1000 mL
$x = 5 \times 10 = 50$
$x = 50$ g or mL of dextrose
PROOF
$5 \times 1000 = 5000$
$100 \times 50 = 5000$

Know   *Want to Know*
0.9 g : 100 mL :: x g : 1000 mL
$x = 0.9 \times 10 = 9$
$x = 9$ g or mL of sodium chloride
PROOF
$100 \times 9 = 900$
$0.9 \times 1000 = 900$

10. *Know*   *Want to Know*
5 g : 100 mL :: x g : 500 mL
$x = 5 \times 5 = 25$
$x = 25$ g or mL of dextrose
PROOF
$5 \times 500 = 2500$
$100 \times 25 = 2500$

Know   *Want to Know*
0.45 g : 100 mL :: x g : 500 mL
$x = 0.45 \times 5 = 2.25$
$x = 2.25$ g or mL of sodium chloride
PROOF
$0.45 \times 500 = 225$
$100 \times 2.25 = 225$

6E (PAGE 160)

1. a. *Know*   *Want to Know*
50 mL : 30 min :: x mL : 60 min
$30x = 50 \times 60 = 3000$
   $x = 100$ mL/hr
PROOF
$30 \times 150 = 3000$
$50 \times 60 = 3000$

b. $\frac{60}{30} \times \frac{50}{1} = \frac{\overset{2}{\cancel{60}}}{\cancel{30}} \times \frac{50}{1} = 100$ gtt/min

2. $\frac{\overset{1}{\cancel{15}}}{\underset{4}{\cancel{60}}} \times \frac{100}{1} = \frac{100}{4} = 25$ gtt/min

3. *Know*   *Want to Know*
150 mL : 60 min :: 250 mL : x min
$150x = 250 \times 60 = 15,000$
   $x = 100$ min = 1.6 hr = 1 hr 36 min
PROOF
$100 \times 150 = 15,000$
$250 \times 60 = 15,000$

4. a. *Know*   *Want to Know*
50 mL : 20 min :: x mL : 60 min
$20x = 50 \times 60 = 3000$
   $x = 150$ mL/hr
PROOF
$20 \times 150 = 3000$
$50 \times 60 = 3000$

b. $\frac{15}{20} \times \frac{50}{1} = \frac{\overset{3}{\cancel{15}}}{\underset{4}{\cancel{20}}} \times \frac{50}{1} = \frac{150}{4} = 37.5$ or 38 gtt/min

5. $\frac{15}{60} \times \frac{100}{1} = \frac{1}{4} \times \frac{100}{1} = \frac{100}{4} = 25$ gtt/min

6. a. $\frac{\overset{2}{\cancel{60}}}{\underset{1}{\cancel{30}}} \times 100 = 200$ gtt/min

b. The infusion device will be set at 200 mL/hr.

Know   *Want to Know*
100 mL : 30 min :: x mL : 60 min
$30x = 100 \times 60 = 6000$
$3\cancel{0}x = 600\cancel{0}$
   $x = 200$ mL/hr

7. a. $\frac{\overset{2}{\cancel{60}}}{\underset{3}{\cancel{90}}} \times 200 = \frac{400}{3} = 133$ gtt/min

b. Set infusion device for 133 mL/hr.

8. Step 1: $\frac{1000}{12} = 83.3$ or 83 mL/hr

   a. Step 2: $\frac{\overset{1}{\cancel{15}}}{\underset{4}{\cancel{60}}} \times 83 = \frac{83}{4} = 20.8$ or 21 gtt/min

   b. The infusion device will be set at 83 mL/hr.

     Know   *Want to Know*
   c. 0.9 g : 100 mL :: x g : 1000 mL

     $x = 0.9 \times 10 = 9$

     $x = 9$ g of sodium chloride (solute)

     PROOF

     $0.9 \times 1000 = 900$

     $100 \times 9 = 900$

9. a. Step 1: $\frac{TV}{TT} = \frac{2000}{8} = 250$ mL/hr

   b. Step 2: $\frac{\overset{1}{\cancel{15}}}{\underset{1}{\cancel{60}}} \times 250 = \frac{250}{4} = 62.5$ or 63 gtt/min

     Know   *Want to Know*
   c. 5 g : 1000 mL :: x g : 2000 mL

     $x = 5 \times 20 = 100$

     $x = 100$ g of dextrose

     PROOF

     $5 \times 2000 = 10,000$

     $100 \times 100 = 10,000$

10. a. $\frac{\overset{3}{\cancel{60}}}{\underset{2}{\cancel{40}}} \times 150 = \frac{450}{2} = 225$ gtt/min is the fastest rate or 225 mL/hr for the infusion device using the microdrip formula

   b. $\frac{60}{60} \times 150 = 150$ gtt/min is the slowest rate. Set infusion device for 150 mL/hr using the microdrip formula

6F (PAGE 161)

1. d. $\frac{20 \text{ gtt}}{30 \text{ min}} \times 50 = \frac{100}{3} = 33$ gtt/min

2. d. *Know*   *Want to Know*

     12 mL : 1 hr :: 150 mL : x hr

     $12x = 150$

     $x = 12.5 = 12$ hr 30 min

     PROOF

     $1 \times 150 = 150$

     $12.5 \times 12 = 150$

3. c. *Know*   *Want to Know*

2500 mL : 24 hr ∷ x mL : 1 hr

$24x = 2500$

$x = 104.16$ mL/hr

PROOF

$2500 \times 1 = 2500$

$24 \times 104.16 = 2500 = 104$ mL/hr

Know   *Want to Know*

15 gtt : 1 mL ∷ x gtt : 104.16 mL   OR $\frac{15}{60} \times 104 = \frac{1560}{60} = 26$ gtt/min

$x = 15 \times 104.16 = 1562$

$x = 1562$ divided by 60 min $= 26$ gtt/min

PROOF

$15 \times 104.16 = 1562$

$1 \times 1562 = 1562$

4. b. *Know*   *Want to Know*

300 mL : 6 hr ∷ x mL : 1 hr

$6x = 300 \times 1 = 300$

$x = 50$ mL/hr mL/hr and microdrip gtt/min are the same $= 50$ gtt/min

PROOF

$300 \times 1 = 300$

$6 \times 50 = 300$

5. d. $\frac{15}{15} \times 50 = 50$ gtt/min

6. b. *Know*   *Want to Know*

25 gtt : 1 min ∷ 10 gtt : x min

$25x = 10$

$x = 0.4$ min $= 1$ mL

PROOF

$25 \times 0.4 = 10$

$1 \times 10 = 10$

Know   *Want to Know*

1 mL : 0.4 min ∷ 1000 mL : x min

$x = 0.4 \times 1000 = 400$

$x = 400$ min divided by 60 $= 6.66$ hr $= 6$ hr 40 min

7. d. *Know*   *Want to Know*

30 gtt : 1 min ∷ 20 gtt : x min

$30x = 20$

$x = 0.66$ min

PROOF

$1 \times 20 = 20$

$30 \times 0.66 = 20$

Know   *Want to Know*
1 mL : 0.66 min :: 500 mL : x min
$x = 0.66 \times 500 = 330$
$x = 330$ min $\div 60 = 5.5$ hr $= 5$ hr 30 min
PROOF
$1 \times 330 = 330$
$0.66 \times 500 = 330$

8. c. *Know*   *Want to Know*
42 gtt : 1 min :: 10 gtt : x min
$42x = 1 \times 10 = 10$
$x = 0.238 = 0.24$ min/mL
PROOF
$1 \times 10 = 10$
$42 \times 0.24 = 10.08 = 10$

Know   *Want to Know*
1 mL : 0.24 min :: 500 mL : x min
$x = 0.24 \times 500 = 120$
$x = 120$ min divided by $60 = 2$ hr
PROOF
$1 \times 120 = 120$
$0.24 \times 500 = 120$
The transfusion was started at 1100 hr. The completion time will be 1300 hr.

9. c. *Know*   *Want to Know*
30 mL : 1 hr :: 500 mL : x hr
$30x = 500$
$x = 16.66$ hr $= 16$ hr 40 min
PROOF
$30 \times 16.6 = 499.8 = 500$
$1 \times 500 = 500$

10. d. $\frac{250}{2} = 125$ mL/hr

Chapter 6 Final: Basic IV Calculations (PAGE 162)

1. 125 mL/hr
   42 gtt/min

2. 21 gtt/min
   Set infusion device at 125 mL/hr.

3. Set infusion device at 83 mL/hr.
   14 gtt/min

4. 150 mL/hr
   150 gtt/min

5. Set infusion device at 83 mL/hr.
   28 gtt/min

6. 125 mL/hr
   42 gtt/min

7. 100 mL/hr
   17 gtt/min

8. Set infusion device at 267 mL/hr.

9. 83 gtt/min

10. 167 gtt/min or 167 mL/hr if infusion device is used

7 Advanced IV Calculations

7A (PAGE 167)

1. b. 9600 μg/hr or 9.6 mg/hr
c. 9900 μg or 9.9 mg/hr
d. 12,000 μg/hr or 12 mg/hr
e. 72,000 μg/hr or 72 mg/hr

2. b. 1 : 1
c. 1 : 10
d. 1 : 2
e. 1 : 2

3. b. $x = 30$ mL/hr (1 : 1 :: 30 : 30)
c. $x = 50$ mL/hr (1 : 10 :: 5 : 50)
d. $x = 6$ mL/hr (1 : 2 :: 3 : 6)
e. $x = 5$ mL/hr (2 : 1 :: 10 : 5)

4. b. (2 : 1 :: 12 : 6) 12 mg/hr
c. (1 : 2 :: 9 : 18) 9 mg/hr
d. (4 : 10 :: 4 : 10) 4 mg/hr
e. (2 : 1 :: 36 : 18) 36 mg/hr

5. b. (1 : 1 :: 9 : 9) 9 mL/hr
c. (2 : 1 :: 20 : 10) 10 mL/hr
d. (1 : 2 :: 1 : 2) 30 mL/hr
e. (8 : 5 :: 8 : 5) 5 mL/hr

7B (PAGE 169)

1.

	mg/hr	μg/hr	mg/min	μg/min
a.	0.050	50	$0.050 \div 60 = 0.0008$	0.8
b.	240	240,000	4	4000
c.	30	30,000	0.5	500
d.	1.2	1200	0.02	20
e.	7.5	7500	0.125	125

2.

	kg	mg/hr	mg/kg/min	μg/kg/min
a.	85	25	$25 \div 85 \div 60 = 0.005$	5
b.	70	$10 \times 70 \times 60 = 42,000$	10	10,000
c.	62	0.37	0.0001	0.1
d.	55	75	0.02	20
e.	48	14.4	0.005	5

3.

	IV Contents	TD : TV Reduced Ratio	HD (mg/hr)	HV (mL/hr)	mg/mL
a.	500 mg/1000 mL	1 : 2	5	10	0.5
b.	250 mg/500 mL	1 : 2	15	30	0.5
c.	400 mg/250 mL	8 : 5	24	15	1.6
d.	500 mg/500 mL	1 : 1	75	75	1
e.	500 mg/250 mL	2 : 1	16	8	2

7C (PAGE 170)

2. a. $1 : 2 :: x$ mg : 15 mL   ($x = 7.5$ mg/hr)
   PROOF
   $1 \times 15 = 15$
   $2 \times 7.5 = 15$
b. 7.5 mg $\times$ 1000 = 7500 μg/hr
c. 7500 μg $\div$ 60 = 125 μg/min
d. 125 μg/min $\div$ 50 kg = 2.5 μg/kg/min

4. a. $4 : 1 :: x$ mg/hr : 10 mL/hr   ($x = 40$ mg)
   PROOF
   $4 \times 10 = 40$
   $10 \times 4 = 40$
b. 40 $\times$ 1000 = 40,000 μg/hr
c. 40,000 μg $\div$ 60 = 666.7 μg/min
d. 666.7 μg/min $\div$ 60 kg = 11.1 μg/kg/min

3. a. $2 : 5 :: x$ mg : 5 mL   ($x = 2$ mg/hr)
   PROOF
   $2 \times 5 = 10$
   $5 \times 2 = 10$
b. 2 mg/hr $\times$ 1000 = 2000 μg/hr
c. 2000 μg/hr $\div$ 60 = 33.3 μg/min
d. 33.3 μg/min $\div$ 55 kg = 0.605 or 0.6 μg/kg/min

5. a. $2 : 1 :: x$ mg : 8 mL/hr   ($x = 16$ mL/hr)
   PROOF
   $2 \times 8 = 16$
   $1 \times 16 = 16$
b. 16 mg $\times$ 1000 = 16,000 μg/hr
c. 16,000 μg/hr $\div$ 60 = 266.7 μg/min
d. 266.7 μg/min $\div$ 79.5 kg = 3.4 μg/kg/min

7D (PAGE 171)

2. a. 1 mg : 1 mL
b. 100 μg $\times$ 60 = 6000 μg/hr
c. 6 mg/hr
d. No, should be 6 mL/hr
e. Notify provider and obtain order to increase.

4. a. 1 mg : 250 mL
b. 5 μg $\times$ 60 = 300 μg/hr or 0.3 mg/hr
c. $1 : 250$ mL $:: 0.3$ mg : x mL
d. $0.3 \times 250 = 75.0$ mL/hr

3. a. 1000 mg : 500 mL = 2 mg : 1 mL
b. 4 mg $\times$ 60 = 240 mg/hr
c. $2 : 1 :: 240 : x = 120$ mL/hr

5. a. 1 mg : 250 mL $:: x$ μg : 50 mL
b. $x = 0.2$ mg/hr
c. 200 μg/hr
d. 200 μg $\div$ 60 = 3.3 μg/min
e. 8-12 μg/min
f. Low; consult with provider

7E (PAGE 173)

2. a. 40-56 mg/hr
b. 45 mg/hr
c. Safe to give
d. $500 : 1000 = 1$ mg/2 mL (1 : 2)
e. $1 : 2 :: 45$ mg : x mL $x = 90$ mL/hr
   PROOF
   $1 \times 90 = 90$
   $2 \times 45 = 90$
f. Safe to infuse at 90 mL/hr

3. a. 7-35 mg/hr
b. $250 : 500 = 1$ mg/2 mL   (1 : 2)
c. $1 : 2 :: x$ mg : 50 mL
   PROOF
   $1 \times 50 = 50$
   $2 \times 25 = 50$
d. 25 mg/hr
e. Safe to give

4. a. 0.5 mg $\times$ 50 = 25 mg/hr maximum
   b. 20 mg/hr is safe for this patient.
   c. 250 mg : 500 mL = 1 : 2
   d. 1 : 2 :: 20 mg : x mL
   PROOF
   1 $\times$ 40 = 40
   2 $\times$ 20 = 40
   e. Infuse at 40 mL/hr

5. a. 7-35 mg/hr
   b. 15 mg/hr is safe dose
   c. 1 : 2 :: 15 : x (x = 30 mL/hr ordered)
   d. 1 : 2 :: x : 50   (x = 25 mg/hr infusing)
   PROOF
   1 $\times$ 50 = 50
   2 $\times$ 25 = 50
   e. 25 mg/hr infusing is unsafe—15 mg/hr ordered; notify MD and obtain order to reduce to 15 mg/hr as ordered originally, which would be at rate of 30 mL/hr. Assess patient for side effects.

7F (PAGE 174)

2. a. 10,000 mU : 1000 mL = 10 : 1
   b. 10 mU : 1 mL :: 1200 mU (hr) : x mL (120) (hr)
   PROOF
   10 $\times$ 120 = 1200
   1 $\times$ 1200 = 1200
   c. Rate should be 120 mL/hr; obtain order to increase.

3. a. 5 : 500 = 1 mg : 100 mL
   b. 10 $\times$ 60 = 600 μg/hr
   c. 0.6 mg/hr
   d. 1 : 100 :: 0.6 mg : x mL
   PROOF
   1 $\times$ 60 = 60
   100 $\times$ 0.6 = 60
   e. x = 60 mL hr for 30 min will deliver 300 μg total as ordered.

4. a. 20 : 500 = 1 : 25
   b. 1 g : 25 mL :: x g : 25 mL/hr
   PROOF
   1 $\times$ 25 = 25
   25 $\times$ 1 = 25
   c. x = 1 g/hr
   d. 2 hr

5. a. 10 U = 10,000 mU
   b. 10 mU : 1 mL
   c. 2 mU $\times$ 60 = 120 mU/hr
   d. 10 : 1 :: 120 : x
   PROOF
   10 $\times$ 12 = 120
   1 $\times$ 120 = 120
   e. x = 12 mL/hr

7G (PAGE 175)

1. a. 65 kg
   b. 3250-13,000 μg/min
   c. 195-780 mg/hr (μg/min $\times$ 60 $\div$ 1000)
   d. (5 g = 5000 mg) 10 : 1 :: x mg : 39 mL
   e. x = 390 mg/hr
   f. 390 $\div$ 60 = 6.5 mg/min
   g. 6500 μg/min
   h. 6500 μg $\div$ 65 kg = 100 μg/kg/min
   i. Safe; continue

3. a. 1000 : 500 = 2 : 1 :: x mg : 50 mL
   b. x = 100 mg/hr
   c. 100 mg $\div$ 60 = 1.66 or 1.7 mg
   d. Safe; continue.

5. a. 125 mg : 125 mL = 1 : 1 :: 15 : 15 mL
   b. Safe; continue infusion.

2. a. 50 mg : 500 mL = 1 mg : 10 mL:: x mg/hr : 6 mL/hr
   b. x = 0.6 mg/hr (600 μg/hr)
   PROOF
   1 $\times$ 6 = 6
   10 $\times$ 0.6 = 6
   c. 1 : 10 :: 0.6 : 6 mL/hr
   d. 0.6 $\div$ 60 = 10 μg/min
   e. Yes
   f. Safe; continue.

4. a. 220 $\div$ 2.2 = 100 kg
   b. 0.3 $\times$ 100 $\times$ 60 = 1800 μg or 1.8 mg/hr
   c. 1 : 5 :: 1.8 mg : x mL x = 9 mL/hr
   d. 15 mL/hr
   e. 3 mg/hr (1 : 5 :: x mg : 15)   (x = 3)
   f. Unsafe; call for order to lower rate to 9 mL/hr.

7H (PAGE 179)

1. a. 5 $\times$ 60 = 300 sec
   300 $\div$ 50 lines = 6 sec/line
   b. 10 mL : 5 min :: x mL : 1 min
   5x = 10
   x = 2 mL/min

3. a. 100 mg : 1 mL :: 900 mg : x mL (x = 9 mL)
   b. 50 mg : 1 min :: 900 mg : x min
   50x = 900
   x = 18 min
   c. 9 mL : 18 min :: x mL : 1 min
   18x = 9
   x = 0.5 mL/min

5. a. 5 mL
   b. 5 $\times$ 60 = 300 sec
   c. 300 $\div$ 25 = 12 sec/line
   d. 5 mL : 5 min :: x mL : 1 min
   5x = 5
   x = 1 mL/min

2. a. 250 μg : 1 mL :: 500 μg : x mL (x = 2 mL)
   b. 10 $\times$ 60 = 600 sec
   c. 600 $\div$ 10 lines — 60 sec/line
   d. 2 mL : 10 min :: x mL : 1 min
   x = 0.2 mL/min

4. a. 10 mg : 1 mL :: 20 mg : x mL   (x = 2 mL)
   b. 2 $\times$ 60 = 120 sec
   c. 120 $\div$ 20 = 6 sec/line
   d. 2 mL : 2 min :: x mL : 1 min
   2x = 2
   x = 1 mL/min

71 (PAGE 181)

1. c

$5 \mu g : 1 \min :: x \mu g : 60 \min$ or

$5 \times 60 = 300 \mu g$ or 0.3 mg/hr

PROOF
$5 \times 60 = 300$
$1 \times 300 = 300$

2. a

$250 \text{ mg} : 1000 \text{ mL} :: x \text{ mg} : 1 \text{ mL}$
TD   TV
$1 \text{ mg} : 4 \text{ mL} :: x \text{ mg} : 1 \text{ mL}$
$x = 0.25 \text{ mg/mL}$

PROOF
$1 \times 1 = 1$
$4 \times 0.25 = 1$

3. a

$1 \text{ g} = 1000 \text{ mg}$
TD   TV
$1000 \text{ mg} : 500 \text{ mL} = 2 : 1$ by
dividing each by the largest
common denominator of 500
or tell ratio at a glance

PROOF
$1000 \text{ mg} : 500 \text{ mL} = 2 : 1 \text{ ratio}$

4. c

Need to determine milligrams
per hour first
$8 \mu g \times 60 \min$ or $480 \mu g/hr$ or
0.48 mg/hr = minimum drug
per hour
TD   TV   HD   HV
$1 \text{ mg} : 250 \text{ mL} :: 0.48 \text{ mg} : x \text{ mL}$
$x = 250 \times 0.48$ or 120 mL/hr needed
to infuse 0.48 mg

PROOF
$1 \times 120 = 120$
$250 \times 0.48 = 120$

5. d

Step 1 total volume to be pushed
$10 \text{ mg} : 1 \text{ mL} :: 30 \text{ mg} : x \text{ ml}$
$x = 3 \text{ mL}$

PROOF
$10 \times 3 = 30$
$1 \times 30 = 30$

Step 2 mL/min
$3 \text{ mL} : 2 \min :: x \text{ mL} : 1 \min$
$2x = 3$ or $x = 1.5 \text{ mL/min}$

PROOF
$3 \times 1 = 3$
$2 \times 1.5 = 3$

6. b

Step 1 Convert milligrams to micrograms or micrograms to milligrams by moving decimals.

0.5 mg = 500 μg OR

250 μg = 0.25 mg

Step 2 Total mL
On Hand

250 μg : 1 mL :: 500 μg : x mL

OR

0.25 mg : 1 mL :: 0.5 mg : x mL

x = 2 mL total volume to be injected over 5 min

PROOF

250 μg : 1 mL :: 500 μg : x mL

$250x$ = 500 or 2 mL

OR $0.25x$ = 0.5 = 2 mL

Step 3 mL/min

2 mL : 5 min :: x mL : 1 min

$5x$ = 2 or 0.4 mL/1 min

PROOF

2 × 1 = 2

5 × 0.4 = 2

7. a

Step 1 Calculate SDR for maintenance for adult

1 mg : 1 min :: x mg : 60 min

x = 60 mg/hr is minimum SDR

6 mg : 1 min :: x mg : 60 min

x = 360 mg/hr is maximum SDR

SDR is 60 − 360 mg/hr.

PROOF

1 × 60 = 60

1 × 60 = 60

PROOF

6 × 60 = 360

1 × 360 = 360

Step 2 Calculate total drug/total volume ratio and ordered drug/hr

TD   TV   HD   HV

1 g : 500 mL = 1000 mg :

500 mL :: x mg : 40 mL

   2 : 1 :: x mg : 40 mL

x = 80 mg/hr being infused

After reduction of TD to TV, the answer can be easily seen.

PROOF

2 × 40 = 80

1 × 80 = 80

8. b

Step 1 Change total drug to milligrams to match hourly drug terms.

TD   TV   HD   HV

1 g : 1000 mL :: 60 mg : x mL

Need to change grams to milligrams by using memorized conversion 1000 mg = 1 g.

TD   TV

1000 mg :: 1000 mL :: 60 mg : x mL

Step 2 Calculate mL/hr infusing

Simplify: reduce the TD/TV ratio and math won't be needed to solve this question.

1 : 1 :: 60 : x mL/hr

$1x$ = 60 x = 60 mL/hr

x = 60 mL/hr

PROOF

1 × 60 = 60

1 × 60 = 60

9. **c**

    TD   HD   HD HV

    20 g : 500 mL :: x g : 30 mL

    $500x = 600 = 1.2$ g/hr

    PROOF

    $20 \times 30 = 600$

    $600 \times 1 = 600$

    1.2 g : 1 hr :: 3 g : x hr

    $1.2x = 3$

    $x = 2.5$ hr or 2 hr 30 min

10. **d**

    2.5 µg $\times$ 70 kg $\times$ 60 min = 10,500 µg/hr needed

    500 µg : 1 mL :: 10,500 µg : x mL

    $500x = 10,500$ $x = 21$ mL/hr flow rate to deliver 10,500 µg/hr

    PROOF

    $500 \times 21 = 10,500$

    $1 \times 500 = 500$

Chapter 7 Final: Advanced IV Calculations (PAGE 183)

1. **a.** 20 kg
   b. 60 mEq
   c. 10 mEq
   d. Safe
   e. 5 mL. Refer to order.
   f. $105 \div 4 = 26.25$ or 26 mL/hr

2. **a.** 15,000 µg (5 µg $\times$ 50 kg $\times$ 60 min)
   b. 7.5 mL (2000 µg : 1 mL :: 15,000 µg : x mL)

3. **a.** 9.6 mg/hr (2 µg $\times$ 80 kg $\times$ 60 min = 9600 µg/hr)
   b. 12 mg/hr (400 mg : 500 mL :: x mg : 15 mL)
      $5x = 4 \times 15 = 60$
      $x = 12$ mg/hr
   c. 12 mL/hr (4 : 5 :: 9.6 : x mL)
      $4x = 48$ $x = 12$ mL/hr
   d. 15 mL/hr infusing
   e. Existing flow rate is too fast. Assess patient for side effects and contact physician for new order.

4. **a.** 50 kg
   b. 100-500 µg/min   (2-10 µg/kg/min)
   c. 200 µg/min   (4 µg/kg/min)
   d. Safe
   e. 4 : 5
   f. 4 : 5 :: x : 15   ($x = 12$ mg/hr)
   g. 4 : 5 :: 12 : x ($x = 15$ mL/hr)
   h. Correct

5. **a.** 0.4 mL
   b. 5 mL
   c. 3 min
   d. $7.2 = 7$ (approximate)
   e. 1.7 mL/min

8 **Parenteral Nutrition**

8A (PAGE 196)

1. Total grams per bag:
% × mL = g/L   g/L × TV/L = g/bag
a. AA 0.055 × 400 = 22 g/L   22 × 1.350 = 29.7 g/bag
b. Dextrose 0.10 × 350 = 35 g/L   35 × 1.350 = 47.25 g/bag
c. Lipids 0.10 × 200 = 20 g/L   20 × 1.350 = 27 g/bag

2. Percentages of concentration per bag:
g/bag ÷ TV = % of concentration
a. AA 29.7 g ÷ 1350 = 2.2%
b. Dextrose 47.25 ÷ 1350 = 3.5%
c. Lipids 27 ÷ 1350 = 2%

3. Percentages for additives per bag:
mEq/L × TV/L = mEq/bag   mEq/bag ÷ TV = % in bag
a. Calcium gluconate 5 × 1.35 = 6.75 mEq/bag   6.75 ÷ 1350 = 0.5% Ca gluconate
b. Magnesium sulfate 10 × 1.35 = 13.5 mEq/bag 13.5 ÷ 1350 = 1% Mg sulfate
c. Potassium chloride 20 × 1.35 = 27 mEq/bag   27 ÷ 1350 = 2% K chloride
d. Sodium chloride 30 × 1.35 = 40.5 mEq/bag   40.5 ÷ 1350 = 3% Na chloride

4. kcal per bag: *Know*
a. CHO 47.25 × 4 = 189   PRO = 4 kcal/g
b. PRO 29.7 × 4 = 118.8   CHO = 4 kcal/g
c. FAT 27 × 9 = 243   FAT = 9 kcal/g
d. Total kcal 550.8

5. mL/hr to set infusion device
$\frac{TV}{TT}$ = mL/hr $\frac{1350}{12}$ = 112.5 = 113 mL/hr

8B (PAGE 198)

1. % × mL = g/L   g/L × TV/L = g/bag
a. 0.085 × 500 = 42.5 g/L AA   42.5 × 1.5 = 63.75 g/bag
b. 0.50 × 500 = 250 g/L DEX   250 × 1.5 = 375 g/bag
c. 0.10 × 250 = 25 g/L LIP   25 × 1.5 = 37.5 g/bag

2. Percentage of concentration
g/bag ÷ TV = % of concentration
a. 63.75 ÷ 1500 = 4.25% AA
b. 375 ÷ 1500 = 25% DEX
c. 37.5 ÷ 1500 = 2.5% LIP

3. Percentage of additives
mEq/L × TV/L = mEq/bag   MmEq/bag ÷ TV = % in bag
a. 5 × 1.5 = 7.5 Calcium gluconate   7.5 ÷ 1500 = 0.5% Ca gluconate
b. 15 × 1.5 = 22.5 magnesium sulfate   22.5 ÷ 1500 = 1.5% $MgSO_4$
c. 8.3 × 1.5 = 12.45 potassium acetate   12.45 ÷ 1500 = 0.83% K acetate
d. 35 × 1.5 = 52.5 potassium phosphate   52.5 ÷ 1500 = 3.5% K phosphate
e. 35 × 1.5 = 52.5 sodium chloride   52.5 ÷ 1500 = 3.5% Na chloride

4. kcal per bag   g/L ×

  a. 63.75 × 4 = 255 kcal PRO   CHO = 4 kcal/g

  b. 375 × 4 = 1500 kcal CHO   PRO = 4 kcal/g

  c. 37.5 × 9 = 337.5 kcal FAT   FAT = 9 kcal/g

  d. Total kcal = 2092.5

5. mL/hr to set infusion device

$$\frac{TV}{TT} = mL/hr \qquad\qquad \frac{1500}{12} = 125 \text{ mL/hr}$$

8C (PAGE 200)

Total grams per bag

1. **Formula: 5 × mL = g/L**   **Formula: g/L × TV/L = g/bag**

  Shortcut method: % × mL = g/L × TV/L = g/bag

  AA 0.10 × 900 = 90 × 1.492 = 134.28 g/bag

  Dex. 0.70 × 430 = 301 × 1.492 = 449 g/bag

Percentage of concentrate per bag

2. **Formula: $\frac{g/bag}{TV}$ = %/bag**

  AA $\frac{134.28}{1492.74}$ = 0.30 = 0.0899 = 9%

  Dex $\frac{449}{1492.74}$ = 0.30 = 30%

Percentage of additives

3. **Formula mEq/L × TV/L = mEq/bag**

  mEq/bag divided by TV = % in bag

  Shortcut method: mEq/L × TV/L divided by TV = % in bag

  a. Sodium chloride 140 × 1.492 = 209 divided by 1492 = 0.14 = 14%

  b. Potassium phosphate 41 × 1.492 = 61 divided by 1492 = 0.040 = 4%

  c. Potassium chloride 43 × 1.492 = 64 divided by 1492 = 0.042 = 4%

  d. Magnesium sulfate 7 × 1.492 = 10 divided by 1492 = 0.007 = 0.7%

  e. Calcium gluconate 7 × 1.492 = 10 divided by 1492 = 0.007 = 0.7%

Total kcal per bag

4. **a.** Protein 134.28 g × 4 = 537 kcal

  b. Carbohydrate 449 g × 4 = 1796 kcal

  c. Total kcal = 2333

5. *Know*   *Want to Know*

  55 mL : 1 hr :: 1492 mL : x hr

  55x = 1 × 1492 = 1492

    x = 27.127 = 27 hr

  PROOF

  55 mL × 27.127 = 1491.9 = 1492

  1 × 1492 = 1492

8D (PAGE 201)

Total grams per bag
1. **Formulas: % × mL = g/L**
   g/L × TV/L = g/bag
   Shortcut method: % × mL = g/L × TV/L = g/bag
   AA 0.08 × 600 = 48 × 1.246 = 59.8 = 60 g/bag
   Dex 0.20 × 600 = 120 × 1.246 = 149.5 = 150 g/bag

Percentage of concentrate per bag
2. **Formula: $\frac{g/bag}{TV}$ = %/bag**
   AA $\frac{60}{1246}$ = 0.048 = 4.8%/bag

   Dex $\frac{150}{1246}$ = 0.120 = 12%/bag

Percentage of additives
3. **Formula: mEq/L × TV/L = mEq/bag**
   mEq/bag divided by TV = %/bag
   Shortcut method: mEq/L × TV/L divided by TV = %/bag
   Sodium chloride 42 × 1.246 = 52.3 divided by 1246 = 0.042 = 4.2%/bag
   Potassium phosphate 26 × 1.246 = 32.3 divided by 1246 = 0.026 = 2.6%/bag
   Potassium acetate 10 × 1.246 = 12.4 divided by 1246 = 0.01 = 1%/bag
   Calcium gluconate 6 × 1.246 = 7.4 divided by 1246 = 0.006 = 0.6%/bag
   Magnesium sulfate 6 × 1.246 = 7.4 divided by 1246 = 0.006 = 0.6%/bag

kcal per bag
4. **Formula: 1 kcal of protein = 4 g; 1 kcal of dextrose = 4 g; 1 kcal of fat = 9 g**
   a. AA 60 × 4 = 240 kcal
   b. CHO 150 × 4 = 600 kcal
   c. Total kcal = 840

5. *Know*   *Want to Know*
   50 mL : 1 hr :: 1246 mL : x hr
   50x = 1 × 1246 = 1246
      x = 24.92   Convert .92 into minutes: 0.92 × 60 = 55 min
      x = 24 hr 55 min
   PROOF
   1 × 1246 = 1246
   50 × 24.92 = 1246

8E (PAGE 202)

1. **d.** $0.085 \times 375 = 31.8 \times 1.500 = 47.8$ g/bag of AA

2. **b.** $\frac{47.8}{1500} = 0.03 = 3\%$ conc. of AA

3. **a.** $0.40 \times 400 = 160 \times 1.450 = 232$ g/bag of dextrose

4. **b.** $\frac{232}{1450} = 0.16 = 16\%$ conc. of dextrose

5. **a.** $0.20 \times 175 = 35 \times 1.200 = 42$ g lipids/bag

6. **b.** $\frac{42}{1200} = 0.035 = 3.5\%$ conc. of lipids

7. **d.** $6 \times 1.350 = 8.1 \div 1350 = 0.006 = 0.6\%$ calcium gluconate

8. **a.** $10 \times 1.258 = 12.5 \div 1258 = 0.01 = 1\%$ magnesium sulfate

9. **c.** $12 \times 1.385 = 16.62 \div 1385 = 0.012 = 1.2\%$ potassium

10. **c.** *Know*   *Want to Know*
    110 mL : 1 hr :: 1275 mL : x hr
    $110x = 1275$
    $x = 11.59$ hr $= 11$ hr 35 min
    PROOF
    $1 \times 1275 = 1275$
    $110 \times 11.59 = 1275$
    IV started at 1800 hr plus 11 hr 35 min = 0535 hr

Chapter 8 Final: Parenteral Nutrition (PAGE 204)

1. **a.** 66.85 g/bag of AA
   b. 267.4 kcal of PRO

2. **a.** 73.62 g/bag of dextrose
   b. 294.48 kcal of CHO

3. **a.** 22.4 g/bag AA
   b. 89.6 kcal of PRO

4. **a.** 212 g/bag dextrose
   b. 848 kcal of dextrose

5. 0.4% potassium chloride

6. 2.5% NaCl

7. 1559 total kcal

8. **a.** 25 g/bag lipids
   b. 225 kcal of fat

9. At 0709 hr the infusion will be completed

10. 11 hr to infuse

9 Insulin

9A (PAGE 214)

1. 27 units
2. 68 units
3. 16 units
4. 44 units
5. 32 units
6. 78 units
7. 42 units
8. 39 units
9. 23 units
10. 18 units

9B (PAGE 216)

1. b
2. a
3. b
4. a
5. a

9C (PAGE 221)

1. Total units: 58
b is correct

2. Total units: 43
a is correct

3. Total units: 23
a is correct

4. Total units: 52
b is correct

5. Total units: 68
a is correct
b insulins are reversed—drawn up incorrectly.

6. 35 units
Peak 0.5 to 1.5 hr

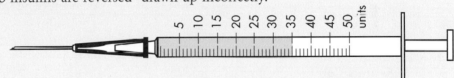

7. 20 units
Onset 15 min

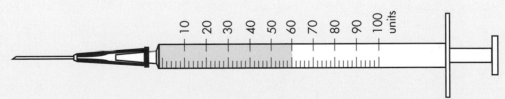

8. 44 units
Peak 6-10 hr
Duration 10-16 hr

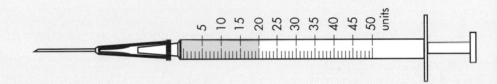

9. 60 units
Duration 12-18 hr

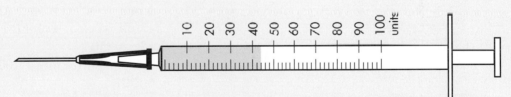

10. 60 units
Peak 6-10 hr
Duration 10-16 hr

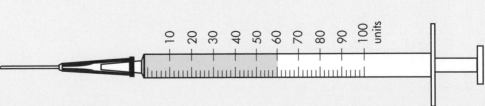

9D (PAGE 227)

1. a. 4 units/hr
   b. 3 units/hr

2. a. *Know*   *Want to Know*
   100 units : 100 mL :: 2.5 units : x mL
   $100x = 100 \times 2.5 = 250$
      $x = 2.5$ mL/hr
   PROOF
   $100 \times 2.5 = 250$
   $100 \times 2.5 = 250$
   b. Change IV rate to 3 mL/hr
   c. 5.5 units

3. 21 total units

4. a. *Know*   *Want to Know*
   50 mL : 100 units :: x mL : 5 units
   $100x = 50 \times 5 = 250$
      $x = 2.5$ mL/hr
   PROOF
   $100 \times 2.5 = 250$
   $50 \times 5 = 250$
   b. 5 units per hour $\times$ 16 hours = 80 units of insulin

5. a. *Know*   *Want to Know*
   100 units : 50 mL :: x units : 3 mL
   $50x = 100 \times 3 = 300$
   $x = 6$ units/hr
   PROOF
   $100 \times 3 = 300$
   $50 \times 6 = 300$
   b. 8 hr $\times$ 6 units per hr = 48 units

6. *Know*   *Want to Know*
   100 units : 150 mL :: 10 units : x mL
   $100x = 150 \times 10 = 1500$
   $100x = 1500$
      $x = 15$ mL/hr = 10 units insulin
   PROOF
   $100 \times 15 = 1500$
   $150 \times 10 = 1500$
   Know   *Want to Know*
   15 mL : 1 hr :: 150 mL : x hr
   $15x = 150$
      $x = 10$ hr to infuse 100 units insulin
   PROOF
   $15 \times 10 = 150$
   $1 \times 150 = 150$

7. *Know*   *Want to Know*
50 mL : 50 units :: x mL : 8 units
$50x = 50 \times 8 = 400$
$50x = 400$
    $x = 8$ mL/hr = 8 units of insulin
PROOF
$50 \times 8 = 400$
$50 \times 8 = 400$
Know   *Want to Know*
8 mL : 1 hr :: 50 mL : x hr
$8x = 50$
    $x = 6.25$ hr to infuse 50 units insulin or
        6 hr 15 min
PROOF
$8 \times 6.25 = 50$
$1 \times 50 = 50$

8. *Know*   *Want to Know*
50 mL : 75 units :: x mL : 100 units
$75x = 50 \times 100 = 5000$
$75x = 66.6 = 67$
    $x = 67$ mL/hr = 100 units
PROOF
$50 \times 100 = 5000$
$75 \times 66.7 = 4995$
Know   *Want to Know*
67 mL : 1 hr :: 50 mL : x hr
$67x = 50$
    $x = 0.74 = 44$ min to infuse
PROOF
$67 \times 0.74 = 49.58$
$1 \times 50 = 50$

9. *Know*   *Want to Know*
100 mL : 120 units :: x mL : 10 units
$120x = 100 \times 10 = 1000$
$120x = 1000$
    $x = 8.33$ mL/hr to deliver 10 units of
        insulin
PROOF
$120 \times 8.33 = 999.6$
$100 \times 10 = 1000$
Know   *Want to Know*
8 mL : 1 hr :: 100 mL : x hr
$8x = 1 \times 100$
$8x = 100$
    $x = 12.5$ hr to infuse 120 units of regular
        insulin or 12 hr 30 min
PROOF
$8 \times 12.5 = 100$
$1 \times 100 = 100$

10. *Know*   *Want to Know*
150 mL : 150 units :: x mL : 12 units
$150x = 150 \times 12$
$150x = 1800$
    $x = 12$ mL/hr to deliver 12 units of insulin
PROOF
$150 \times 12 = 1800$
$12 \times 150 = 1800$
Know   *Want to Know*
12 mL : 1 hr :: 150 mL : x hr
$12x = 150$
    $x = 12.5$ hr to infuse 150 units of regular
        insulin or 12 hr 30 min
$12 \times 12.5 = 150$
$1 \times 150 = 150$

9E (PAGE 231)

1. d. 4 units
Know   *Want to Know*
250 mL : 100 units :: 10 mL : x units
$250x = 100 \times 10 = 1000$
   $x = 4$ units/hr
PROOF
$250 \times 4 = 1000$
$100 \times 10 = 1000$

3. c. 3 mL/hr
Know   *Want to Know*
100 units : 100 mL :: 3 units : x mL
$100x = 100 \times 3 = 300$
   $x = 3$ mL/hr
PROOF
$100 \times 3 = 300$
$100 \times 3 = 300$

5. a. 50 mL/hr
Know   *Want to Know*
500 mL : 100 units :: x mL : 10 units
$100x = 500 \times 10 = 5000$
   $x = 50$ mL/hr
PROOF
$100 \times 50 = 5000$
$500 \times 10 = 5000$

6. c. Humulin R

7. d. 24 hr

8. b. 6-12 hr

9. d. is peakless

10. b. bedtime

2. b. 25 hr
Know   *Want to Know*
4 units : 1 hr :: 100 units : x hr
$4x = 100$
 $x = 25$ hr
PROOF
$1 \times 100 = 100$
$4 \times 25 = 100$

4. b. 2.5 units/hr
Know   *Want to Know*
30 units : 12 hr :: x units : 1 hr
$12x = 30$
   $x = 2.5$ units/hr
PROOF
$30 \times 1 = 30$
$12 \times 2.5 = 30$
a. 4 mL/hr
50 mL : 12 hr :: x mL : 1 hr
$12x = 50$
   $x = 4.16 = 4$ mL/hr
PROOF
$50 \times 1 = 50$
$12 \times 4.16 = 4.9$

Chapter 9 Final: Insulin (PAGE 232)

1. 15 units
   b

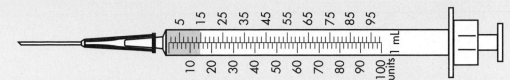

2. Sliding scale
   Give 8 units.

3. 16 units Humulin R
   30 units Humulin N
   Total amount is 46 units.

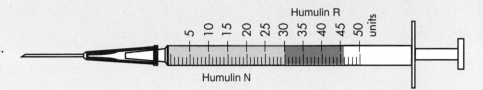

4. 18 units Humalog
   b is easier to read

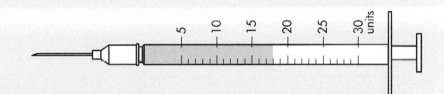

5. 15 units Humulin

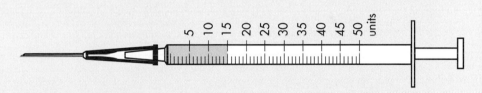

6. 20 mL/hr = 10 units
   25 hr to infuse. An IV solution can only hang for 24 hr (CDC guidelines).

7 15 mL/hr to infuse 6 units insulin
   16.6 hr to infuse = 16 hr 36 min

8. 20 mL/hr to infuse 8 units insulin
   12.5 hr to infuse = 12 hr 30 min

9. 14 mL/hr to infuse 7 units insulin
   14.2 hr to infuse = 14 hr 12 min

10. 45 mL/hr to infuse 9 units insulin
   11.1 hr to infuse = 11 hr 6 min

10 Anticoagulants

10A (PAGE 239)

1. *Know*   *Want to Know*

10,000 units : 1 mL :: 7000 units : x mL

$10x = 7$

$x = 0.7$ mL

PROOF

$1 \times 7000 = 7000$

$10,000 \times 0.7 = 7000$

2. *Know*   *Want to Know*

20,000 units : 1 mL :: 15,000 units : x mL

$20x = 15$

$x = 0.75$ mL

PROOF

$1 \times 15,000 = 15,000$

$20,000 \times 0.75 = 15,000$

3. *Know*   *Want to Know*

20,000 units : 1 mL :: 8000 units : x mL

$20x = 8$

$x = 0.4$ mL

PROOF

$20 \times 0.4 = 8$

$1 \times 8 = 8$

4. *Know*   *Want to Know*

20,000 units : 1 mL :: 17,000 units : x mL } use the 20,000 units/mL strength

$20x = 17$

$x = 0.85$ mL

PROOF

$1 \times 17 = 17$

$20 \times 0.85 = 17$

5. *Know*   *Want to Know*

10,000 IU : 1 mL :: 7500 IU : x mL

$100x = 75$

$x = 0.75$ mL Fragmin

PROOF

$1 \times 75 = 75$

$100 \times 0.75 = 75$

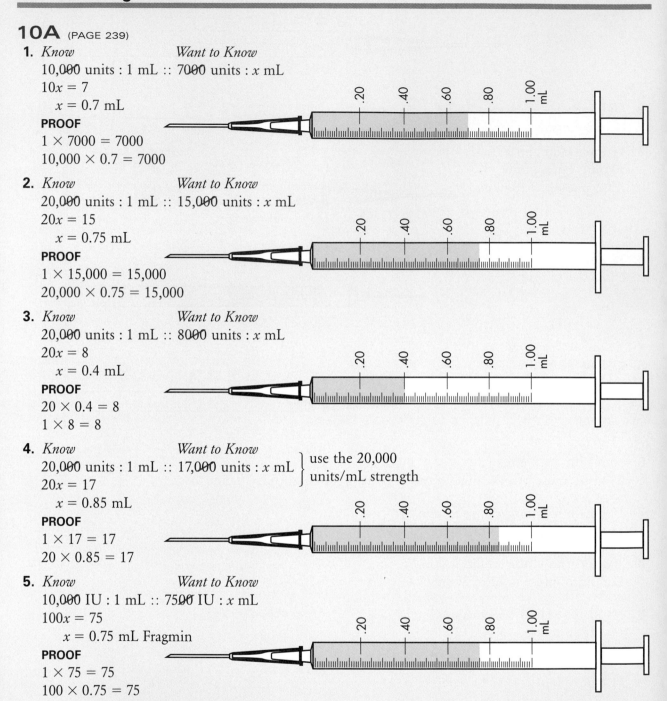

6. *Know*   *Want to Know*
1000 units : 1 mL :: 750 units : x mL
100Øx = 75Ø
     $x = 0.75$ mL
PROOF
$1000 \times 0.75 = 750$
$1 \times 750 = 750$

7. *Know*   *Want to Know*
10ØØ units : 1 mL :: 8ØØ units : x mL
$10x = 8$
     $x = 0.8$ mL
PROOF
$10 \times 0.8 = 8$
$1 \times 8 = 8$

8. *Know*   *Want to Know*
5ØØØ units : 1 mL :: 3ØØØ units : x mL
$5x = 3$
     $x = 0.6$ mL
PROOF
$1 \times 3 = 3$
$5 \times 0.6 = 3$

9. *Know*   *Want to Know*
10 units : 1 mL :: x units : 10 mL
$x = 10 \times 10 = 100$
$x = 100$ units in the vial

Know   *Want to Know*
10 units : 1 mL :: 5 units : x mL
$10x = 5$
     $x = 0.5$ mL
PROOF
$1 \times 5 = 5$
$10 \times 0.5 = 5$

10. *Know*   *Want to Know*
10Ø units : 1 mL :: 5Ø units : x mL
$10x = 5$
     $x = 0.5$ mL
PROOF
$1 \times 5 = 5$
$10 \times 0.5 = 5$

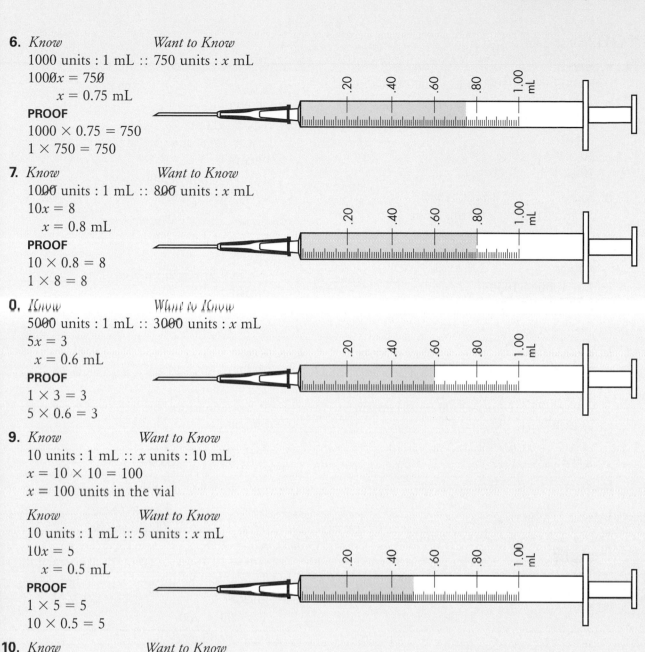

10B (PAGE 243)

1. a. *Know*   *Want to Know*
20,000 units : 1000 mL :: 1000 units : x mL
$20x = 1000$
$\quad x = 50$ mL/hr = 1000 units heparin
PROOF
$20 \times 50 = 1000$
$1000 \times 1 = 1000$

b. *Know*   *Want to Know*
50 mL : 1 hr :: 1000 mL : x hr
$50x = 1000$
$\quad x = 20$ hr
PROOF
$1 \times 1000 = 1000$
$50 \times 20 = 1000$

3. a. *Know*   *Want to Know*
20,000 units : 1000 mL :: 1500 units : x mL
$200x = 15,000$
$\quad x = 75$ mL/hr = 1500 units heparin
PROOF
$200 \times 75 = 15,000$
$100 \times 15 = 15,000$

b. *Know*   *Want to Know*
75 mL : 1 hr :: 1000 mL : x hr
$75x = 1000$
$\quad x = 13.33$ hr or 13 hr, 20 min
PROOF
$1 \times 1000 = 1000$
$75 \times 13.33 = 999.75$

5. a. *Know*   *Want to Know*
10,000 units : 500 mL :: 1200 units : x mL
$100x = 6000$
$\quad x = 60$ mL/hr
PROOF
$500 \times 12 = 6000$
$100 \times 60 = 6000$

b. *Know*   *Want to Know*
60 mL : 1 hr :: 500 mL : x hr
$60x = 500$
$\quad x = 8.33$ hr or 8 hr 20 min
PROOF
$60 \times 8.33 = 499.8$
$1 \times 500 = 500$

2. a. $\frac{1000}{12} = 83.3$ or 83 mL/hr

b. *Know*   *Want to Know*
20,000 units : 12 hr :: x units : 1 hr
$12x = 20,000$
$\quad x = 1666$ units/hr
PROOF
$20,000 \times 1 = 20,000$
$12 \times 1666 = 19,992$

c. *Know*   *Want to Know*
83 mL : 1 hr :: 750 mL : x hr
$83x = 750$
$\quad x = 9$ hr remaining
PROOF
$1 \times 750 = 750$
$83 \times 9 = 747$

4. a. *Know*   *Want to Know*
10,000 units : 15 hr :: x units : 1 hr
$15x = 10,000$
$\quad x = 666$ units /hr
PROOF
$15 \times 666 = 9990$
$10,000 \times 1 = 10,000$

b. $\frac{1000}{15} = 66.6$ or 67 mL/hr

c. *Know*   *Want to Know*
67 mL : 1 hr :: 700 mL : x hr
$67x = 700$
$\quad x = 10.45$ hr or 10 hr 27 min remaining
The IV will be infused at 1727 hr.
PROOF
$1 \times 700 = 700$
$67 \times 10.45 = 700$

6. a. *Know*   *Want to Know*
50,000 units : 1000 mL :: 2000 units : x mL
$50x = 2000$
$\quad x = 40$ mL/hr
PROOF
$50 \times 40 = 2000$
$1000 \times 2 = 2000$

b. *Know*   *Want to Know*
40 mL : 1 hr :: 1000 mL : x hr
$40x = 1000$
$\quad x = 25$ hr
PROOF
$1 \times 1000 = 1000$
$40 \times 25 = 1000$

7. a. *Know*   *Want to Know*

25,000 units : 500 mL :: 1000 units : x mL

$25x = 500$

$x = 20$ mL/hr

PROOF

$25 \times 20 = 500$

$500 \times 1 = 500$

b. *Know*   *Want to Know*

20 mL : 1 hr :: 500 mL : x hr

$20x = 500$

$x = 25$ hr

PROOF

$1 \times 500 = 500$

$20 \times 25 = 500$

8. a. *Know*   *Want to Know*

25,000 units : 500 mL :: 1300 units : x mL

$250x = 6500$

$x = 26$ mL/hr

PROOF

$26 \times 250 = 6500$

$500 \times 13 = 6500$

b. *Know*   *Want to Know*

26 mL : 1 hr :: 500 mL : x hr

$26x = 500$

$x = 19.23$ hr or 19 hr 14 min

PROOF

$1 \times 500 = 500$

$26 \times 19.23 - 499.98$

9. a. *Know*   *Want to Know*

25,000 units : 250 mL :: 1800 units : x mL

$250x = 4500$

$x = 18$ mL/hr

PROOF

$250 \times 18 = 4500$

$250 \times 18 = 4500$

b. *Know*   *Want to Know*

18 mL : 1 hr :: 250 mL : x hr

$18x = 250$

$x = 13.88$ hr or 13 hr 53 min

PROOF

$1 \times 250 = 250$

$18 \times 13.8 = 248.4$

10. a. *Know*   *Want to Know*

20,000 units : 250 mL :: 1000 units : x mL

$20x = 250$

$x = 12.5$ mL/hr or 13 mL/hr

PROOF

$20 \times 12.5 = 250$

$250 \times 1 = 250$

b. *Know*   *Want to Know*

13 mL : 1 hr :: 250 mL : x hr

$13x = 250$

$x = 19.23$ hr or 19 hr 14 min

PROOF

$1 \times 250 = 250$

$13 \times 19.2 = 249.8$

10C (PAGE 245)

1. c. *Know*   *Want to Know*
120 IU : 1 kg :: x IU : 84 kg
$x = 120 \times 84 = 10{,}080$
$x = 10{,}080$ IU of Fragmin
PROOF
$120 \times 84 = 10{,}080$
$1 \times 10{,}080 = 10{,}080$

2. b. *Know*   *Want to Know*
25,000 IU : 1 mL :: 10,080 : x mL
$25{,}000x = 10{,}080$
$x = 0.4$ mL
PROOF
$1 \times 10{,}080 = 10{,}080$ (units can be rounded up or down)
$0.4 \times 25{,}000 = 10{,}000$

3. c. *Know*   *Want to Know*
1 kg : 2.2 lb :: x kg : 132 lb
$2.2x = 132$
$x = 60$ kg
PROOF
$1 \times 132 = 132$
$2.2 \times 60 = 132$

d. *Know*   *Want to Know*
120 IU : 1 kg :: x IU : 60 kg
$x = 60 \times 120$
$x = 7200$ IU q12h
PROOF
$1 \times 7200 = 7{,}200$
$60 \times 120 = 7{,}200$

4. a. *Know*   *Want to Know*
10,000 IU : 1 mL :: 7200 IU : L : x mL
$10{,}000x = 7200$
$x = 0.72 = 0.7$ mL
PROOF
$7200 \times 1 = 7200$
$10{,}000 \times 0.72 = 7200$

5. a. *Know*   *Want to Know*
80 units : 1 kg :: x units : 73 kg
$x = 80 \times 73 = 5840$
$x = 5840$ units of heparin
PROOF
$1 \times 5840 = 5840$
$80 \times 73 = 5840$

6. d. *Know*   *Want to Know*
18 units : 1 kg :: x units : 80 kg
$x = 18 \times 80 = 1440$
$x = 1440$ units/hr
PROOF
$1 \times 1440 = 1440$
$18 \times 80 = 1440$

d. *Know*   *Want to Know*
1000 mL : 20,000 units :: x mL : 1440 units
$20{,}000x = 1000 \times 1440 = 1{,}440{,}000$
$x = 72$ mL/hr
PROOF
$1000 \times 1440 = 1{,}440{,}000$
$72 \times 20{,}000 = 1{,}440{,}000$

7. b. *Know*   *Want to Know*
1000 mL : 25,000 units :: x mL : 3000 units
$25,000x = 3,000,000$
$25x = 120$ mL/hr
PROOF
$25 \times 120 = 3000$
$1000 \times 3 = 3000$

9. a. 220 divided by 2.2 = 100 kg
   d. *Know*   *Want to Know*
120 IU : 1 kg :: x IU : 100 kg
$x = 120 \times 100 = 12,000$
$x = 12,000$ IU Fragmin
PROOF
$1 \times 12,000 = 12,000$
$100 \times 120 = 12,000$

8. d. *Know*   *Want to Know*
10,000 units : 500 mL :: 500 units : x mL
$10,000x = 250,000$
$x = 25$ mL/hr
PROOF
$25 \times 10,000 = 250,000$
$500 \times 500 = 250,000$

10. c. *Know*   *Want to Know*
25,000 IU : 1 mL :: 12,000 IU : x mL
$25,000x = 12,000$
$x = 0.48$ mL
PROOF
$1 \times 12,000 = 12,000$
$25,000 \times 0.48 = 12,000$

Chapter 10 Final: Anticoagulants (PAGE 247)

1. 0.8 mL

3. 0.2 mL using the 10,000 U/mL strength or
0.4 mL using the 5000 U/mL strength

5. 0.8 mL

7. 30 mL/hr
16 hr, 40 min

9. 42 mL/hr
1458 U/hr

2. 0.25 mL

4. 0.35 mL using the 20,000 U/mL strength or
0.7 mL using the 10,000 U/mL strength

6. 17.5 mL/hr or 18 mL/hr
27 hr, 42 min

8. 42 mL/hr
1041.6 U/hr

10. 100 mL/hr via infusion device
10 hr to infuse

11 Children's Dosages

11A (PAGE 253)

1. a. Estimate: 7 kg
   Actual: 6.4 kg
   b. Estimate: 6 kg
   Actual: 12.1 lb (2 steps)
           5.5 kg
   c. Estimate: 5 kg
   Actual: 4.5 kg
   d. Estimate: 28 lb
   Actual: 30.8 lb
   e. Estimate: 20 lb
   Actual: 22 lb

2. a. 150 mg $\times$ 3 = 450 mg
   b. 200 mg $\times$ 4 = 800 mg
   c. 400 μg $\times$ 6 = 2400 μg or 2.4 mg
   d. 50 mg $\times$ 3 = 150 mg
   e. 750 μg $\times$ 2 = 1500 μg or 1.5 mg

3. a. 1 g or 1000 mg/4 = 250 mg
   b. 750 mg/3 = 250 mg
   c. 2 g or 2000 mg/4 = 500 mg
       2 g or 2000 mg/6 = 333.3 mg
   d. 16 g a day/2 = 8 g
       16 g a day/4 = 4 g
   e. 500 mg/4 = 125 mg

4. a. 10 $\times$ 5 = 50 mg
   b. 5 $\times$ 7.3 = 36.5 mg (low dose)
       8 $\times$ 7.3 = 58.4 mg (high dose)
       SDR is 36.5 to 58.4 mg.
   c. 8 lb = approximately 4 kg estimated
   Step 1: 8 lb = 3.6 kg actual
   Step 2: *Low dose:* 6 $\times$ 3.6 = 21.6 mg
           High dose: 8 $\times$ 3.6 = 28.8 mg
       SDR is 21.6 to 28.8 mg.
   d. 5 lb, 8 oz = approximately 2.5 kg
   Step 1: *oz to lb:* 8 oz/16 = 0.5 lb
   Step 2: *lb to kg:* 5.5 lb/2.2 = 2.5 kg
   Step 3: *Low dose:* 3 $\times$ 2.5 = 7.5 mg
           High dose: 6 $\times$ 2.5 = 15 mg
       SDR is 7.5 to 15 mg.
   e. 4 lb, 6 oz = approximately 2 kg
   Step 1: *oz to lb:* 6 oz/16 = 0.37 or 0.4 lb
   Step 2: *lb to kg:* 4.4 lb/2.2 = 2 kg
   Step 3: *Low dose:* 200 μg $\times$ 2 = 400 μg or
           0.4 mg
           High dose: 400 μg $\times$ 2 = 800 μg or
           0.8 mg
       SDR is 400 to 800 μg or 0.4 to 0.8 mg.

5. a. 36 to 54 mg (2 $\times$ 18 = 36) (3 $\times$ 18 = 54)
   b. 12 to 18 mg (36 $\div$ 3) (54 $\div$ 3)
   c. 150 mg/day; 50 mg per dose
       (50 $\times$ 3)   (150 $\div$ 3)
   d. Unsafe to give. Overdose ordered. Hold and clarify promptly with the physician.

11B (PAGE 254)

1. a. Estimated wt in kg: 12.5 kg
 b. Actual wt in kg: 11.54 or 11.5 kg (25.4/2.2)
 c. SDR for this child: 115 to 345 mg/day
  $10 \times 11.5 = 115$ mg
  $30 \times 11.5 = 345$ mg
 d. Dose ordered: 100 mg tid or 300 mg/day
 e. Evaluation and decision: Safe to give

3. a. Estimated wt in kg: 10 kg
 b. Actual wt in kg: 9.09 or 9.1 kg
 c. SDR for this child: 18.2 to 36.4 mg/day
  $2 \times 9.1 = 18.2$ mg
  $4 \times 9.1 = 36.4$ mg
 d. Dose ordered: 50 mg daily
 e. Evaluation and decision: Hold and clarify promptly (overdose)

5. a. Estimated wt in kg: 2.5 kg
 b. Actual wt in kg: 2.27 or 2.3 kg
 c. SDR for this child: 23-46 μg/day
  $10 \times 2.3 = 23$ μg
  $20 \times 2.3 = 46$ μg
 d. Dose ordered: 0.03 mg $\times$ 4 = 0.12 mg/day or 120 μg/day
 e. Evaluation and decision: Hold and clarify promptly (overdose)

2. a. Estimated wt in kg: 16.5 kg
 b. Actual wt in kg: 15 kg
 c. SDR for this child: 1500 to 3000 μg/day or 1.5 to 3 mg/day
  15×100 μg = 1500 μg or 1.5 mg
  15×200 μg = 3000 μg or 3 mg
 d. Dose ordered: 0.5 mg tid or 1.5 mg/day
 e. Evaluation and decision: Safe to give

4. a. Estimated wt in kg: 42.5 kg
 b. Actual wt in kg: 38.63 or 38.6 kg
 c. SDR for this child: 386 mg to 579 mg/day in divided doses
 d. Dose ordered: 100 mg q6h or $100 \times 4 = 400$ mg/day
 e. Evaluation and decision: Safe to give

11C (PAGE 257)

1. 0.15 m^2
$10 \times 0.15 = 1.5 \text{ mg}$

2. 0.20 m^2
$15 \times 0.2 = 3 \text{ mg}$

3. 0.27 m^2
$5 \times 0.27 = 1.35 \text{ mg}$

4. $4 \times 10 = 40 \text{ mg}$

5. $15 \times 6 = 90 \text{ mg}$

6. $5 \times 10 = 50 \text{ mg}$

7. $10 \times 1.8 = 18 \text{ mg}$

8. 2.72 kg
$2 \times 2.72 = 5.4 \text{ mg}$

9. $\frac{60 \times 100}{3600} = 1.66$
$\sqrt{1.66} = 1.29 \text{ m}^2$

10. $\frac{70 \times 12}{3131} = 0.268$
$\sqrt{0.268} = 0.517 = 0.52 \text{ m}^2$

11D (PAGE 258)

1. a. Estimated wt in kg: 7 kg
  b. Actual wt in kg: 6.36 or 6.4 kg
  c. SDR for this child: 0.13 to 0.32 mg/day
    $0.02 \times 6.4 = 0.128 \text{ mg}$
    $0.05 \times 6.4 = 0.32 \text{ mg}$
  d. Dose ordered: 150 µg $\times$ 2 = 300 µg/day
    or 0.3 mg/day
  e. Evaluation and decision: Safe to give

2. a. SDR for this child: 4.0 to 6.4 mg qid
    $5 \times 0.8 \text{ m}^2 = 4.0 \text{ mg}$
    $8 \times 0.8 \text{ m}^2 = 6.4 \text{ mg}$
  b. Dose ordered: 4 mg qd
  c. Evaluation and decision: Safe to give

3. a. Estimated wt in kg: 9.5 kg
  b. Actual wt in kg: 8.63 or 8.6 kg
  c. SDR for this child: 0.86 to 2.6 mg in
    2 divided doses or 800 to 2600 µg in
    2 divided doses
    $0.1 \times 8.6 = 0.86 \text{ mg}$ or 0.9 mg
    $0.3 \times 8.6 = 2.58$ or 2.6 mg
  d. Dose ordered: 2500 µg bid or 2.5 mg $\times$
    2 = 5 mg/day
  e. Evaluation and decision: Hold and clarify
    promptly (overdose)

4. a. Estimated wt in kg: 4.5 kg
  b. Actual wt in kg: 4.09 or 4.1 kg
  c. SDR for this child: 4.1 to 20.5 µg/day
    $1 \times 4.1 = 4.1 \text{ µg}$
    $5 \times 4.1 = 20.54 \text{ µg}$
  d. Dose ordered: 0.01 mg or 10 µg qd
  e. Evaluation and decision: Safe to give

5. a. Estimated wt in kg: 13 kg
  b. Actual wt in kg: 11.8 kg
  c. SDR: 1000 to 2000 mg in
    4 divided doses
  d. Dose ordered: 500 mg $\times$ 4 or 2000 mg
  e. Evaluation and decision: Safe to give

11E (PAGE 259)

1. a. Estimated wt in lb: 14×2 or 28 lb
b. Actual wt in lb: 30.8 lb
c. SDR for this child: For 24 to 35 lb, 1 tsp
d. Dose ordered: 160 mg
e. Evaluation and decision: Safe to give
f. Give: 1 tsp or 5 mL (80 mg per $\frac{1}{2}$ tsp)

2. a. Estimated wt in kg: 27.5 kg
b. Actual wt in kg: 25 kg
c. SDR for this child: 750 to 1250 mg/day in 4 divided doses
$30 \times 25 = 750$
$50 \times 25 = 1250$
d. Dose ordered: $300 \times 4 = 1200$ mg/day
e. Evaluation and decision: Safe to give
f. Give 7.5 mL
Have   *Want to Have*
200 mg : 5 mL :: 300 mg : x mL
$\frac{200}{200}x = \frac{1500}{200}$ (5 × 300)
$x = 7.5$ mL
PROOF
$200 \times 7.5 = 1500$
$1 \times 1500 = 1500$

3. a. SDR for this child:
$10 \times 0.5 \times 4 = 20$ mg/day
b. Dose ordered: 20 mg/day
c. Evaluation and decision: Safe to give
d. Give 1 tab

4. a. SDR for this child: 400 to 800 mg/day in 3 to 4 divided doses
b. Dose ordered in mg:
0.25 g = 250 mg × 3 = 750 mg/day
Have   *Want to Have*
1 g : 1000 mg :: 0.25 g : x mg
$x = 1000 \times 0.25$ or 250 mg
PROOF
$1 \times 250 = 250$
$1000 \times 0.25 = 250$
c. Evaluation and decision: Safe to give
d. Give 12.5 mL
Have   *Want to Have*
100 mg : 5 mL :: 250 mg : x mL
$\frac{100}{100}x = \frac{1250}{100}$ (5 × 250)
$x = 12.5$ mL
PROOF
$100 \times 12.5 = 1250$
$5 \times 250 = 1250$

5. a. Estimated wt in kg: 13
b. Actual wt in kg: 12.3 kg
c. SDR for this child: 492 mg/day or 164 mg tid
d. Dose ordered: 180 mg/dose or 540 mg/day
e. Evaluation and decision: Slight overdose. Hold and clarify promptly.
f. Not applicable

11F (PAGE 262)

1. a. Estimated wt in kg: 16 kg
  b. Actual wt: 14.7 kg (2 steps)
  Have   *Want to Have*
  16 oz : 1 lb :: 5 oz : x lb
  $\frac{\cancel{16}}{\cancel{16}}x = \frac{5}{16}$
    $x = 0.312$ or 0.3 lb
  Child weighs 32.3 lb ÷ 2.2 = 14.68
  or 14.7 kg
  c. SDR for this child: 14.7 to 32.3 mg q4h
    $1 \times 14.7 = 14.7$ mg
    $2.2 \times 14.7 = 32.34$ mg = 32.3 mg
  d. Dose ordered: 30 mg
  e. Evaluation and decision: Safe to give
  f. Give 0.4 mL
  Have   *Want to Have*
  75 mg : 1 mL :: 30 mg : x mL
  $\frac{\cancel{75}}{\cancel{75}}x = \frac{30}{75}$
    $x = 0.4$ mL
  PROOF
  $75 \times 0.4 = 30$
  $1 \times 30 = 30$

3. a. Estimated wt: 8.5 kg
  b. Actual wt: 8 kg (2 steps)
  Have   *Want to Have*
  16 oz : 1 lb :: 9 oz : x lb
  $\frac{\cancel{16}}{\cancel{16}}x = \frac{9}{16}$
    $x = 0.56$ or 0.6 lb
  Child weighs 17.6 lb ÷ 2.2 or 8 kg
  c. SDR for this child: between 7 and 9 kg,
  0.2 mg
  d. Dose ordered: 0.2 mg
  e. Evaluation and decision: Safe to give
  f. Give 0.5 mL
  Have   *Want to Have*
  0.4 mg : 1 mL :: 0.2 mg : x mL
  $\frac{\cancel{0.4}}{\cancel{0.4}}x = \frac{0.2}{0.4}$ (1×0.2)
    $x = 0.5$ mL
  PROOF
  $0.4 \times 0.5 = 0.2$
  $1 \times 0.2 = 0.2$

2. a. Estimated wt: 27 kg
  b. Actual wt: 25.2 kg (2 steps)
  Have   *Want to Have*
  16 oz : 1 lb :: 8 oz : x lb
  $16x = 8$
    $x = 0.5$ lb   Child weighs 55.5 lb ÷ 2.2
                    or 25.2 kg
  c. SDR for this child: 2.52 to 5.04 mg q4h
    $0.1 \times 25.2 = 2.52$ mg
    $0.2 \times 25.2 = 5.04$ mg
  d. Dose ordered: 5 mg IM
  e. Evaluation and decision: Safe to give
  f. Give 0.5 mL
  Have   *Want to Have*
  10 mg : 1 mL :: 5 mg : x mL
  $\frac{\cancel{10}}{\cancel{10}}x = \frac{5}{10}$
    $x = 0.5$ mL
  PROOF
  $10 \times 0.5 = 5$
  $1 \times 5 = 5$

4. a. Estimated wt : 3.5 kg
  b. Actual wt : 3.2 kg (1 step)
  c. SDR for this child: 320 to 640 mg/day
  (based on 3.2 kg wt)
  d. Dose ordered: 1000 mg/day
  e. Evaluation and decision: Overdose. Hold
  and clarify promptly. Also ask whether IV
  route is preferred.
  f. Not applicable.

5. a. Estimated wt: 75 ÷ 2 or 37.5 kg
  b. Actual wt: 75 ÷ 2.2 or 34.1 kg (1 step)
  c. SDR for this child: 1705 to 3410 mg day in
  4 divided doses
    $50 \times 34.1 = 1705$ mg
    $100 \times 34.1 = 3410$ mg
  d. Dose ordered: 1500×3 or 4500 mg/day
  e. Evaluation and decision: Ordered $3 \times$ day
  and is recommended qid. Total dose exceeds
  recommendation.
  Hold and clarify promptly (overdose)
  f. Not applicable

11G (PAGE 266)

1. a. Estimated wt in kg: 31 kg
   b. Actual wt in kg: 28.18 or 28.2 kg
   c. SDR for this child: 28.2 to 84.6 kg q24h
   d. Dose ordered: 65 mg IV stat
   e. Evaluation and decision: Safe to give
   f. Volume to be administered, if applicable:
      Give 1.5 mL
      130 mg : 3 mL :: 65 mg : x mL
      $130x = 195$
      $x = 1.5$ mL
      PROOF
      $130 \times 1.5 = 195$
      $3 \times 65 = 195$

2. a. Estimated wt in kg: 27.5 kg
   b. Actual wt in kg: 25 kg
   c. SDR for this child: 25 to 150 mg
      (1 to 6 mg/kg)
      $1 \times 25 = 25$
      $6 \times 25 = 150$
   d. Dose ordered: 25 mg IV stat
   e. Evaluation and decision: Safe to give
      (The initial dose must not exceed the
      lowest dose in the SDR.)
   f. Give 2.5 mL
      Have   *Want to Have*
      40 mg : 4 mL :: 25 mg : x mL
      $\dfrac{\cancel{40}}{\cancel{40}} = \dfrac{10\cancel{0}(4 \times 25)}{4\cancel{0}}$
      $x = 2.5$ mL
      PROOF
      $40 \times 2.5 = 100$
      $4 \times 25 = 100$

3. a. Estimated wt in kg: 17 kg
   b. Actual wt in kg: 15.45 or 15.5 kg
   c. SDR for this child: 775 to 1550 mg/day
      divided by 3 and 4 or 516 mg/max individ-
      ual dose
   d. Dose ordered: 0.3 g or 300 mg q6h =
      1200 mg total dose per day
   e. Evaluation and decision: Safe to give
   f. First dilution. Mix Zinacef with 9 mL and
      withdraw 3.6 mL
      Have   *Want to Have*
      750 mg : 9 mL :: 300 mg : x mL
      $\dfrac{\cancel{750}}{\cancel{750}}x = \dfrac{2700}{750}$
      $x = 3.6$ mL to be further diluted to
         20 mL and administered on an
         IV infusion pump with a volume-
         control device. (Add diluent to equal
         20 mL.)
      PROOF
      $750 \times 3.6 = 2700$
      $9 \times 300 = 2700$
   g. Infuse at 40 mL/hr for 30 min
      Have   *Want to Have*
      20 mL : 30 min :: x mL : 60 min
      $30x = 1200$
      $x = 40$ mL/hr
      PROOF
      $20 \times 60 = 1200$
      $30 \times 40 = 1200$

4. a. Estimated wt in kg: 28 kg
   b. Actual wt in kg: 25.45 or 25.5 kg
   c. SDR for this child: 229.5 mg/day or
      76.5 q8h
   d. Dose ordered: 60 mg q8h or 180 mg/day
   e. Evaluation and decision: Safe to give. Slight
      underdose. Give and clarify.
   f. Amount withdrawn from vial: Give 6 mL
      Have   *Want to Have*
      20 mg : 2 mL :: 60 mg : x mL
      $\dfrac{2\cancel{0}x}{2\cancel{0}} = \dfrac{12\cancel{0}}{4\cancel{0}}$
      $x = 6$ mL
   g. Flow rate in mL/hr on pump, if applicable:
      Further dilute to 50 mL and administer at
      50 mL/hr for 60 minutes.

5. a. Estimated wt in kg: 13 kg
   b. Actual wt in kg: 11.81 or 11.8 kg
   c. SDR for this child: 590 to 5900 mg divided
      by 4 doses = 1475 mg maximum unit dose
      $50 \times 11.8 = 590$
      $500 \times 11.8 = 5900$
   d. Dose ordered: 2 g or 2000 mg q6h
   e. Evaluation and decision: Hold and clarify
      promptly (overdose)
   f. Not applicable
   g. Not applicable

11H (PAGE 269)

1. a. Estimated wt in kg: 17 kg
   b. Actual wt in kg: $34 \div 2.2 = 15.45$ or 15.5 kg
   c. SDR for this child: 310 mg $\div$ 3 or 103.3 mg tid
   d. Dose ordered: 100 mg $\times$ 3 or 300 mg/day
   e. Evaluation and decision: Safe to give, but clarify (very slight underdose)
   f. Give 2 mL
   Have   *Want to Have*
   250 mg : 5 mL :: 100 mg : x mL
   $250x = 500$
   $x = 2$ mL
   PROOF
   $250 \times 2 = 500$
   $5 \times 100 = 500$

2. a. Estimated wt in kg: 35 kg
   b. Actual wt in kg: 31.81 or 31.8 kg
   c. SDR for this child: 5×31.8 or 159 mg in 2 or 3 divided doses
   d. Dose ordered: 75 mg bid $75 \times 2 = 150$ mg per day
   e. Evaluation and decision: Safe to give, but clarify (very slight underdose)
   f. Give 11.25 or 11.3 mL
   Have   *Want to Have*
   100 mg : 15 mL :: 75 mg : x mL
   $100x = 1125$
   $x = 11.25$ or 11.3 mL
   PROOF
   $100 \times 11.25 = 1125$
   $15 \times 75 = 1125$

3. a. Estimated wt in kg: 24.5 kg
   b. Actual wt in kg: 22.27 or 22.3 kg
   c. SDR for this child: 89.2 to 111.5 µg/day po 44.6 to 55.75 µg/day IV ($\frac{1}{2}$ po dose)
   $4\ \mu g \times 22.3 = 89.2\ \mu g$
   $5\ \mu g \times 22.3 = 111.5\ \mu g$
   d. Dose ordered: 0.1 mg (100 µg) IV q AM
   Have   *Want to Have*
   1 mg : 1000 µg :: 0.1 mg : x µg
   $x = 1000 \times 0.1 = 100$ µg
   e. Evaluation and decision: Hold and clarify promptly (overdose for IV administration)
   f. Not applicable

4. a. Estimated wt in kg: 33 kg
   b. Actual wt in kg: 30 kg
   c. SDR for this child: 30 to 66 mg
   $1 \times 30 = 30$
   $2.2 \times 30 = 66$
   d. Dose ordered: 35 mg
   e. Evaluation and decision: Safe to give
   f. Give 0.7 mL
   Have   *Want to Have*
   50 mg : 1 mL :: 35 mg : x mL
   $\frac{50}{50}x = \frac{35}{50}$
   $x = 0.7$ mL
   PROOF
   $50 \times 0.7 = 35$
   $1 \times 35 = 35$

5. a. Estimated wt in lb: 27 lb
   b. Actual wt in lb: 29.92 or 30 lb
   c. SDR for this child: 40 mg/0.6 m^2 = 24 mg/day
   d. Dose ordered: 30 mg/day
   e. Evaluation and decision: Hold and clarify (overdose)
   f. Not applicable

6. a. Estimated wt in kg: 11 kg
   b. Actual wt in kg: 10 kg
   c. SDR for this child: 500 to 1000 mg/day in 4 divided doses (250 mg each max)
   d. Dose ordered: 250 mg IV q6h
   e. Evaluation and decision: Safe to give
   f. Give 12.5 mL
   Have   *Want to Have*
   1000 mg : x mL :: 20 mg : 1 mL
   $\frac{20}{20}x = \frac{1000}{20}$
   $x = 50$ mL
   1000 mg : 50 mL :: 250 mg : x mL
   $\frac{1000}{1000}x = \frac{12,500}{1000}$
   $x = 12.5$ mL

7. a. Estimated wt in kg: 3 kg
  b. Actual wt in kg: 2.72 or 2.7 kg
  c. SDR for this child: Up to 8.1 mEq q24h
      $3 \times 2.7 = 8.1$
  d. Dose ordered: 0.9 mEq q8h or 2.7 q24h
  e. Evaluation and decision: Safe to give; monitor lab potassium values for therapeutic range, and assess patient's heart rate, rhythm, and muscle tone. May be underdosed.
  f. Add 0.45 mL KCl to compatible IV and mix well
      Have   *Want to Have*
      2 mEq : 1 mL :: 0.9 mEq : x mL

      $\frac{2}{2}x = \frac{0.9}{2} = 0.45$ mL

      PROOF
      $2 \times 0.45 = 0.9$
      $1 \times 0.9 = 0.9$

9. a. Draw up 0.2 mL po in a 1 mL syringe. Remove the needle first. Administer along the inside of the cheek.
  b. Use enclosed dropper.
      Have   *Want to Have*
      80 mg : 0.8 mL :: 20 mg : x mL

      $\frac{80}{80}x = \frac{16}{80}$

      $x = 0.2$ mL
      PROOF
      $80 \times 0.2 = 16$
      $0.8 \times 20 = 16$

8. a. Estimated wt in kg: 15.5 kg
  b. Actual wt in kg: 14.09 or 14.1
  c. SDR for this child: Up to 1410 mg in 2 doses or 705 mg dose
      $100 \times 14.1 = 1410$
  d. Dose ordered: 600 mg IV q12h or 1200 mg/day
  e. Evaluation and decision: Safe to give
  f. Use 6 mL after reconstituting
      Have   *Want to Have*
      100 mg : 1 mL :: 600 mg : x mL

      $\frac{100}{100}x = \frac{600}{100}$

      $x = 6$ mL
      PROOF
      $100 \times 6 = 600$
      $1 \times 600 = 600$
  g. Infuse for 30 min at 60 mL/hr
      Have   *Want to Have*
      30 mL : 30 min :: x mL : 60 min

      $\frac{30}{30}x = \frac{1800}{30}$

      $x = 60$ mL/hr
      PROOF
      $30 \times 60 = 1800$
      $60 \times 30 = 1800$

10. a. Estimated wt in kg: 13 kg
  b. Actual wt in kg: 12 kg
  c. SDR for this child: 240 to 480 mg day
  d. Dose ordered: 360 mg/day
  e. Evaluation and decision: Safe to give
  f. Give 4.8 mL
      Have   *Want to Have*
      125 mg : 5 mL :: 120 mg : x mL

      $\frac{125}{125}x = \frac{600}{125} = 4.8$ mL

      PROOF
      $125 \times 4.8 = 600$
      $5 \times 120 = 600$

11I (PAGE 274)

1. b
This is a *two-step* problem.
Estimated wt in kg: 25 kg
Step 1:
2.2 lb : 1 kg :: 50 lb : x kg
x = 50/2.2 or 22.7 kg
Step 2:
20 mg : 1 kg :: x mg : 22.7 kg
x = 20 × 22.7 or 454 mg

PROOF
2.2 × 22.7 = 49.94 or 50
1 × 50 = 50
PROOF
20 × 22.7 = 45
1 × 454 = 454

2. c
30 mg : 1 m^2 :: x mg : 1.20 m^2
x = 30 × 1.20 or 36 mg

PROOF
30 × 1.20 = 36
1 × 36 = 36

3. b
5 mL = 1 tsp
5 mL : 1 tsp :: x mL : 1.5 tsp
x = 7.5 mL
Measure 7.5 mL

PROOF
5 × 1.5 = 7.5
1 × 7.5 = 7.5

4. c
This is a *three-step* problem.
Estimated wt in kg: 25/2 or 12.5 kg
Step 1:
2.2 lb : 1 kg :: 25 lb : x kg
x = 25/2.2 or 11.4 kg
Step 2:
2 mg : 1 kg :: x mg : 11.4 kg
x = 2 × 11.4 or 22.8 mg *low safe dose*
Step 3:
5 mg : 1 kg :: x mg : 11.4 kg
x = 57 mg *maximum safe dose*
30 mg is within SDR of 22.8 mg to 57 mg.

PROOF
2.2 × 11.4 = 25
1 × 25 = 25
PROOF
2 × 11.4 = 22.8
1 × 22.8 = 22.8
PROOF
5 × 11.4 = 57
1 × 57 = 57

5. d
Estimated wt: 5.5/2 or 2.5 kg
Step 1: lb to kg
2.2 lb : 1 kg :: 5.5 lb : x kg
2.2x = 5.5x = 2.2 kg = 2.5 kg
Step 2: SDR
40 mg : 1 kg :: x mg : 2.5 kg
x = 40 × 2.5   or   100 mg/day
Compare the SDR with the order. 125 mg order exceeds 100 mg recommended
dose. Clarify with the physician promptly and document promptly.

PROOF
2.2 × 2.5 = 5.5
1 × 5.5 = 5.5
PROOF
40 × 2.5 = 100
1 × 100 = 100

6. **a**

Estimated wt: 55/2 or 27.5 kg

Step 1: lb to kg

2.2 lb : 1 kg :: 55 lb : x kg

2.2x = 5.5

x = 25 kg

PROOF

2.2 × 25 = 55

1 × 55 = 55

Step 2: SDR

2 mg : 1 kg :: x mg : 25 kg

x = 2 × 25 or 50 mg *low safe dose*

PROOF

2 × 25 = 50

1 × 50 = 50

Compare low SDR with the order. They are equal for the q8h (tid) order.
No need to calculate high safe dose. Give the medication.

7. **b**

Estimated wt: 6/2 or 3 kg

This is a *three-step* problem

Step 1: lb to kg

2.2 lb : 1 kg :: 55 lb : x kg

2.2x = 55

x = 25 kg

PROOF

2.2 × 25 = 55

1 × 55 = 55

Step 2: SDR

5 mg : 1 kg :: x mg : 6 kg

x = 5 × 6 or 30 mg

PROOF

5 × 6 = 30

1 × 30 = 30

Compare the SDR with the order. 30 mg/2 = 15 mg bid. The order is
15 mg bid. The order is safe.

Step 3: Calculate the unit dose.

30 mg : 5 mL :: 15 mg : x mL

30x = 75x = 2.5 mL

PROOF

30 × 2.5 = 75

5 × 15 = 75

Give 2.5 mL using a syringe to measure, if necessary.

8. **d**

1000 μg = 1 mg

500 μg = 0.5 mg

200 μg = 0.2 mg

Metric equivalents

Estimate: You want to give *more than double* the 10 mL dose.

Have   *Want to Have*

200 μg : 10 mL :: 500 μg : x mL

$\dfrac{200x}{200} = \dfrac{5000}{200}$

x = 25 mL

PROOF

200 × 2.5 = 500

1 × 500 = 500

9. d

Estimated wt in kg: 29 kg

Step 1: lb to kg   **PROOF**

2.2 lb : 1 kg :: 58 lb : x kg $2.2 \times 26.36 = 57.92$ or 58

$2.2x = 58$ $1 \times 58 = 58$

$x = 26.36$ kg or 26.4 kg (to *nearest tenth*)

Step 2: low SDR

Low safe dose range is 1 mg/kg or 26.4 mg.

No math is needed for low safe dose range.

The order is for 30 mg; therefore continue and calculate high SDR.

Step 3: High SDR   **PROOF**

2.2 mg : 1 kg :: x mg : 26.4 kg $2.2 \times 26.4 = 58.08$

$x = 2.2 \times 26.4$ or 58.08 or 58.2 mg $1 \times 58.08 = 58.08$

The order for 30 mg is within the SDR of 26.4 mg to 58.2 mg unit dose.

(Step 3 Dose Calculation)   **PROOF**

You want to give more than 25 mg or 1 mL $25 \times 1.2 = 30$

25 mg : 1 mL :: 30 mg : x mL $1 \times 30 = 30$

$\dfrac{25x}{25} = \dfrac{30}{25}$

$x = 1.2$ mL

10. b

Estimated wt in kg is 15 kg.

lb to kg   **PROOF**

2.2 : 1 kg :: 30 : x kg $2.2 \times 13.6 = 29.92$

$\dfrac{2.2x}{2.2} = \dfrac{30}{2.2}$ $1 \times 30 = 30$

$x = 13.6$

SDR   **PROOF**

25 mg : 1 kg :: x mg : 13.6 kg $25 \times 13.6 = 340$

$x = 25 \times 13.6$ or 340 mg day in *4 divided* doses $1 \times 340 = 340$

or 85 mg per dose

50 mg = 2 times the 25 mg dose of 680 mg/day high safe dose per day

Decision: Hold the order. The drug is supposed to be given 4 times a day, not 3 times a day; and the amount ordered, 750 mg per day, exceeds the recommended safe dose of 680 mg per day

Chapter 11 Final: Children's Dosages (PAGE 276)

1. a. Estimated wt in kg: 21 kg
  b. Actual wt in kg: 19.09 or 19.1 kg
  c. SDR for this child: 477.5 to 955 mg/day in 4 divided doses
  d. Dose ordered: 200 mg × 4 or 800 mg/day
  e. Evaluation and decision: Safe to give
  f. Give 8 mL.

3. a. SDR for this child: 150 mg maximum in 24 hr in divided doses
  b. Dose ordered: 25 mg × 4 or 100 mg/day
  c. Evaluation and decision: Safe to give
  d. Dose to be administered: 2 tsp or 25 mg per dose

5. a. Estimated wt in kg: 17.5 kg
  b. Actual wt in kg: 15.9 kg
  c. SDR for this child: 0.3 mg (for 12 to 26 kg child)
  d. Dose ordered: 0.3 mg
  e. Safe to give.
  f. Give 0.75 mL in anterolateral thigh.

7. a. Actual wt in kg: 15.9 kg
  b. SDR for this child: 95.4 to 119.3 mg/day
  c. Dose ordered: 35 × 3 or 105 mg/day
  d. Evaluation and decision: Safe to give
  e. Dose after reconstitution: 35 mL
  f. IV flow rate on device: 70 mL/hr for $\frac{1}{2}$ hr

9. a. BSA in m²: 1.10 m²
  b. SDR for this child: Up to 44 mg/day
     1.10 × 10 × 4 = 44
  c. Dose ordered: 40 mg/day
  d. Evaluation and decision: Safe to give
  e. Give 2 tab.

2. a. Actual wt in kg: 19.09 or 19.1 kg
  b. SDR for this child: 573 to 955 mg/day in 4 divided doses
  c. Dose ordered: 175 mg × 4 or 700 mg/day
  d. Evaluation and decision: Safe to give
  e. Give 4.4 mL.

4. a. SDR for this child: 400 to 800 mg/day
  b. Dose ordered: 2000 mg/day
  c. Evaluation and decision: Overdose. Hold and clarify promptly.
  d. Dose to be administered: Not applicable

6. a. Actual wt in kg: 15.9 kg
  b. SDR for this child: 318 to 636 mg/day
  c. Dose ordered: 500 mg × 3 or 1500 mg
  d. Evaluation and decision: Overdose. Hold and clarify promptly.
  e. Dose to be administered: Not applicable

8. a. Actual wt in kg: 15.9 kg
  b. SDR for this child: 0.795 or 0.8 to 1.6 mg q4h
  c. Dose ordered: 5 mg q4h
  d. Evaluation and decision: Hold and clarify promptly (overdose).
  e. Not applicable

10. a. Estimated wt in lb: 36 lb
  b. Actual wt in lb: 39.6 lb
  c. SDR for this child: $1\frac{1}{2}$ tsp for children weighing 36 to 47 lb
  d. Dose ordered: 240 mg or $1\frac{1}{2}$ tsp
  e. Evaluation and decision: Safe to give
  f. Give $1\frac{1}{2}$ tsp or 7.5 mL
  g. The enclosed measuring cup

12 Dimensional Analysis

12A (PAGE 283)

1. *Know*   *Want to Know*

$$x \text{ mL} = \frac{1 \text{ mL}}{500 \text{ mg}} \times \frac{800 \text{ mg}}{1 \text{ L}} = \frac{800}{500} = 1.6 \text{ mL}$$

2. *Know*   *Want to Know*

$$x \text{ tabs} = \frac{1 \text{ tab}}{400 \text{ mg}} \times \frac{1000 \text{ mg}}{1 \text{ g}} \times \frac{0.8 \text{ g}}{1 \text{ L}} = \frac{800}{400} = 2 \text{ tablets}$$

3. *Know*   *Want to Know*

$$x \text{ gtt/min} = \frac{20 \text{ gtt}}{1 \text{ mL}} \times \frac{125 \text{ mL}}{60 \text{ min}} = \frac{2500}{60} = 41.6 = 42 \text{ gtt/min}$$

4. *Know*   *Want to Know*

$$x \text{ mL} = \frac{1 \text{ mL}}{50 \text{ mg}} \times \frac{35 \text{ mg}}{1 \text{ L}} = \frac{35}{50} = 0.7 \text{ mL}$$

5. *Know*   *Want to Know*

$$x \text{ mL} = \frac{5 \text{ mL}}{200 \text{ mg}} \times \frac{250 \text{ mg}}{1 \text{ L}} = \frac{1250}{200} = 6.25 \text{ mL}$$

6. *Know*   *Want to Know*

$$x \text{ mL} = \frac{5 \text{ mL}}{200 \text{ mg}} \times \frac{750 \text{ mg}}{1 \text{ L}} = \frac{3750}{200} = 18.75 \text{ mL}$$

7. *Know*   *Want to Know*

$$x \text{ mL} = \frac{1 \text{ L}}{1000 \text{ mL}} \times \frac{1260}{1 \text{ L}} = \frac{1260}{1000} = 1.26 \text{ L}$$

8. *Know*   *Want to Know*

$$x \text{ mL} = \frac{2 \text{ mL}}{250 \text{ mg}} \times \frac{300 \text{ mg}}{1 \text{ L}} = \frac{600}{250} = 2.4 \text{ mL}$$

9. *Know*   *Want to Know*

$$x \text{ mL} = \frac{1 \text{ mL}}{250 \text{ mg}} \times \frac{400 \text{ mg}}{1 \text{ L}} = \frac{400}{250} = 1.6 \text{ mL}$$

10. *Know*   *Want to Know*

$$x \text{ mL} = \frac{1.2 \text{ mL}}{500 \text{ mg}} \times \frac{700 \text{ mg}}{1 \text{ L}} = 1.2 \times \frac{700}{1} \times 500 = \frac{840}{500} = 1.7 \text{ mL}$$

12B (PAGE 286)

1. *Know*   *Want to Know*

$$x \text{ mL} = \frac{1000 \text{ mL}}{20,000 \text{ units}} \times \frac{1000 \text{ units}}{1 \text{ hr}} = \frac{1,000,000}{20,000} = 50 \text{ mL/hr}$$

2. *Know*   *Want to Know*

$$x \text{ units/hr} = \frac{20,000 \text{ units}}{1000 \text{ mL}} \times \frac{50 \text{ mL}}{1 \text{ hr}} = \frac{1,000,000}{1000} = 1000 \text{ units/hr}$$

3. *Know*   *Want to Know*

$$x \text{ mg/hr} = \frac{400 \text{ mg}}{500 \text{ mL}} \times 60 \text{ mL/hr} = \frac{24,000}{500} = 48 \text{ mg/hr}$$

4. *Know*   *Want to Know*

$$x \text{ mL/hr} = \frac{1000 \text{ mL}}{30 \text{ units}} \times \frac{2 \text{ units}}{1 \text{ hr}} = 66.6 = 67 \text{ mL/hr}$$

5. a. *Know*   *Want to Know*

$$x \text{ mL/hr} = \frac{1000 \text{ mL}}{24 \text{ hr}} \times \frac{1 \text{ hr}}{1} = \frac{1000}{24} = 41.6 = 42 \text{ mL/hr}$$

b. *Know*   *Want to Know*

$$x \text{ units/hr} = \frac{42 \text{ mL}}{1 \text{ hr}} \times \frac{50 \text{ units}}{1000 \text{ mL}} = \frac{2100}{1000} = 2.1 \text{ units/hr}$$

6. a. *Know*   *Want to Know*

$$x \text{ mL/hr} = \frac{250 \text{ mL}}{12 \text{ hr}} \times \frac{1 \text{ hr}}{1} = \frac{250}{12} = 20.8 = 21 \text{ mL/hr}$$

b. *Know*   *Want to Know*

$$x \text{ units/hr} = \frac{21 \text{ mL}}{1 \text{ hr}} \times \frac{30 \text{ units}}{250 \text{ mL}} = \frac{630}{250} = 2.5 \text{ units/hr}$$

7. a. *Know*   *Want to Know*

$$x \text{ mL/hr} = \frac{250 \text{ mL}}{8 \text{ hr}} \times \frac{1 \text{ hr}}{1} = \frac{250}{8} = 31.2 = 31 \text{ mL/hr}$$

b. *Know*   *Want to Know*

$$x \text{ mg/hr} = \frac{31 \text{ mL}}{1 \text{ hr}} \times \frac{300 \text{ mg}}{250 \text{ mL}} = \frac{9300}{250} = 37.2 \text{ mg/hr}$$

8. a. *Know*   *Want to Know*

$$x \text{ mL/hr} = \frac{1000 \text{ mL}}{12 \text{ hr}} \times \frac{1 \text{ hr}}{1} = \frac{1000}{12} = 83.3 = 83 \text{ mL/hr}$$

b. *Know*   *Want to Know*

$$x \text{ mEq/hr} = \frac{83 \text{ mL}}{1 \text{ hr}} \times \frac{20 \text{ mEq}}{100 \text{ 0 mL}} = \frac{1660}{1000} = 1.66 \text{ mEq/hr}$$

9. *Know*   *Want to Know*

$$x \text{ hr} = \frac{1000 \text{ mL}}{1} \times \frac{15 \text{ gtt}}{1 \text{ mL}} \times \frac{1 \text{ min}}{20 \text{ gtt}} \times \frac{1 \text{ hr}}{60 \text{ min}} = \frac{15,000}{1} \times 20 \times 60 = \frac{15,000}{1200} = 12.5 = 12 \text{ hr } 30 \text{ min}$$

10. *Know*   *Want to Know*

$$x \text{ hr} = \frac{1000 \text{ mL}}{1} \times \frac{1 \text{ hr}}{120 \text{ mL}} = \frac{1000}{120} = 8.33 = 8 \text{ hr } 20 \text{ min}$$

12C (PAGE 287)

1. a. *Know*   *Want to Know*

$$x \, \mu g/min = \frac{1 \, kg}{2.2 \, lb} \times \frac{190 \, lb}{1} \times \frac{3 \, \mu g}{min/1 \, kg} = \frac{570}{2.2} = 259 \, \mu g/min$$

b. *Know*   *Want to Know*

$$x \, mL/hr = \frac{60 \, min}{1 \, hr} \times \frac{259 \, \mu g}{1 \, min} \times \frac{1 \, mg}{1000 \, \mu g} \times \frac{250 \, mL}{30 \, mg} = \frac{3,885,000}{30,000} = 129.5 = 130 \, mL/hr$$

c. *Know*   *Want to Know*

$$x \, gtt/min = \frac{259 \, \mu g}{1 \, min} \times \frac{1 \, mg}{1000 \, \mu g} \times \frac{250 \, mL}{30 \, mg} \times \frac{60 \, gtt/min}{1 \, mL} = \frac{3,885,000}{30,000} = 129.5 = 130 \, gtt/min$$

2. a. *Know*   *Want to Know*

$$x \, \mu g/min = \frac{5 \, \mu g/min}{1 \, kg} \times \frac{110 \, kg}{1} = 550 \, \mu g/min$$

b. *Know*   *Want to Know*

$$x \, mL/hr = \frac{60 \, min}{1 \, hr} \times \frac{550 \, \mu g}{1 \, min} \times \frac{1 \, mg}{1000 \, \mu g} \times \frac{250 \, mL}{200 \, mg} = \frac{8,250,000}{200,000} = 41.2 = 41 \, mL/hr$$

3. a. *Know*   *Want to Know*

$$x \, \mu g/min = \frac{1 \, kg}{2.2 \, lb} \times \frac{160 \, lb}{1} \times 6 \, \mu g/min = \frac{960}{2.2} = 436 \, \mu g/min$$

b. *Know*   *Want to Know*

$$x \, mL/hr = \frac{60 \, min}{1 \, hr} \times \frac{436 \, \mu g}{1 \, min} \times \frac{1 \, mg}{1000 \, \mu g} \times \frac{500 \, mL}{800 \, mg} = \frac{13,080,000}{800,000} = \frac{1308}{80} = 16.35 = 16 \, mL/hr$$

4. a. *Know*   *Want to Know*

$$x \, mL/hr = \frac{1000 \, mL}{12 \, hr} \times \frac{1 \, hr}{1} = \frac{1000}{12} = 83.3 = 83 \, mL/hr$$

b. *Know*   *Want to Know*

$$x \, units/hr = \frac{10,000 \, units}{12 \, hr} \times \frac{1 \, hr}{1} = \frac{10,000}{12} = 833.3 \, units/hr$$

5. *Know*   *Want to Know*

$$x \, hr = \frac{1350 \, mL}{1} \times \frac{1 \, hr}{112 \, mL} = \frac{1350}{112} = 12 \, hr$$

6. *Know*   *Want to Know*

$$x \, gtt/min = \frac{1000 \, mL}{4 \, hr} \times \frac{20 \, gtt}{1 \, mL} \times \frac{1 \, hr}{60 \, min} = \frac{20,000}{240} = 83 \, gtt/min$$

7. *Know*   *Want to Know*

$$x \, gtt/min = \frac{500 \, mL}{1.5 \, hr} \times \frac{12 \, gtt}{1 \, mL} \times \frac{1 \, hr}{60 \, min} = \frac{6000}{90} = 66.6 = 67 \, gtt/min$$

8. *Know*   *Want to Know*

$$x \, gtt/min = \frac{500 \, mL}{1} \times \frac{10 \, gtt}{1 \, mL} = \frac{5000}{120} = 41.6 = 42 \, gtt/min$$

9. *Know*   *Want to Know*

$$x \, mL = \frac{2000 \, mL}{24 \, hr} \times \frac{1 \, hr}{1} = \frac{2000}{24} = 83.3 = 83 \, mL/hr$$

10. *Know*   *Want to Know*

$$x \, mL/hr = \frac{1000 \, mL}{6 \, hr} \times \frac{1 \, hr}{1} = \frac{1000}{6} = 166.6 = 167 \, mL/hr$$

12D (PAGE 289)

1. c. *Know*   *Want to Know*

$$x \, (\text{SDR}) = \frac{5 \text{ kg}}{1} \times \frac{10 \text{ mg}}{1 \text{ kg}} = \frac{50}{1} = 50 \text{ mg}$$

a. Yes. 50 mg is the maximum dose for a 5 kg child. The dose ordered is one dose of 25 mg.

2. d. *Know*   *Want to Know*

$$x \text{ kg} = \frac{1 \text{ kg}}{2.2 \text{ lb}} \times \frac{8 \text{ lb}}{1} = \frac{8}{2.2} = 3.6 \text{ kg}$$

b. *Know*   *Want to Know*

$$x \text{ mg (low dose)} = \frac{6 \text{ mg}}{1 \text{ kg}} = \frac{3.6 \text{ kg}}{1} = 21.6 = 22 \text{ mg}$$

a. *Know*   *Want to Know*

$$x \text{ mg (high dose)} = \frac{8 \text{ mg}}{1 \text{ kg}} \times \frac{3.6 \text{ kg}}{1} = 28.8 = 29 \text{ mg}$$

3. d. *Know*   *Want to Know*

$$x \text{ mL} = \frac{2.5 \text{ mL}}{80 \text{ mg}} \times \frac{250 \text{ mg}}{1} = 2.5 \times \frac{240}{80} = \frac{600}{80} = 7.5 \text{ mL}$$

4. b. *Know*   *Want to Know*

$$x \text{ mL} = \frac{1 \text{ g}}{1000 \text{ mg}} \times \frac{1 \text{ mL}}{0.5 \text{ g}} \times \frac{600 \text{ mg}}{1} = \frac{600}{500} = 1.2 \text{ mL}$$

5. c. *Know*   *Want to Know*

$$x \text{ hr} = \frac{1300 \text{ mL}}{1} \times \frac{1 \text{ hr}}{112 \text{ mL}} = \frac{1330}{112} = 11.87 = 11 \text{ hr } 52 \text{ min}$$

a. 2000 hr + 12 hr = 0800 hr

6. a. *Know*   *Want to Know*

$$x \text{ mL/hr} = \frac{1000 \text{ mL}}{12 \text{ hr}} \times 1 = \frac{1000}{12} = 83.3 - 83 \text{ mL/hr}$$

d. *Know*   *Want to Know*

$$x \text{ units/min} = \frac{50,000 \text{ units}}{12 \text{ hr}} \times \frac{1 \text{ hr}}{60 \text{ min}} = \frac{50,000}{720} - 69.4 - 69 \text{ units/min}$$

7. a. *Know*   *Want to Know*

$$x \text{ kg} = \frac{1 \text{ kg}}{2.2 \text{ lb}} \times \frac{40 \text{ lb}}{1} = \frac{40}{2.2} = 18 \text{ kg}$$

c. *Know*   *Want to Know*

$$x \text{ mg (low dose)} = \frac{30 \text{ mg}}{1 \text{ kg}} \times \frac{18 \text{ kg}}{1} = 540 \text{ mg}$$

c. *Know*   *Want to Know*

$$x \text{ mg (high dose)} = \frac{50 \text{ mg}}{1 \text{ kg}} \times \frac{18 \text{ kg}}{1} - 50 \times \frac{18}{1} = 900 \text{ mg}$$

8. d. *Know*   *Want to Know*

$$x \text{ mL/hr} = \frac{500 \text{ mL}}{40 \text{ units}} \times \frac{3 \text{ units}}{1 \text{ hr}} = \frac{1500}{40} = 37.5 = 38 \text{ mL/hr}$$

9. d. *Know*   *Want to Know*

$$x \text{ kg} = \frac{1 \text{ kg}}{2.2 \text{ lb}} \times \frac{195 \text{ lb}}{1} = \frac{195}{2.2} = 88.6 = 89 \text{ kg}$$

b. *Know*   *Want to Know*

$$x \text{ units/min} = \frac{89 \text{ kg}}{1} \times \frac{0.5 \text{ units/min}}{1 \text{ kg}} = 44.5 = 45 \text{ units/min}$$

c. *Know*   *Want to Know*

$$x \text{ mL/hr} = \frac{45 \text{ units}}{1 \text{ min}} \times \frac{60 \text{ min}}{1 \text{ hr}} \times \frac{500 \text{ mL/hr}}{20,000 \text{ units}} = \frac{1,350,000}{200,000} = 67.5 = 68 \text{ mL/hr}$$

10. b. *Know*   *Want to Know*

$$x \text{ mL/hr} = \frac{1000 \text{ mL}}{60,000 \text{ units}} \times \frac{5000 \text{ units}}{1 \text{ hr}} = \frac{5000}{60} = 83.3 = 83 \text{ mL/hr}$$

Chapter 12 FINAL: Dimensional Analysis (PAGE 289)

1. 0.75 mL

2. 1.6 mL

3. 1.3 mL

4. a. 4.0 mL
   b. 300 mg/24 hr

5. 20 tablets of 500 mg scored tablets needed for 10 days

6. 5600 units of Heparin for an IV bolus dose

7. 13 gtt/min

8. 33 gtt/min

9. 150 gtt/min

10. a. 11.3 kg
   b. 1130 μg is the low SDR.
   c. 2260 μg is the high SDR.
   d. Yes, 1500 μg/day is a safe order.

◼ Multiple Choice Final (PAGE 293)

1. d	**2.** c	**3.** a	**4.** c
5. b	**6.** c	**7.** b; d	**8.** a
9. c	**10.** a	**11.** b	**12.** c, d
13. a	**14.** d	**15.** d	**16.** a; d
17. d	**18.** a	**19.** c	**20.** c; d

◼ Comprehensive Final (PAGE 301)

1. 2 tab

2. 1 tab

3. 7.5 mL

4. 2 cap

5. 1.25 mL

6. 10 mg; 2 tabs

7. 24 mg/hr; 24,000 μg/hr; 5 μg/kg/min; flow rate is correct

8. Error: 0845 Dose given 45 minutes after prior dose. Order stated q4h intervals prn. Current Actions: Prescribe complete bed rest for patient, assess mental status and vital signs, notify supervising nurse/charge nurse and physician immediately, and obtain orders for medication to reverse.

Establish a patent IV line according to hospital policy in case emergency care may be needed.

Have crash cart close at hand. Document the error and to whom reported, patient evaluations, and all interventions and continue to make the above assessments and evaluate. Fill out incident report. Continue to assess and evaluate patient q 10-15 min until patient is stabilized. Then gradually extend assessment time.

Prevention: prn and stat medications need to be charted as soon as possible after administration. Nurse A needed to report to Nurse B orally when her patients were due for their next prn medications. Nurse B needed to state she was too busy to care for additional patients beyond her own caseload. Nurse B needed to check record carefully to see when last medication for pain was given. Nurse B needed to ask patient when last medication for pain was received. (This is a recommended double check but not always reliable. The accuracy of response depends on the patient's mental status.)

9. **a.** Total milliliters to be injected: 2 mL
   b. Total time in seconds: 120
   c. Seconds per calibration: 12
   d. 1 mL/min for 2 min

10. **a.** Estimated wt in kg: 4.5
    b. Actual wt in kg: 4.09 = 4.1
    c. SDR: 2.1 to 4.1 mg
    d. Dose ordered: 3 mg
    e. The dose ordered is within the SDR.
    f. Give 0.3 mL.

11. 19 g/bag amino acids
    29 g/bag carbohydrates
    14 g/bag lipids

12. 76 protein kilocalories
    116 carbohydrate kilocalories
    126 fat kilocalories
    Total kilocalories = 318

13. 6 units of Lantus

14. 0.8 IU Fragmin

15. 50 mL/hr
    20 hr to infuse

16. 75 mL/hr
    75 gtt/min

17. 250,000 units/mL
    Give 1.6 mL
    500,000 units/mL
    Give 0.8 mL

18. 70 mL/hr

19. Add 2 mL of diluent
    4 vials per 24 hr

20. 21 gtt/min
    83 mL/hr on infusion device

Index

24-hour clock. *See* Clock
24-hour dose, SDR, 259, 266

A

AA. *See* Amino acids
Abbott. *See* ADD-VANTAGE
    System
Abdominal surgery, recuperation,
    246
Access locks, flushing, 139
Acetaminophen. *See* Children's
    Tylenol
  suspension liquid, order
    calculation, 274
Activity level, 224
Additives, 195
  percentage, 192, 200
  volume, 193
ADD-VANTAGE System (Abbott)
  100 mL, 5% dextrose, 155f
  usage. *See* Medication
Administration. *See* Medication
  procedures, 46
  records. *See* Medication
    administration records
  six rights. *See* Drugs
  times, 60
Admission data, 51
Admixtures. *See* Fats; Intravenous
    piggyback
Advanced intravenous (IV)
    calculations
  critical thinking exercises, 183
  final, 183-184
    answer key, 376
  multiple-choice practice, 181-182
    answer key, 374-376
  objectives, 163
  practice, worksheet, 167-168
    answer key, 370
Agency policy, 51
Alcohol. *See* Sweetened alcohol

Allergies, 240. *See also*
    Cephalosporins; Penicillin
  reaction, 104
  reconfirming. *See* Patients
All-in-one formula, 191
Alprazolam. *See* Xanax
Ambulatory infusion device. *See*
    CADD-Prizm VIP
    ambulatory battery-operated
    infusion device; MedFlo
    postoperative gain
    management system
    ambulatory infusion device
Ambulatory patients, 157
Amicar order, 5 g, 161
Amino acids (AA)
  amount, calculation, 200
  concentration, percentage, 196,
    198, 200, 201
  grams, calculation, 196, 198, 201
  usage, 189, 190
Aminophylline
  500 mg (1000 mL D5W), 165f
  usage. *See* Infusion
    worksheet. *See* Intravenous
    calculations
Aminophylline order
  15 mg/hr, 173
  20 mg/hr, 173
  45 mg/hr, 173
  50 mL/hr, 173
  250 mg, 181
  300 mg, 286
Amoxicillin
  clavulanate potassium, oral
    suspension (label). *See*
    Augmentin
  oral suspension, label. *See* Amoxil
Amoxil (amoxicillin), 329
Amoxil (amoxicillin, oral
    suspension) label
  80 mL, 269f
  100 mL, 57f, 103f, 109f, 261f,
    273f, 279f
  calculation, 261, 279

Ampicillin (injection)
  1 g IV, order, 295
  label
    1 g, 121f, 125f, 135f, 263f,
     272f, 285f
    125 mg, 119f, 130f
Ampicillin order
  500 mg, 159
  calculation, 300 mg, 282-283
  suspension, calculation, 275
Ampicillin, usage. *See* Polycillin
Ampules, usage. *See* Medication
Analgesia. *See* Patient-controlled
    analgesia
Analgesic tablets, label. *See* Aspirin
Anaphylactic shock reaction, 125
Anisindione (Miradon), 244
Answer key, 309
Antecubital region vein, 138
Antibiotics
  powder form, 265
  usage, 140
Anticoagulants. *See* Injectable
    anticoagulants; Oral
    anticoagulants
  critical thinking exercises, 246
  dosage. *See* Therapeutic
    anticoagulant dosage
  final, 247-248
    answer key, 391
  multiple-choice practice,
    worksheet, 245-246
    answer key, 390-391
  objectives, 235
Antidotes, 138
Antihistamine, 125
Antiinfectives, administration, 125
Antineoplastic drugs, 255, 280
Antipyretic tablets, label. *See* Aspirin
Apothecary equivalents. *See* Unit
    dose
Apothecary measurements
  approximate equivalents, 97t
  comparison, worksheet, 97-99
    answer key, 346

Page numbers followed by f indicate figures, t, tables, and b, boxes

411

Apothecary system, 97-98
Aqueous penicillin, order, 160
Aqueous suspensions, 54
Arthritis, 102
Aspirin
  analgesic/antipyretic tablets, label,
    99f
  calculation, 67
Atenolol order, 0.025 g, 88
Atrial fibrillation, 248
Atropine order, 0.4 mg IM stat, 100
Atropine sulfate
  IM order, 0.3 mg, 278
  injection, label (20 ml), 92f, 103f,
    263f, 278f, 295f
Augmentin (amoxicillin clavulanate
    potassium, oral suspension)
    label, 108f, 112f
AZT (zidovudine) order, 0.2 g, 100

B

Bacteriostatic agent, usage, 114
Bacteriostatic water, 114, 119
Bag
  concentration percentage, 192
  kilocalories (Kcal) per, 192
  total grams per, 190-192
Bar code IDs, 51
BD-Safety-LOK syringe, 89f
Bedside Monitoring Blood Glucose
    (BMBG), 206, 225f, 227f
Benadryl Allergy Liquid
    (diphenhydramine HCl)
    label (25 mg), 277f
Benzyl alcohol, 114
BG. *See* Blood glucose
Biaxin PO order, 100 mg, 291
Bleeding, incidence, 238
Blood glucose (BG)
  flow sheet, 225f. *See also* Insulin
  levels, 224, 225f, 230, 304. *See also*
    Premeal blood glucose level
    scenario, 232
Blood (pint), usage, 161
Blood samples, withdrawal, 139f
BMBG level, 227
Body mass, adequacy, 128
Body surface area (BSA)
  BSA-based (mg/kg) dosages,
    comparison (worksheet), 257
  answer key, 394
  calculation, 260
    mathematical formula, usage,
      255-256
  dosages, 250

Body surface area (BSA) *(Continued)*
  estimation, West nomogram, 256f
    method (mg/m^2), 255-263
Body weight, 224
  dosages, 250
Bolus administration
  recommended rate, 176f
  syringe, usage. *See* Direct IV
    administration
Bretylium tosylate, 183
Bruising, 241
BSA. *See* Body surface area

C

CADD-Prizm VIP ambulatory
    battery-operated infusion
    device, 157f
Calcium chloride, order, 179
Calcium gluconate, 192, 195
  additive, 202
  percentage, 200
Calculation. *See* Advanced
    intravenous calculations;
    Dosages; Drop factor
    calculations; Insulin;
    Intravenous calculations
  critical thinking exercises. *See*
    Metric system calculations
  device. *See* Sigma 8000 automatic
    dose-related calculation
    device
  mathematical formula, usage. *See*
    Body surface area
  physician order. *See* Total
    Parenteral Nutrition
  usage, worksheet. *See* Obstetrics
  worksheet. *See* Central Parenteral
    Nutrition; Infusion devices;
    Intravenous insulin;
    Intravenous push; Peripheral
    Parenteral Nutrition; Solute
    g/mL
Capsules, 54, 55f. *See also* Extended-
    release capsules
  supply values, 72
Carbamazepine. *See* Tegretol
Carbenicillin disodium.
    See Geopen
Carbenicillin, usage, 136
Cardiac surgery, 236, 245
Cardizem (diltiazem HCl)
  label, 52f
  order, 15 mg/hr, 175
Caregivers, protection, 153
Carpuject syringe, 117f

Cartridge. *See* Pre-filled sterile
    cartridge/needle
Catheter. *See* Peripheral inserted
    central catheter
  type, 152f
Cefadyl (sterile cephapirin sodium)
  IM order, 600 mg, 289
  label (1 g), 121f, 124f, 128f, 285f,
    307f
Cefazolin order
  1 g, 159
  200 mL, 162
Cefobid (cefoperazone sodium)
    label
  1g, 119f, 131f
  2g, 120f, 130f
Cefoperazone sodium, label. *See*
    Cefobid
Ceftazidime, injection (label). *See*
    Tazicef
Ceftriaxone sodium. *See* Rocephin
Cefuroxime sodium. *See* Zinacef
Central Parenteral Nutrition (CPN),
    189
  calculations, worksheet, 196-197
    answer key, 377
  label, sample, 200f
  solution, 202
Cephalexin (oral suspension), 53f,
    276f
Cephalosporins, allergies, 277
Cephalothin (1 g), order, 160
CHF. *See* Congestive heart failure
Children
  dosage, calculation, 257-258
  intramuscular medications, 262-
    263
    answer key, 396
  oral medications, 259-261
    answer key, 395
  safe dose range (SDR), practice
    (worksheet), 254, 258
    answer key, 393, 394
  SDR
    estimation, 276, 298
    recommendation, 251
  subcutaneous medications, 262-
    263
    answer key, 396
  weight, 267-273, 276-280
    estimation, 250, 276
Children, dosages
  calculator practice, worksheet, 253
    answer key, 392
  critical thinking exercises, 276

Children, dosages (Continued)
  final, 276-280
    answer key, 403
  multiple-choice practice,
    worksheet, 400-402
  objectives, 249
  worksheet, 269-273
    answer key, 398-399
Children, intravenous (IV)
    medications, 264-268
  reconstitution/dilution/flow rate
    information, 264-266
  worksheet, 266-268
    answer key, 397
Children's Tylenol (acetaminophen)
  Elixir, 259f
  Suspension liquid, 280f
Chlorothiazide. See Diuril
Chlorpromazine HCl. See Thorazine
Cimetidine
  order, 0.45 g, 88
  tablets, label (400 mg), 102f,
    283f
Claforan IM order, 500 mg, 294
Cleocin Phosphate (sterile solution),
    label, 94f
Clinoril order, 800 mg, 83
Clock. See Conversion clock
  timing (24-hour), 58-59
    example, 59f
Closures (20 mm), 155f
Clotting factors, activation, 244
Codeine phosphate injection, label,
    99f
Common denominator, 6
  determination. See Fractions
  usage, 9
Common fractions
  change. See Decimals
  difference, 15
Compazine (prochlorperazine/
    prochlorperazine maleate)
  label, 92f
  order, 25 mg, 100
Comprehensive final, 301-307
  answer key, 409-410
Computer-generated MAR, sample.
    See PRN orders
Concentrated drops, differentiation,
    260
Concentration, percentages, 196-
    198, 200-202
Confined patients, 157
Congestive heart failure (CHG),
    162, 276

Container
  total amount, 56-58
  total dose, 78
  total volume, 78-79
Contaminated needles, 153
Continuous infusion, 156. See also
    Dextrose (5%) in water
Continuous IV, 176
Continuous IV therapy, 243
Continuous therapeutic range,
    maintenance, 245
Controlled substances, monitoring,
    49f
Conversion clock, 98f
Coumadin. See Warfarin
  dose range, 244f
CPN. See Central Parenteral
    Nutrition
Critical care intravenous (IV) orders,
    evaluation (worksheet), 171-
    172
  answer key, 371
Crystal form, usage, 135
Crystals. See Medication
    powders/crystals
  dilution. See Vials
Cup. See Measuring; Medication
  liquid measure. See Medicine
  usage. See Medicine

D

D5LR, 307
D5W. See Aminophylline; Dextrose
    (5%) in water
Dalteparin. See Fragmin
Decimal fractions, 15
Decimal points
  aligning, 18-19
  placement, 22
Decimal system, 71
Decimals
  addition, 18
    worksheet, 18
    worksheet, answer key, 313
  change. See Fractions
  common fractions, change, 25
    worksheet, 25
    worksheet, answer key, 317
  comparison, worksheet, 17
    answer key, 312
  conversion. See Percentages
  division, 20-23
    worksheet, 22-23
    worksheet, answer key,
    314-316

Decimals (Continued)
  movement. See Metric
    conversions
  multiplication, 20
    worksheet, 20
    worksheet, answer key, 313-314
  percentages, change, 28
  place, 33. See also Dividend
    decimal place
  calculation, 26
  movement, 28
  usage, 23, 25
  presence. See Divisor
  products, rounding, 27
    worksheet, 27
    worksheet, answer key, 318
  rounding, 26-27
    worksheet, 27
    worksheet, answer key, 318
  subtraction, 19
    worksheet, 19
    worksheet, answer key, 313
  usage, 28-30
  value, 15-16
    worksheet, 16
    worksheet, answer key, 312
  worksheet, 29
    answer key, 318
Deep vein thrombosis (DVT), 236,
    245
  prevention, 237
Delivery. See Dextrose; Prefilled
    cartridges; Prefilled syringe
  modes, 156-157. See also Total
    Parenteral Nutrition
  sets. See Intravenous delivery sets
Deltasone tablets (10 mg), label,
    271f
Deltoid muscle, usage (caution),
    262
Demerol (meperidine HCl) order,
    35 mg, 100
Denominator. See Common
    denominator
  determination. See Fractions;
    Lowest common
    denominator
  division, 7
Depo-Provera (sterile aqueous
    suspension, sterile
    medroxyprogesterone acetate
    suspension) label, 96f
Desyrel order, 75 mg, 83
Dexamethasone tablets, label,
    104f

Dextrose
  50 mL, 155f
  concentration, percentage, 196, 198, 200, 201
  dextrose (10%) / sodium chloride (0.9%) injection, label, 147f
  grams, calculation, 196, 198, 200
  percentage, calculation, 200
Dextrose (5%). *See* ADD-VANTAGE System
  bag, 149f
  delivery, 188
  injection. *See* Dopamine
    bag, 149f, 306f
    label, 149f. *See also* Lactated Ringer's Injection
  sodium chloride (0.9%) injection
    bag, 151f
    label, 147f, 151f
  sodium chloride (0.45%) injection
    bag, 151f
    label, 147f, 151f
Dextrose (5%) in water (D5W), 139, 171-175
  abbreviations, 146
  continuous infusion, 145
  infusion, 140, 144
  order
    2000 mL, 160
    3000 mL, 162
    calculation, 287
Dextrose injection (5%), label, 146f
Diabetes
  flow sheet, 229f
  management, label, 304f
  medications. *See* Oral diabetes medications
  mellitus, 206
  type, 224
Diapers, calculation, 43
Diaphragm, center, 176f
Diaphragm-plunger, pushing, 116f
Diazepam. *See* Valium
DIC, 236
Diclofenac sodium, labels. *See* Voltaren
Dicloxacillin sodium capsules (500 mg), label, 278f
Digitoxin order, 0.2 mg, 83
Digoxin
  elixir (usage), critical thinking exercise, 276
  label. *See* Lanoxin
  order, 0.5 mg, 177-179

Dilantin (extended phenytoin sodium capsules), 176
  label, 86f, 104f
  order, 0.2g, 87
Dilaudid (hydromorphone HCl), label, 92f, 93f
Diltiazem HCl. *See* Cardizem
Diluents, 116f
  adding, 109, 114, 119-121
    amount, 129-131
  administering, 134
  amount, 138
  calculations, 133-135
  container, holding, 156f
  need, 125
  types, 114
  usage, 125-127
  withdrawal, 115
Dilution
  information. *See* Children
  usage, 133
  verification, 50
Dimensional analysis, 36, 282-283
  final, 291
    answer key, 408
  objectives, 281
Direct IV (bolus) administration, syringe (usage), 176-178
Direct IV medications, Freedom 60 syringe infusion device system (usage), 179f
Dispensing charts, 243
Disposable syringe, usage, 230
Dissolution, delay, 54
Distilled water, amount (usage), 110
Diuril (chlorothiazide) order, 0.05 g, 87
Dividend decimal place, 20
Division, indication, 36
Divisor
  decimal, presence, 21
  examination, 20
  whole number, conversion, 22
Dobutamine order
  2.5 μg/kg/min, 182
  5 μg/kg/min, 183
  100 μg/min, 171
  calculation, 288
Dobutrex
  HCl order, 297
  HCl Solution (20 mg), label, 297f
  order, 150 mg, 161

Documentation, 46
Dopamine
  Dopamine hydrochloride / dextrose (5%) injection (200 mg), label, 184f, 303f
  HCl, order, 288
Dopamine order. *See* Intropin
  2 μg/kg/min, 184
  4 μg/kg/min, 184
  200 μg/min, 171
Dosages. *See* Body weight; Children; Surface area
  calculations, 50, 126
    accuracy, 46, 50
  packages. *See* Unit dose
  range. *See* Coumadin
  reconstitution, practice (worksheet). *See* Parenteral dosages
  reconstitution/administering. *See* Intravenous drugs
  rounding. *See* Medication dosages
Dose. *See* Container; Fractional dose
  amount, 111
  calculation, 94. *See also* Drugs
  difference. *See* Unit dose
  errors. *See* Total dose
  measures. *See* Single-dose measures
  medication. *See* Single-dose medication
  package. *See* Single-dose package; Unit dose
  preparation. *See* Multidose preparation
  problems. *See* Metric dose problems
  rate. *See* Safe dose rate
  reconstitution. *See* Intramuscular doses
  strength discrepancy. *See* Ordered dose
  vials. *See* Multidose vials; Single-dose vials
Dose/flow rate adjustments, 164
Drop factor, 264f, 284
  calculations, 140-141, 144
Dropper. *See* Medicine
Drops
  differentiation. *See* Concentrated drops
  rounding, 74
Drops per minute (by manufacturer), 141f, 142

Drops/min, calculation, 287-290
Drugs
    administration
        accuracy, 46
        six rights, 61-65
    amount, 185
    dose, calculation, 165-167
    flow rate, change, 167
    forms. *See* Liquids; Oral drug
        forms; Solid drug forms
    formula. *See* Titrated infusions
    orders, matching, 61
    overload injury, patient
        protection, 60
    preparation, accuracy, 46
    prioritization. *See* Emergency
        drugs; Stat drugs
    rates, worksheet. *See* Intravenous
        drug rates
    references. *See* Pediatric drug
        references
    sensitivity, 125
    strength, maintenance, 54
    substance, 54
    vials, attachment. *See*
        Unreconstituted drug vial
DVT. *See* Deep vein thrombosis
Diphenhydramine HCl. *See*
        Benadryl Allergy Liquid
Dyphylline elixir. *See* Lufyllin

E

Electrolytes, 77
Electronic infusion
    devices, 156-158, 157f. *See also*
        Intravenous electronic
        infusion device
        setting, 159
    pump, volume control device,
        264f
Elixirs, 54
    differentiation, 260
Emergency drugs,
        prioritization, 61
Emulsions, 54
    admixture. *See* Fats
Enoxaparin. *See* Lovenox
Enteric-coated tablets, 54, 55f
Entry errors, avoidance, 60
Entry site, 154
Epinephrine, usage, 125
Equivalence, maintenance, 7, 8
Equivalency tables, 84
Equivalent fractions
    change, higher terms (usage), 8
    fractions, change, 7

Errors. *See* Medication errors;
        Ounces conversion;
        Pounds conversion
    avoidance, 178. *See also* Entry
        errors
    documentation, 52
    factors, contribution, 246
    reduction, 51
EryPed 400, label.
        See Erythromycin
        Ethylsuccinate
Erythromycin Ethylsuccinate
    oral suspension (200 mg)
        calculation, 289
        label, 80f, 108f, 113f, 132f,
            260f, 277f, 284f
        order, calculation, 260
    suspension (EryPed 400), label,
        251f
Esmolol hydrochloride order,
        39 mL/hr, 175
Expiration date, 52, 52f, 117. *See also*
        Medication
Extended care facilities, 156
Extended phenytoin sodium
        capsules, label.
        See Dilantin
Extended-release capsules, 55f
Extracts, usage, 55. *See also* Fluid
        extracts

F

Fast-acting insulin, 210
    mixtures, 211
Fats
    emulsions, admixture, 195
    usage, 54
Femur, compound fracture, 278
Ferrous sulfate tablets, label, 99f
Fibrillation. *See* Atrial fibrillation;
        Ventricular fibrillation
Final. *See* Comprehensive final;
        Multiple-choice final
Flow rates, 138, 172. *See also*
        Pre-set flow rate; Volume
        control device
    adjustment. *See* Dose/flow rate
        adjustments
    calculations. *See* Two-step IV flow
        rate calculations
    change. *See* Drugs
    consultation, 164
    formula. *See* Titrated infusions
    information. *See* Children
    worksheet. *See* Intravenous flow
        rates

Fluid
    amounts, 262
    extracts, usage, 55
    restriction, 164
Fluoxetine hydrochloride. *See*
        Prozac
Flushing ranges. *See* Intermittent
        flushing ranges
Foscavir order, 200 mL, 160
Fractional dose, 61
Fractions. *See* Decimal fractions
    calculation. *See* Reduced
        fraction
    change. *See* Decimals;
        Equivalent fractions
    common denominator,
        determination, 6-7
    decimals, change, 24
        worksheet, 24
        worksheet, answer key, 316
    difference. *See* Common
        fractions
    division, 31
    numerator, sum, 5
    percentages, change, 28
    reduction, lowest terms, 1, 7-8
    usage, 4, 28-30
    value, 13-14
        worksheet, 14
        worksheet, answer key, 312
    worksheet, 29
        answer key, 318
Fractions/mixed numbers
    addition, 8-9
        worksheet, 9
        worksheet, answer key, 310
    division, 12-13
        worksheet, 13
        worksheet, answer key, 311
    multiplication, 11-12
        worksheet, 12
        worksheet, answer key, 311
    subtraction, 10-11
        worksheet, 11
        worksheet, answer key, 310-311
Fragmin (dalteparin), 237
    9.5 mL multidose vial, 238f, 240f,
        305f
    order
        18,000 units, 296
        calculation, 237, 240, 245-246
    single-dose prefilled syringes,
        237f
Freedom 60 syringe infusion device
        system, 264f
    usage. *See* Direct IV medications

Furosemide, 176
  injection, label (40 mg/4 mL),
    267f, 304f
  order
    20 mg, 180
    30 mg, 181

G

Garamycin order (50 mg),
    calculation, 275
Gemfibrozil tablets, label.
    See Lopid
Generic name, 52f, 56, 57-58, 117
Gentamicin
  bag (60 mg), 306f
  order, 160
    100 mL, 144
Gentamycin order, 80 mg, 291
Geopen (carbenicillin disodium)
  IM order, 1 g, 299
  label (5 g), 268f
Glipizide order, 5000 μg, 88
Glucagon emergency kit, usage,
    206f
Glucophage (metformin
    hydrochloride tablets)
  label, 85f
  order, calculation, 233
Glucose tablets, 206
Grains (gr), confusion, 99
Grams
  change, 76
  conversion, 71, 282
Granules, 54
Gravity flow
  calibration, 141f
  IV piggyback, 154f
Gravity infusion, microdrip tubing,
    264f
Gravity IV, 74
Gravity piggyback infusions, 154
Gtt/min, calculations, 143-145, 162

H

Halcion (triazolam)
  order, 125 μg, 87
  tablets, label, 96f
HD/HV ratio. *See* Hourly
    drug/hourly volume ratio
Hematocrit level, 243
Hematoma development, 238
Hemodialysis, 236
Heparin. *See* Intravenous heparin;
    Titrated heparin
  flush, injection, 242
  half-life, 236, 237

Heparin *(Continued)*
  injections. *See* Subcutaneous
    heparin injections
  IV bolus, 291
  IV flushes, 242
  lock, 242. *See also* Intermittent
    heparin lock; Saline/heparin
    lock
    flush solution, label, 242f. *See
      also* Hepflush
  order, calculation, 238-241, 245-
    248
  resistance, 241
  titration, 245
Heparin order
  10,000 units, 288
  20,000 units, 290
  50,000 units, 289
Heparin sodium
  injection, usage, 236
  IV, bolus, 245
  units, calculation, 243-244
Heparin sodium injection, label
  1,000 USP, 241f
  5,000 USP, 238f, 241f, 247f
  10,000 USP, 239f, 240f, 247f
  20,000 USP, 239f, 240f, 247f, 286
Heparin sodium IV (10,000 units),
    297
Hepatitis B vaccine, label, 54f
Hepflush*-10 (Heparin lock flush
    solution), label (10 mL), 78f,
    242f
High-use floor stock, monitoring,
    49f
Home infusion pharmacy, label,
    193f
Hospitals
  bed, calculation, 43
  pharmacies, 264
  protocol, 242
Hourly drug/hourly volume
    (HD/HV) ratio, 165, 169
  calculation, 170-175
Household designations, 97
Household measurements
  approximate equivalents, 97t
  comparison, worksheet, 97-99
    answer key, 346
Household system, 97-98
Household utensils, substitution, 55
Huff cap, 138
Humalog insulin
  clarity, 226f
  lispro injection (10 mL), label,
    210f

Humalog insulin *(Continued)*
  order, calculations, 223,
    232-233
  vials, 209f
Human insulin
  calculations, 227-228
  order, calculation, 226
  production, 207
Humulin
  50/50 (human insulin isophane
    suspension / human insulin
    injection) label (10 mL),
    211f
  70/30 (human insulin isophane
    suspension / human insulin
    injection)
    label (10 mL), 211f
    order, calculation, 223
  U (Ultralente) human insulin,
    label (10 mL), 211f, 217f
Humulin L (Lente) human insulin
    zinc suspension
  label (10 mL), 210f, 218f
  order, calculation, 223, 233
  vials, 209
Humulin N (NPH)
  60 units, order, 219
  human insulin (10 mL), 210f,
    217f
  multidose vials. *See* Intermediate-
    acting insulin
  order, calculation, 223, 232
Humulin R (Regular)
  15 units, order, 219
  air, injection, 219f
  calculations, 228, 232-233, 286,
    296
  insulin
    (30 units). *See* U-100 Humulin
      R insulin
    human injection, label (10
      mL), 79f, 210f, 216f,
      306f
  order, calculation, 223
Hydrocortisone sodium succinate
    (injection), label. *See* Solu-
    Cortef
Hydromorphone HCl, label. *See*
    Dilaudid
Hydroxyzine hydrochloride. *See*
    Vistaril
Hyperglycemia, 195
Hyperlipemia, 248
Hypoglycemia, 206
Hypokalemia, 183
Hypothyroidism, 275

I

IA. *See* Intraarterial
Ibuprofen. *See* Motrin
Illness, acute phases, 226
IM. *See* Intramuscular
Imipramine pamoate.
    See Tofranil-PM
Immobilized patients, 236
Improper fractions, 33
    change, 1. *See also* Mixed
        numbers; Whole numbers
    mixed numbers, change, 5
        worksheet, 5
        worksheet, answer key, 309-310
    numerator, 4
Infants, injection site, 262f
Infants' Tylenol (concentrated
        drops), label, 82f, 273f
Infusion. *See* Continuous infusion;
        Gravity piggyback infusions;
        Intermittent infusion;
        Intravenous infusions;
        Piggyback; Titrated infusions
    aminophylline, usage, 165f
    microdrip tubing. *See* Gravity
        infusion
    pumps, volume control device.
        See Electronic infusion
    time, calculation, 161
    worksheet. *See* Solutions
Infusion devices. *See* Electronic
        infusion; Insulin; Pressure-
        flow infusion device
    calculations worksheet, 160
        answer key, 366-367
    programmable. *See* Sigma
        international 6000
        programmable infusion
        device
    setting, 196, 198
    usage, 142. *See also* Direct IV
        medications
Injectable anticoagulants, 236-242
Injections. *See* Subcutaneous
        heparin injections
    giving. *See* Intramuscular
        injections
    port, 176f
    sites, 51. *See also* Infants; Insulin
        massage, 238
    worksheet. *See* Subcutaneous
        injections
INR. *See* International Normalized
        Ratio
Insert needle. *See* Syringes
Inservice, allotment, 43

Inside numbers, multiplication, 37,
        38, 40
Insulin, 206. *See also* Fast-acting
        insulin; Intermediate-acting
        insulin; Intravenous insulin;
        Long-acting insulin
    30 units. *See* U-100 Humulin R
        insulin
    amount, determination, 225f
    blood glucose flow sheet, 225f
    change. *See* Pork insulin
    chart, 209t
    clarity, 210
    clumps, 226f
    contamination, 220
    critical thinking exercises, 232
    deficiency, 206
    dosages, 219
    drawing up, 220
    drip, 295
    final, 232-233
        answer key, 385
    glargine. *See* Lantus
    infusion
        chart, 227f
        devices, 230
    injection, 206
        areas, 207f
        sites, 207
    mixing, 210, 219-223, 219f
        worksheet, 221-223
        worksheet, answer key, 381
    multiple-choice practice,
        worksheet, 231
        answer key, 384
    name, 213
    objectives, 205
    orders, 213, 224
    pens, 208f
    production. *See* Human insulin
    resistance, 206, 224
    route, 213
    sliding scale calculations, 224-225
    syringes, 208f, 212. *See also* U-100
        insulin
        calculation, 43
        calibration, 212
        types, 207-209. *See also* U-100
            insulin
        units, number, 213
Insulin, single-dose measures
    practice, worksheet, 216-218
        answer key, 381
    worksheet, 214-215
        answer key, 381
Integrilin, 244

Intensive care units, 253
InterLink IV Access System, 153f
Intermediate-acting insulin, 210,
        219
    (Humulin N), multidose vials, 49f
    mixtures, 211
Intermittent flushing ranges, 139t
Intermittent heparin lock, 176
Intermittent infusion, 158
Intermittent IV therapy, 243
International Normalized Ratio
        (INR), 244, 245
International System of Units (SI),
        70
International time, 58, 65
Intraarterial (IA) lines, 236
Intramuscular (IM) doses,
        reconstitution, 119
Intramuscular (IM) injections,
        giving, 116
Intramuscular (IM) medications. *See*
        Children
Intramuscular (IM) preparation, 53
Intramuscular (IM) use, 126, 271,
        275
Intravenous (IV) administration,
        syringe (usage). *See* Direct IV
        administration
Intravenous (IV) bags
    percentage numbers, 146
    solute, percentage, 146
Intravenous (IV) calculations, 139-
        142. *See also* Advanced
        intravenous calculations
    aminophylline, usage (worksheet),
        173
        answer key, 371-372
    critical thinking exercises, 162
    final, 162
        answer key, 369
    multiple-choice practice,
        worksheet, 161
        answer key, 367-369
    objectives, 137
    practice, worksheet, 144-145
        answer key, 361-363
    usage, worksheet. *See* Obstetrics
    worksheet, 143
        answer key, 361
Intravenous (IV) delivery sets, 152-
        160
Intravenous (IV) drugs
    dosages, reconstitution/
        administering, 155f
    rates, worksheet, 169
        answer key, 370

Intravenous (IV) electronic infusion
device, 73
Intravenous (IV) flow
rates, worksheet, 169
sheet, 152f
Intravenous (IV) flushes, 242
Intravenous (IV) heparin, 243
calculations, worksheet, 243-244
answer key, 388-389
Intravenous (IV) infusions, 138
pump, 279
Intravenous (IV) insulin, 226-229
calculations, worksheet, 227-228
answer key, 382
Intravenous (IV) lines. *See* Occlude
IV line; Peripheral IV lines
types, 138-139
Intravenous (IV) medications. *See*
Children
Freedom 60 syringe infusion
device system, usage. *See*
Direct IV medications
Intravenous (IV) orders, evaluation
(worksheet). *See* Critical care
intravenous orders
Intravenous (IV) practice problems,
worksheet, 175
answer key, 373
Intravenous (IV) pumps, 139
Intravenous (IV) push, 176
calculations, worksheet, 179-180
answer key, 373
medications, timing methods,
176-178
Intravenous (IV) set, 167
primary set (roller clamp), 153f
Intravenous (IV) solutions
abbreviations, 146
dilution, 264
usage, 265
Intravenous (IV) systems. *See*
Needleless IV systems
Intravenous (IV) therapy. *See*
Continuous IV therapy;
Intermittent IV therapy
MAR, example, 152f
Intravenous piggyback (IVPB), 155f,
231. *See also* Gravity flow;
Premixed frozen IVPBs
admixtures, 155
infusions (50 mL), 154f
Intropin (dopamine), order, 166
Isoniazid tablets, label (100 mg),
104f, 301f
Iso-osmotic sterile solution, 154

Isoproterenol hydrochloride, order.
See Isuprel
Isotonic saline, 242
Isuprel (isoproterenol
hydrochloride), 5 μg/min
(order), 172, 181
IV. *See* Intravenous
IV rate. *See* Positional IV rate
IVPB. *See* Intravenous piggyback

K

Kantrex (300 mg), order, 160
KCl. *See* Potassium chloride
Keflin (sodium cephalothin)
order
1g/mL, 291
2 g, 160
usage, 135, 136
Ketoacidosis, 230
Kilocalories (Kcal), 195
calculation, 196, 198, 200-202
per bag. *See* Bag
Kilograms, change, 76

L

Labels. *See* Medication labels
reading. *See* Liquids
reconstitution. *See* Medication
validation, physician order. *See*
Total Parenteral Nutrition
Lactated Ringer's Injection
bag, 149f, 150f
dextrose (5%) injection
bag, 149f, 307f
label, 149f
label, 79f, 150f
Lactated Ringer's solution, order,
144
Lanoxin (Digoxin)
0.125 mg, order, 101
capsule, 80f
injection, label, 104f
IV push 0.5 mg, order, 181
label, 79f
order, 83, 87, 100
tablet (125 μg), 81f
label, 81f, 294f
Lantus (insulin glargine), 209f
15 units, order, 231
administering, 231
injection, label (100 units/mL),
211f
mixing, caution, 211
L-Dopa (levodopa), 2 g (order), 100
Lente vials. *See* Humulin L

Leucovorin Calcium tablets
label (5 mg), 260f, 280f, 302f
order, calculation, 260
Leukemia, 274
Levodopa. *See* L-Dopa
Levothyroxine sodium, tablets. *See*
Synthroid
Lid protector, removal, 116f
Lidocaine
addition, 114
order
4 mg/min, 172
500 mL, 181
Lighted Matrix Drawer, 49f
Lincocin (lincomycin hydrochloride
injection)
IM order, 0.3g, 298
label (300 mg/mL), 65f, 95f, 298f
Lines, types. *See* Intravenous lines
Lipids
administration, 195
concentration, 189, 192
percentage, 196, 198
solutions, 195
usage, 196-198
Liposyn II (fat emulsion), usage. *See*
Parenteral nutrition
Liquid medications
administering, practice
(worksheet), 108-113
answer key, 347-350
measurement, 106-113
practice, worksheet, 108-113
reconstitution, practice
(worksheet), 108-113
single-dose package, 55f
Liquids
amount, addition, 267
drug forms, 54-56
labels, reading, 82
measure. *See* Medicine cup
sedimentation, checking, 48
Liters
calculation. *See* Milliliters
change, 76
rounding. *See* Milliliters
Long-acting insulin, 211
Long-term care centers, 155
Lopid (gemfibrozil) tablets, label, 886f
Lopressor, 329
label, 56f
Lorabid (loracarbef, oral suspension)
label
100 mg, 110f, 131
200 mg, 111f, 117f, 284f

Lovenox (enoxaparin), 237
    order, calculation, 238
Lowest common denominator, 31
    determination, 1, 6, 10
    usage, 8
Lufyllin (dyphylline elixir) label
    (473 mL), 270f
Luminal (sodium injection,
    phenobarbital sodium
    injection), label, 98f,
    266f

M

Macro drip, 141f
Magnesium sulfate, 192, 195
    additive, 202
    percentage, 200
Magnesium sulfate order
    2 g/hr, 174
    25 mL/hr, 174
    30 mL/hr, 182
Markers, schedule, 178
MARs. *See* Medication
    administration records
Mathematics
    final (test), 33-34
        answer key, 320-321
    foundation, 331
    multiple-choice practice,
        worksheet, 31-32
        answer key, 320
    objectives, 3
    self-assessment, 1-2
        answer key, 309
µg/min, calculation, 287-290
Measurement, metric system, 55
Measuring
    cup, 106f
    teaspoon, 74f
MedFlo postoperative gain
        management system
        ambulatory infusion
        device, 157f
Medication. *See* Children; Oral
        diabetes medications
    administration, 51, 242
        ADD-VANTAGE system,
            usage, 156f
        days, 61
    amount, 128
        questioning, 84
        tolerance, 120
    ampules, usage, 50f
    assembling, ADD-VANTAGE
        system (usage), 156f

Medication *(Continued)*
    calculation problems, solving, 75
    carts, 48
    cup, 103
    dissolving, 115
    documentation, 51-52
    dropper, 56f
    effects, 52
    evaluation, 52
    expiration date, 331
    history, 125
    ID, carrying, 61
    incident report, 60
        example, 64f
    interventions, 52
    measurement, 97. *See also* Liquid
        medications
    orders, 65
        discrepancy, 84
        verification/interpretation, 46
    packaging, 48-50
    physical properties, 114
    placement. *See* Volume control
        device
    preparation, 48
        reference, 50
    problems, 75
        worksheet. *See* One-step oral
            medication problems
    reconstitution, 114. *See also*
        Liquid medications
    refusal, 51f
    reporting, 51-52
    supplies, 46
        control, 226
    tablets, supply values, 72
    time given, data, 60
    timing methods. *See* Intravenous
        push medications
    type, 53f
    utensils, 55
    vials, usage, 50f
Medication administration records
        (MARs), 123f
    date, 60
    example. *See* Intravenous
        therapy
    interpretation, worksheet, 61
        answer key, 330
    prioritization, 60
    reconfirming, 48
    sample, 62f, 123f, 203f, 237f.
        See also PRN orders
    understanding, 60-61
    usage, 303

Medication dosages
    calculation, 17
    infusion, worksheet. *See* Solutions
    rounding, 26, 73-74
    units/milliequivalents,
        understanding (worksheet),
        77-79
        answer key, 335
Medication errors
    avoidance, 46-52
    critical thinking exercises, 67-68,
        101
    multiple-choice practice,
        worksheet, 65-66
        answer key, 330-331
    objective, 45
    reduction, 156
    reporting, 60
Medication labels, 50, 289
    interpretation, 52-58
    multiple-choice practice,
        worksheet, 65-66
        answer key, 330-331
    objectives, 45
    reading/understanding, 46
    reconstitution, 117
    worksheet, 56-58
        answer key, 329
Medication powders/crystals
    critical thinking exercises, 132
    final, 133-136
        answer key, 359-360
    multiple-choice practice,
        worksheet, 130-132
        answer key, 357-359
    objectives, 105
Medication records
    critical thinking exercises, 67-68
    multiple-choice practice,
        worksheet, 65-66
        answer key, 330-331
    objectives, 45
    verification, 50
Medication-related problem, 52, 65
Medicine
    cup
        liquid measure, 55f
        usage, 106f
    dropper, 74f
    withdrawal, syringe (usage), 74f
Medley Medication Safety System,
        157f
Medrol. *See* Solu-Medrol
    methylprednisolone tablets, label,
        95f

Meniscus, 55, 106f
Mental status, 51
Meperidine HCl, 176
Meperidine (HCL injection), label
 50 mg/mL, 271f, 294f
 75 mg/mL, 91f, 92f, 103f, 185f,
 262f
Meperidine HCl order
 10 mg, 180
 35 mg. *See* Demerol
 calculation, 275
mEq/L, 77
mEq/mL, 77
Metformin hydrochloride tablets,
 label. *See* Glucophage
Methotrexate order, 3.3 mg/m², 297
Methotrexate sodium, order
 calculation, 274
Methylprednisolone
 sodium succinate (injection),
 label. *See* Solu-Medrol
 tablets, label. *See* Medrol
Metoprolol tartrate, 329
Metric conversions, decimals
 (movement), 71-72
 worksheet, 72
 answer key, 332
Metric conversions, usage, 80
Metric dose problems, 75
Metric equivalents. *See* Unit dose
 problems, 75
 usage, 85
 worksheet. *See* One-step metric
 equivalents
Metric measurements, 71t
 approximate equivalents, 97t
 comparison, worksheet, 97-99
 answer key, 346
Metric one-step calculations, 75
Metric one-step oral problems,
 worksheet, 94-96
Metric one-step parenteral
 problems, worksheet,
 94-96
 answer key, 344-345
Metric one-step ratio, 75
Metric oral one-step practice
 problems, worksheet, 83
 answer key, 336
Metric oral two-step problems,
 worksheet, 85-88
 answer key, 337-340
Metric parenteral mixes, worksheet,
 91-94
 answer key, 342-344
Metric prefixes, 71t

Metric system, 55, 70-71. *See also*
 Measurement
Metric system calculations
 critical thinking exercises, 101
 final (test), 102-104
 answer key, 347
 multiple-choice practice,
 worksheet, 100
 answer key, 347
 objectives, 69
Metric two-step oral problems,
 worksheet, 94-96
Metric two-step parenteral
 problems, worksheet, 94-96
 answer key, 344-345
Metric values, 71t
Mg/Kg
 method, 250-252
 orders, comparison, 257
 problems, solving (steps), 250-252
Mg/Lb orders, comparison, 257
Mg/M². *See* Body surface area
MI, 236
Microdrip, 141f, 162
 order, 145
 set, 141
 tubing, 164. *See also* Gravity
 infusion
Micrograms
 change, 76
 conversion, 71
 milligrams, difference, 169
Midanterolateral thigh, site
 preference, 262, 262f
Military time, 58, 65
Milliequivalents, understanding
 (worksheet). *See* Medication
Milligrams
 change, 76
 conversion, 71
Milliliters
 adding/administering, 108-113
 calculation, 91
 per hour, 139
 rounding, 73
Milliunit, 77
Mini-Bag Plus Container, 155f
Minoxidil tablets, label, 103f
Miradon. *See* Anisindione
Mixed numbers
 addition. *See* Fractions/mixed
 numbers
 change, 11. *See also* Improper
 fractions
 division. *See* Fractions/mixed
 numbers

Mixed numbers *(Continued)*
 improper fractions, change, 4-5
 worksheet, 5
 multiplication. *See*
 Fractions/mixed numbers
 subtraction. *See* Fractions/mixed
 numbers
Mixing options, 128
Mix-o-vial directions, 116f
mL/hour. *See* Pump
 calculations, 143-145, 287-290
Morphine sulfate (MS) injection
 label
 10 mg/ml, 94f, 263f, 279f
 15 mg/mL, 298f
 order, 5 mg, 298
Motrin (ibuprofen) tablets, label,
 95f
MS. *See* Morphine sulfate
Multidose preparation, 53f
Multidose vials, 118, 246. *See also*
 Intermediate-acting insulin;
 Regular insulin
 calculation, 44
Multiple-choice final, 293-299
 answer key, 409
Multiple-dose vial, 117

N

Naloxone HCl injection label
 (400 µg/mL), 293f
Naproxen order, 0.5 g, 88
Nearest hundredth, rounding, 74
Nearest tenth, rounding, 73
Nebcin (tobramycin sulfate)
 IV order, 60 mg, 298
 label (20 mg/2 mL), 268f, 279f,
 298f
Needle. *See* Contaminated needle;
 Pre-filled sterile
 cartridge/needle;
 Syringes
 lengths, 262
 size, 152f
 withdrawal, 219f
Needleless IV systems, 153, 153f
Needleless resealable valves, 138
Nembutal (0.1 g), order, 100
Nipride (sodium nitroprusside),
 order, 175
Nitroglycerin (10 µg/min), order,
 175
Nitroprusside sodium order, 30 mg,
 287
Nitrostat (Nitroglycerin) tablets,
 label, 98f

Norepinephrine order
  1 mg in 250 mL of N/S, 181
  50 mL/hr infusion, 172
Normal saline (NS)
  0.9% bag, 148f
  0.45% bag, 148f
  abbreviations, 146
  order
    250 mL, 160
    calculation, 286
  usage, 114, 144, 180, 226
Nosebleeds, 241
Novolin L (Lente)
  human insulin zinc suspension
    (10 mL), 210f, 220f
  order, 20 units, 220
Novolin R (Regular)
  human insulin injection (10 mL),
    210f, 216f, 220f
  multidose vials. See Regular
    insulin
  order, 10 units, 220
NPH vials, 209f
NPO, 62, 188, 331
NS. See Normal saline
Numerator, 28
  addition, 8
  division, 7
  sum. See Fractions
Nurse-activated piggyback systems,
    155-156
Nursing
  considerations. See Total
    Parenteral Nutrition
  process, usage, 274
Nutrition. See Parenteral nutrition
  calculations, worksheet. See Central
    Parenteral Nutrition;
    Peripheral Parenteral Nutrition
  tubing. See Total Parenteral
    Nutrition

O

Obstetrics, IV calculations usage
    (worksheet), 174
  answer key, 372
Occlude IV line, 176f
ODMs. See Oral diabetes
    medications
Oils, usage, 54
One-step calculation,
    determination, 84, 94-96
One-step metric equivalents
  problems, 76
  worksheet, 76
    answer key, 332-334

One-step metric proportion
    calculations, 75-83
One-step metric ratio calculations,
    75-83
One-step oral medication problems,
    worksheet, 80-82
  answer key, 335
Oral anticoagulants, 244
Oral diabetes medications (ODMs),
    230
Oral drug forms, 54-56. See also
    Solid oral drug forms
Oral liquid medicine.
    See Syringes
Oral medications. See Children
  problems, worksheet. See One-
    step oral medication
    problems
Oral one-step practice problems,
    worksheet. See Metric
    oral one-step practice
    problems
Oral syringes, 107f. See also Prefilled
    oral syringe
Oral two-step problems, worksheet.
    See Metric oral two-step
    problems
Ordered amount, withdrawal, 265
Ordered dose
  dilution, 122
  SDR, limits, 264
  strength discrepancy, 73
Orders
  clarification, 48
  critical thinking exercises, 67-68,
    101
  expiration, 61
  matching. See Drugs
  multiple-choice practice, 65-66
  nurse, initialing, 47f
  objectives, 45
  rechecking, 51, 73
  safety, 165
  verification/interpretation. See
    Medication
Osteomyelitis, 124
Ounces conversion, errors, 252
Outside numbers, multiplication,
    37, 38, 40
Overdose, 269, 275
  orders, calculation (caution),
    262
  symptoms, 241
Oxacillin sodium
  dilution, sterile water (usage),
    115f

Oxacillin sodium (Continued)
  injection, label
    1 g, 129f
    500 mg, 115f, 118f, 124f, 125f,
      133f, 263f
Oxytocin. See Pitocin

P

Pancreas, stimulation, 230
Parenteral dosages, reconstitution
    practice (worksheet), 118-122
  answer key, 350-353
  worksheet, 124-128
  answer key, 354-356
Parenteral mixes, worksheet. See
    Metric parenteral mixes
Parenteral Nutrition (PN)
  calculations, 284
    worksheet. See Central Parenteral
      Nutrition; Peripheral
      Parenteral Nutrition
  critical thinking exercises, 204
  final, 204
    answer key, 380
  formula, 204
  Liposyn II (fat emulsion), usage,
    190f
  multiple-choice practice,
    worksheet, 202-203
    answer key, 380
  objectives, 187
  solution
    order, calculation, 289
    total volume, 202
  tubing. See Total Parenteral
    Nutrition
Partial thromboplastin time (PTT)
  levels, 236
  results, 245
  tests, 237
Patient safety, 46
  critical thinking exercises, 67-68
  implications, 257
  multiple-choice practice, 65-66
  objective, 45
Patient-care setting, 168
Patient-controlled analgesia (PCA),
    157
Patients. See Ambulatory patients;
    Confined patients;
    Immobilized patients
  allergies, reconfirming, 51, 61
  assessment, 46
  feedback, 51
  ID, 60
    carrying, 61

Patients *(Continued)*
  intervention/follow-up, 46
  muscle mass, assessment, 120
  overdosing, avoidance, 74
  protection, 46. *See also* Drugs
  record, clarification, 48
  response, 166
  surname, 61
  weight, 170, 184
PCA. *See* Patient-controlled
  analgesia
PCN label, sample, 201f
PE. *See* Pulmonary embolus
Pediatric drug references, 264
Pediatric IV
  dilutions/administration
  rates, 267
Pediatric IV drug references,
  consultation, 267
Pediatric medication
  administration, 251
  orders, references (checking), 250
Pediatric units, 253
Penicillin
  allergies, 277
  order. *See* Aqueous penicillin
    600,000 units, 291
Penicillin G potassium injection
  label, one million units, 118f,
    126f, 133f. *See also* Pfizerpen
  order, 132
    five million units, 306
Percent number, 28
Percentage of concentration per bag.
  See Bag
Percentages
  change. *See* Decimals; Fractions
  decimals, conversion, 28
  finding, 30
    worksheet, 30
    worksheet, answer key, 319
  usage, 28-30
    worksheet, 29
    answer key, 318
Percocet, calculation, 68
Peripheral arterial embolization, 248
Peripheral central line, 201f
Peripheral inserted central catheter
  (PICC), 138, 139f
Peripheral IV lines, 138, 242
Peripheral Parenteral Nutrition
  (PPN), 189
  calculation, worksheet, 198-199
    answer key, 377-378
  order, 204
    solution, 288

Petechiae, 241
Pfizerpen (penicillin G potassium,
  injection) label
  five million units, 78f, 127f,
    134f, 306f
  one million units, 120f, 122f,
    128f, 129f, 283f
Pharmacology reference, 50
Phenobarbital
  order, 83
  Sodium injection, label. *See*
    Luminal
Phenytoin oral suspension, order
  suspension, 275
Phenytoin sodium
  capsules, label. *See* Dilantin
  IV loading dose, order, 179
Physical trauma, 262
Physician order. *See* Total Parenteral
  Nutrition
  checking, 190
  handwritten order, 47f
  sample, 191f, 194f, 197f, 199f
PICC. *See* Peripheral inserted
  central catheter
Piggyback
  infusions, 159
    50 mL. *See* Intravenous
      piggyback
  medications, 154
  order, 161
  port. *See* Primary set
  premixed IVs, 154-155
  systems. *See* Nurse-activated
    piggyback systems
Pitocin (oxytocin) order
  2 mU/min, 174
  20 mU/min, 174
Plain tablets, 54, 55f
Plants, concentrated alcoholic
  liquid extract, 55
PN. *See* Parenteral Nutrition
Pneumonia, 133
Polycillin (ampicillin), usage,
  135
Pork insulin, change, 207
Portal site, 153
Positional IV rate, 142
Postoperative patient, nausea,
  102
Potassium acetate, additive, 202
Potassium chloride (KCl)
  30 mEq (syringe), 183
  label (40 mEq), 79f, 183f,
    272f
  percentage, 200

Potassium chloride (KCl) order
  10 mEq, 183
  20 mEq, 83
  elixir (20 mEq), 100
Potassium phosphate, 192, 195
  percentage, 200
Pounds, conversion, 282
  errors, 252
Powdered drug, usage, 116f
Powders, 54. *See also* Medication
  powders/crystals
  accuracy. *See* Reconstituted
    powder
  dilution. *See* Vials
  form. *See* Antibiotics
  volume, 115
PPN. *See* Peripheral Parenteral
  Nutrition
Prednisone, calculation, 68
Preferred routes, 164
Prefilled cartridges, delivery, 116
Prefilled oral syringe, 259f
Pre-filled sterile cartridge/needle,
  117f
Prefilled syringe. *See* Fragmin
  delivery, 116
Premeal blood glucose level, 230
Premixed frozen IVPBs, 155
Premixed IVs. *See* Piggyback
Preparation
  directions, 53
  instructions, 52
Prepared syringe, calibrated
  increments, 176
Pre-set flow rate, 158
Pressure-flow infusion device, 158
Preventive therapy, 104
Primary set
  piggyback port, 153f
  roller clamp. *See* Intravenous set
PRN cap, 138
PRN orders, 62
  computer-generated MAR,
    sample, 63f
Procainamide hydrochloride. *See*
  Pronestyl
Procanbid (Procainamide HCl),
  label, 85f
Prochlorperazine. *See* Compazine
Promethazine HCl tablets, label,
  102f
Pronestyl (procainamide
  hydrochloride) order
  40 mL/hr, 182
  50 mL/hr, 175
  60 mg/hr, 182

Proportion. *See* Ratio/proportion
  calculations. *See* One-step metric
    proportion calculations;
    Two-step metric proportion
    calculations
  conversions, usage, 80
  equivalents, usage, 85
  final (test), 44
    answer key, 329
  multiple-choice practice,
    worksheet, 43
    answer key, 328
  objectives, 35
  practice problems, solving, 37-40
    worksheet, 38-40
    worksheet, answer key, 322-325
  problems, 75
  setup, 40-42
    worksheet, 41-42
    worksheet, answer key, 325-328
  usage, 42-44, 259, 266, 276
Proprietary name, 117
Protamine sulfate
  antagonist, 243
  usage, 236
Prothrombin (PT) test, 244
Prozac liquid (fluoxetine
    hydrochloride oral solution)
    label (20 mg/5mL), 301f
Pruritic rash, 277
PT. *See* Prothrombin
PTT. *See* Partial thromboplastin time
Pulmonary embolus (PE), 236, 245,
    248
  prevention, 237
Pump. *See* Electronic infusion;
    Intravenous pumps
  setting, mL/hour, 192
Push calculations, worksheet. *See*
    Intravenous push
    calculations
Push medications, timing methods.
    See Intravenous push
    medications

Q

Qualified resources, usage, 46
Quinidine sulfate (0.3 g), order, 100

R

Ratio
  calculations. *See* One-step metric
    ratio calculations; Two-step
    metric ratio calculations
  conversions, usage, 80
  equivalents, usage, 85

Ratio *(Continued)*
  expression (fractions), 36
    worksheet, 36
    worksheet, answer key, 321
  final (test), 44
    answer key, 329
  multiple-choice practice,
    worksheet, 43
    answer key, 328
  objectives, 35
  setup, 40-42
    worksheet, 41-42
    worksheet, answer key, 325-328
  usage, 42-44, 56-58. *See also*
    Written ratio
Recombinant DNA technology,
    207
Reconstituted parenteral dosages.
    See Parenteral dosages
Reconstituted powder, accuracy, 116
Reconstitution, 285. *See also*
    Medication labels
  directions, 119
  information. *See* Children
  label, 119f
  practice. *See* Liquid medications;
    Parenteral dosages
Records. *See* Medication records
Reduced fraction, calculation, 140
Regular insulin
  clarity, 226f
  intravenous use, 226
  (Novolin R), multidose vials
    (10 mL), 49f
Regular vials, 209f
Renal status, 224
Resuscitation equipment, 125
Rifadin (rifampin capsules), 329
  label, 57f, 78f, 85f
Rifampin, 329
Ringer's lactate order, 500 mL, 286,
    287, 290
Rocephin (Ceftriaxone sodium,
    injection) label
  1 g, 272f, 296
  500 mg, 126f
Roller clamp. *See* Intravenous set
Route. *See* Insulin; Preferred routes
  usage, 65

S

Safe dose rate (SDR), 104, 173-175.
    See also 24-hour dose; Unit
    dose
  applicability, determination,
    171-172

Safe dose rate (SDR) *(Continued)*
  calculation, 250, 253-254, 262-
    263, 269-274
  estimation. *See* Children
  evaluation, 165
  limits. *See* Ordered dose
  ordered dosage, comparison, 251
  practice, worksheet. *See* Children
  recommendation, 166. *See also*
    Children
  usage, 263, 276-280, 287-290
Saline lock, 138
Saline/heparin lock, 138f
Scored tablets, 54, 55f, 81, 291. *See
    also* Unscored tablets
Septicemia, 262
Sequential numbering system, 58
Serum potassium levels, 195
Shelf life, 117-119, 125-127
SI. *See* International System of
    Units; Système International
    d'Unités
Side effects, 52
Sigma 8000 automatic dose-related
    calculation device, 189f
Sigma international 6000
    programmable infusion
    device, 189f
Single-dose measures, worksheet. *See*
    Insulin
Single-dose medication, 48
Single-dose package. *See* Liquid
    medications
Single-dose vials, 53f
  label, 119f
Six rights. *See* Drugs
Skin integrity, 51
Sliding scale calculations. *See*
    Insulin
Sodium bicarbonate, label, 53f
Sodium cephalothin, usage. *See*
    Keflin
Sodium chloride, 192, 195. *See also*
    Dextrose
  0.9% injection
    bag, 148f
    label, 148f, 305f
  0.45% injection label/bag, 148f
  order, 288, 291
  percentage, 200
Sodium nitroprusside. *See* Nipride
Solid drug forms, 54
Solid oral drug forms, 55f
Solu-Cortef (hydrocortisone sodium
    succinate, injection) label
    (250 mg), 95f, 285f

Solu-Medrol (methylprednisolone sodium succinate injection) label, 95f

Solute g/mL (calculations), worksheet, 160
answer key, 366-367

Solute percentage. *See* Intravenous bags

Solutions
abbreviations. *See* Intravenous solutions
concentration, 132
medication dosages, infusion (worksheet), 170-171
answer key, 371

Standard Infusion Insulin Drip Rate chart, 229f, 231

Start time, 178

Stat drugs, prioritization, 61

Sterile aqueous suspension. *See* Depo-Provera

Sterile cephapirin sodium, label. *See* Cefadyl

Sterile medroxyprogesterone acetate suspension, label. *See* Depo-Provera

Sterile solution. *See* Iso-osmotic sterile solution

Sterile ticarcillin disodium, injection. *See* Ticar

Sterile water
addition, 57, 128-130, 193
dilution, 177, 266
injection, 115
usage, 118, 120, 124, 185. *See also* Oxacillin Sodium

Sterility, ensuring, 116

Stools, 241

Storage
conditions, 117
direction, 58
instructions, 52

Strength-reconstitution directions, 117

Streptomycin sulfate, 329

Streptomycin sulfate injection, label
2.5 mL, 58f
5.0 g, 130f

Subcutaneous cannula, tubing (securing), 230

Subcutaneous heparin injections, 236, 238

Subcutaneous injections
sites, 236f
worksheet, 239-242
answer key, 386-387

Subcutaneous medications. *See* Children

Sure-Med Unit Dose Center, 49f

Surface area, 256f. *See also* Body surface area

Suspensions. *See* Aqueous suspensions

Swallowing ability, 51, 65

Sweetened alcohol, 54

Synthroid (levothyroxine sodium tablets), label
50 µg, 293f
175 µg, 78f, 81f, 96f
200 µg, 270f

Synthroid (levothyroxine sodium tablets), order, 83
calculation, 275

Syringes. *See* BD-Safety-LOK syringe; Carpuject syringe; Insulin; Oral syringes; Tubex blunt Pointe sterile cartridge unit

1 mL
0.01 mL increments, 89f
example, 74f
3 mL (0.1 mL increments), 89f
5 mL (0.2 mL increments), 89f
10 mL (0.2 mL increments), 89f
30-unit syringes, 208f, 212f, 213f
50-unit syringes, 208f, 212f, 213f
100-unit syringes, 208f, 212f, 213f, 219f
administering, 127
amounts, measuring/reading, 89-99
calculation, 133-136, 232-233, 238-242, 381-387
calibrated increments. *See* Prepared syringe
calibrations, 91-94, 116, 177-180, 219-220
usage, 74
examination, 89
filling, 106f
insert needle, 176f
markings, 73
oral liquid medicine, 55f
ordered amount, 216f-218f
pump, 264f
single-dose. *See* Fragmin single-dose prefilled syringes
sizes/calibrations, comparison, 89f
total capacity, calculation, 90f
total volume, calculation, 91f-94f
types. *See* U-100 insulin

Syringes *(Continued)*
units, measurement, 214-215, 221-223
usage, 118-122, 124-128, 341-344, 352-360. *See also* Disposable syringe; Medicine
volume practice, worksheet, 90
answer key, 341

Système International d'Unités (SI), 70

T

Tablets. *See* Enteric-coated tablets; Glucose tablets; Plain tablets; Scored tablets; Unscored tablets

Tazicef (ceftazidime injection) label, 119f

TD/TV ratio. *See* Total drug/total volume ratio

Teaspoon. *See* Measuring

Tegretol (carbamazepine) label (100 mg/5 ml), 261f
calculation, 261

Terbutaline (10 µg/min), order, 174

Tetracycline HCl, 329
capsules, 58f
order, 250 mg, 88

Theo-dur (450 mg), order, 83

Therapeutic anticoagulant dosage, 243

Therapeutic range, maintenance, 245. *See also* Continuous therapeutic range

Thorazine (Chlorpromazine HCl) injection, label (10 mL multi-dose vial), 303f

Three-in-one formula, label, 200f

Three-in-one solution, 189

Three-in-one TPN solution, 204

Ticar (sterile ticarcillin disodium injection) label (1 g), 127f, 129f, 134f

Ticarcillin disodium, injection. *See* Ticar

Time limit, 117

Titrated heparin, 245

Titrated infusions, 164-167
flow rate
formula, 165-167
requirement, 165
hourly drug formula, 165-167
problems, solving, 165

Titration schedule, 304f

Tobramycin sulfate. *See* Nebcin
Tofranil-PM (imipramine pamoate)
   capsules, label (75 mg),
   302f
Total dose
   difference. *See* Unit dose
   error, 53
Total drug/total volume (TD/TV)
   ratio, 164
   calculation, 170-175
   reduction, calculation, 167-168
Total grams per bag. *See* Bag
Total Parenteral Nutrition (TPN),
   158, 188-195
   bag, 188f
      label, 193f
   calculation (example), physician
      order, 191f, 194f
   delivery mode, 158
   increase, 192
   label validation, physician order,
      193
   nursing considerations, 195
   order, 204
   solution, calculation, 296
   tubing, 158
Total Volume (TV)
   calculation. *See* Syringes
   preparation, 93
   ratio. *See* Total drug/total volume
      ratio
   usage, 202
TPN. *See* Total Parenteral
      Nutrition
Trade name, 52f, 56, 57
Treat-to-Target FPG, label, 304f
Triazolam. *See* Halcion
Tridil, infusion rate, 161
Tuberculosis, risk, 104
Tubex blunt Pointe sterile cartridge
      unit, 89f
TV. *See* Total Volume
Two-step calculation, determination,
      84, 94-96
Two-step formula, writing, 144
Two-step IV flow rate calculations,
      140
Two-step metric proportion
      calculations, 84-88
Two-step metric ratio calculations,
      84-88
Tylenol. *See* Children's Tylenol;
      Infants' Tylenol
   calculation, 66, 67
   differences, 331
   elixir order, 240 mg, 289

U
U-100 Humulin R insulin (30 units),
      213
U-100 insulin
   syringes, types, 212
   types, 210
Ulcers, 102
Unit dose, 52, 52f, 53f
   apothecary equivalents, 98
   calculation, 65
   checking, 61
   excess, 269
   form, 56, 57
   metric equivalents, 98
   packages, 49f
   SDR, 259, 266
   total dose, difference, 50, 61
Units, understanding (worksheet).
      See Medication
Units/hr, calculation, 287-290
Unreconstituted drug vial,
      attachment, 156
Unscored tablets, 73, 81
Urinary tract infection (UTI), 133
Utensils, substitution. *See*
      Household utensils
UTI. *See* Urinary tract infection

V
Valium (Diazepam) order
   0.01 g, 87
   5 mg, 83
Vancocin HCl (Vancomycin
      hydrochloride, oral
      suspension) label (1 g), 110f,
      112f
Vastus lateralis muscle, 262f
V-Cillin K (125 mg), order
      calculation, 274
Vegetables, concentrated alcoholic
      liquid extract, 55
Veins, condition, 189
Velosulin BR (Buffered Regular)
      human insulin injection
      label (10 mL), 210f
   usage, 230
Ventricular fibrillation, 183
Ventrogluteal muscle, site
      preference, 262
Verbal orders, avoidance, 48
Vials. *See* Humalog insulin;
      Humulin L; Multiple-dose
      vial
   attachment. *See* Unreconstituted
      drug vial
   crystals, dilution, 115-117

Vials *(Continued)*
   powders, dilution, 115-117
   rechecking, 156f
   total volume, 79
   usage, 121. *See also* Medication
Vistaril (hydroxyzine
      hydrochloride), label, 91f,
      93f
Vital signs, 51
Vitamin B_{12} order, 1000 μg, 100
Vitamin K, activity (inhibition),
      244
Voltaren (diclofenac sodium)
   labels, 102f
   order, 450 mg, 83
Volume control device. *See*
      Electronic infusion
   flow rate, 266
   medication, placement, 265
   usage, 164, 264
Volume equivalents, 97t

W
Warfarin (Coumadin), 244
Water solution, 54
Weight
   dosages. *See* Body weight
   equivalents, 97t
   estimation, 253-254. *See also*
      Children
   measurement, 146
   usage, 263
West nomogram, 255. *See also* Body
      surface area
   usage, 257
Whole numbers
   borrowing, 10
   conversion. *See* Divisor
   improper fractions, change, 4-5
      worksheet, 5
      worksheet, answer key, 309
   multiplication, 5
Written ratio, usage, 259, 266, 276

X
Xanax (alprazolam) tablets, label,
      94f

Z
Zantac tablets, label (300 mg),
      301f
Zeros, elimination, 84
Zidovudine. *See* AZT
Zinacef (cefuroxime sodium)
      injection, label (750 mg),
      267f